Medical robotics

Related titles:

Joint replacement technology (ISBN 978-1-84569-245-2)

Biomaterials for spinal surgery (ISBN 978-1-84569-986-4)

Minimized cardiopulmonary bypass techniques and technologies (ISBN 978-1-84569-800-3)

Details of these books and a complete list of titles from Woodhead Publishing can be obtained by:

- visiting our web site at www.woodheadpublishing.com
- contacting Customer Services (e-mail: sales@woodheadpublishing.com; fax: +44 (0) 1223 832819; tel.: +44 (0) 1223 499140 ext. 130; address: Woodhead Publishing Limited, 80, High Street, Sawston, Cambridge CB22 3HJ, UK)
- in North America, contacting our US office (e-mail: usmarketing@woodheadpublishing.com; tel.: (215) 928 9112; address: Woodhead Publishing, 1518 Walnut Street, Suite 1100, Philadelphia, PA 19102-3406, USA

If you would like e-versions of our content, please visit our online platform: www.woodheadpublishingonline.com. Please recommend it to your librarian so that everyone in your institution can benefit from the wealth of content on the site.

We are always happy to receive suggestions for new books from potential editors. To enquire about contributing to our Biomaterials series, please send your name, contact address and details of the topic/s you are interested in to laura.overend@woodheadpublishing.com. We look forward to hearing from you.

The Woodhead team responsible for publishing this book:
Commissioning Editor: Laura Overend
Publications Coordinator: Lucy Beg
Project Editor: Cathryn Freear
Editorial and Production Manager: Mary Campbell
Production Editor: Adam Hooper
Copyeditor: Janice Gordon
Proofreader: George Moore
Cover Designer: Terry Callanan

Woodhead Publishing Series in Biomaterials: Number 51

Medical robotics

Minimally invasive surgery

Edited by

Paula Gomes

WOODHEAD PUBLISHING

Oxford Cambridge Philadelphia New Delhi

Published by Woodhead Publishing Limited,
80 High Street, Sawston, Cambridge CB22 3HJ, UK
www.woodheadpublishing.com
www.woodheadpublishingonline.com

Woodhead Publishing, 1518 Walnut Street, Suite 1100, Philadelphia, PA 19102-3406, USA

Woodhead Publishing India Private Limited, G-2, Vardaan House, 7/28 Ansari Road, Daryaganj, New Delhi – 110002, India
www.woodheadpublishingindia.com

First published 2012, Woodhead Publishing Limited

British Library Cataloguing in Publication Data
A catalogue record for this book is available from the British Library.

Library of Congress Control Number: 2012946143

ISBN 978-0-85709-130-7 (print)
ISBN 978-0-85709-739-2 (online)
ISSN 2049-9485 Woodhead Publishing Series in Biomaterials (print)
ISSN 2049-9493 Woodhead Publishing Series in Biomaterials (online)

The publisher's policy is to use permanent paper from mills that operate a sustainable forestry policy, and which has been manufactured from pulp which is processed using acid-free and elemental chlorine-free practices. Furthermore, the publisher ensures that the text paper and cover board used have met acceptable environmental accreditation standards.

Typeset by Replika Press Pvt Ltd, India
Printed by TJ International Ltd, Padstow, Cornwall, UK

Contents

	Contributor contact details	*ix*
	Woodhead Publishing Series in Biomaterials	*xiii*
	Introduction	*xix*
1	Introduction to robot-assisted minimally invasive surgery (MIS) V. Vitiello, K.-W. Kwok and G.-Z. Yang, The Hamlyn Centre for Robotic Surgery, Imperial College London, UK	1
1.1	Introduction	1
1.2	Minimally invasive surgery and robotic integration	2
1.3	Definitions and development of surgical robotic systems	4
1.4	Perceptual docking for synergistic control	25
1.5	Conclusions and future trends	32
1.6	References	34
2	Localization and tracking technologies for medical robotics N. Glossop, Queen's University, Canada	41
2.1	Introduction	41
2.2	Requirements for position sensors	42
2.3	Dynamic referencing	46
2.4	Types of position sensors	46
2.5	Future trends	57
2.6	Conclusion	57
2.7	References	57
3	Robotics for neurosurgery T. L. Cossetto, K. Zareinia and G. R. Sutherland, University of Calgary, Canada	59
3.1	Introduction to neurosurgical progression	59
3.2	The evolution of neurosurgical robots	61
3.3	Maintaining operator control	64

3.4 Human–machine interface (HMI) 65
3.5 Future trends: informatic surgery 74
3.6 Conclusion 75
3.7 Acknowledgments 75
3.8 References 76

4 Robotic systems for cardiovascular interventions 78
M. A. Zenati and M. Mahvash, Harvard Medical School, USA

4.1 Introduction 78
4.2 Heart conditions and the evolving role of cardiac surgeons and cardiologists 78
4.3 Surgical robot requirements and availability for cardiovascular interventions 81
4.4 Proposed novel robots for cardiovascular interventions 82
4.5 Future trends 87
4.6 Sources of further information and advice 88
4.7 References 88

5 Robotics in orthopaedic surgery 90
A. Hodgson, UBC Mechanical Engineering, Canada

5.1 Introduction 90
5.2 Existing orthopaedic robotic systems 92
5.3 Evaluation of impact of orthopaedic surgical robots 95
5.4 Conclusion 108
5.5 References 110

6 Robotic-assisted knee replacement surgery 113
C. Plaskos, OMNIlife Science, Inc., USA, J. A. Koenig, Winthrop University Hospital, USA and C. E. Ponder, Oklahoma Sports and Orthopedics Institute, USA

6.1 Introduction 113
6.2 Apex robotic technology (ART) 126
6.3 Clinical experience 138
6.4 Conclusions and future trends 152
6.5 Acknowledgments 153
6.6 References 153

7 Robotics in ear, nose and throat (ENT) surgery 159
B. Bell, M. D. Caversaccio and S. Weber, University of Bern, Switzerland

7.1 Introduction 159
7.2 Telemanipulators in ENT 160
7.3 Image-guided interventions 167

7.4 Computer numerical control (CNT) 172
7.5 Conclusions 180
7.6 References 181

8 Robotic-assisted vitreoretinal surgery 185
H. C. M. Meenink, R. Hendrix, G. J. L. Naus, M. J. Beelen, H. Nijmeijer and M. Steinbuch, Eindhoven University of Technology, The Netherlands, E. J. G. M. van Oosterhout, Catherina Hospital Eindhoven, The Netherlands and M. D. de Smet, Montchoisi Clinic, Switzerland and University of Amsterdam, The Netherlands

8.1 Introduction 185
8.2 Requirements for vitreoretinal surgery 187
8.3 Master console 193
8.4 Slave robot 198
8.5 Results 203
8.6 Conclusions and future trends 206
8.7 Acknowledgments 207
8.8 References 208

9 Robotics for minimally invasive surgery (MIS) and natural orifice transluminal endoscopic surgery (NOTES) 210
J. Reynoso, A. Meyer, J. Unnirevi and D. Oleynikov, University of Nebraska Medical Center, USA

9.1 Introduction 210
9.2 Minimally invasive surgery (MIS) 211
9.3 Natural orifice transluminal endoscopic surgery (NOTES) 216
9.4 Future trends and conclusions 221
9.5 References 223

10 Mesoscale mobile robots for gastrointestinal minimally invasive surgery (MIS) 224
J. L Gorlewicz, R. J. Webster III and P. Valdastri, Vanderbilt University, USA

10.1 Introduction 224
10.2 Commercial gastrointestinal wireless capsule endoscopes 225
10.3 Robotic capsule modules 227
10.4 Future trends in mobile surgical devices 242
10.5 Conclusion 243
10.6 References 244

11 Real-time software platform using MRI for *in vivo* navigation of magnetic microrobots 252
K. Belharet, D. Folio and A. Ferreira, Laboratoire PRISME, Ecole Nationale Supérieure d'Ingénieurs de Bourges, France

11.1 Introduction 252
11.2 Magnetic resonance imaging (MRI) navigation 254
11.3 Microrobot navigation 259
11.4 Conclusions and future trends 271
11.5 Sources of further information and advice 272
11.6 References 273

12 Robotic surgery and ethical challenges 276
N. Sharkey and A. Sharkey, University of Sheffield, UK

12.1 Introduction 276
12.2 Types of robotic surgery 278
12.3 The patient experience of robotic surgery 279
12.4 The marketing of robotic surgery 280
12.5 Comparing robotic surgery with other types of surgery 282
12.6 The need for training 283
12.7 Costs versus benefits 285
12.8 Ethical issues relating to remotely operated surgery 286
12.9 The automated hospital 288
12.10 Conclusions 289
12.11 References 289

Index *293*

Contributor contact details

(* = main contact)

Editor

Paula Gomes
Cambridge Consultants
Science Park
Milton Road
Cambridge
CB4 0DW
UK

E-mail: mpsfgomes@gmail.com

Chapter 1

V. Vitiello, K.-W. Kwok and G.-Z. Yang*
The Hamlyn Centre for Robotic Surgery
Level 4, Bessemer Building
Imperial College London
London
SW7 2AZ
UK

E-mail: g.z.yang@imperial.ac.uk

Chapter 2

Neil Glossop
School of Computing
557 Goodwin Hall
Queen's University
Kingston, Ontario
K7L 3N6
Canada

E-mail: neilglossop@gmail.com

Chapter 3

Tyler Cossetto
Research Assistant
Department of Clinical Neurosciences
University of Calgary
Health Research Innovation Centre
3280 Hospital Drive NW
Calgary, Alberta
T2N 4Z6
Canada

Kourosh Zareinia
Postdoctoral Fellow
Department of Clinical Neurosciences
University of Calgary
Health Research Innovation Centre
3280 Hospital Drive NW
Calgary, Alberta
T2N 4Z6
Canada

Garnette R Sutherland*
Professor of Neurosurgery
Department of Clinical Neurosciences
University of Calgary
Health Research Innovation Centre
3280 Hospital Drive NW
Calgary, Alberta
T2N 4Z6
Canada

E-mail: garnette@ucalgary.ca

Chapter 4

Marco A. Zenati*
Professor of Surgery, Harvard Medical School
Chief of Cardiac Surgery
VA Boston Healthcare System
Cardiac Surgery
1400 VFW Parkway
West Roxbury, MA
USA

E-mail: Marco_Zenati@hms.harvard.edu

Mohsen Mahvash
Instructor of Surgery, Harvard Medical School
VA Boston Healthcare System
Cardiac Surgery,
1400 VFW Parkway
West Roxbury, MA
USA

E-mail: mahvash@hms.harvard.edu

Chapter 5

Antony Hodgson
UBC Mechanical Engineering
6250 Applied Science Lane
Vancouver BC
V6T 1Z4
Canada

E-mail: ahodgson@mech.ubc.ca

Chapter 6

Christopher Plaskos*
Chief Technology Officer
OMNIlife Science, Inc.
50 O'Connel Way #10
East Taunton
MA 02718
USA

E-mail: cplaskos@omnils.com

Jan A. Koenig
Advanced Orthopedic Specialists
2000 North Village Avenue, Suite 306
Rockville Centre
NY 11570
USA

Corey E. Ponder
Oklahoma Sports and Orthopedics Institute
13800 Benson Rd. Suite 201
Edmond
OK 73013
USA

Chapter 7

Brett Bell
ARTORG Center for Biomedical Engineering
University of Bern
Murtenstrasse 50
CH-3010
Bern
Switzerland

Marco D. Caversaccio
Chairman and Director of Department of ENT
Head and Neck Surgery, Inselspital
University of Bern
Freiburgstrasse
CH-3010 Bern
Switzerland

Stefan Weber*
Director
ARTORG Center for Biomedical Engineering
University of Bern
Murtenstrasse 50
CH-3010
Bern
Switzerland

E-mail: Stefan.Weber@artorg.unibe.ch

Chapter 8

H. C. M. Meenink*, R. Hendrix, G. J. L. Naus, M. J. Beelen, H. Nijmeijer and M. Steinbuch
Eindhoven University of Technology
P.O. Box 513
5600 MB
Eindhoven
The Netherlands

E-mail: h.c.m.meenink@tue.nl

E. J. G. M. van Oosterhout
Catherina Hospital Eindhoven
Eindhoven
The Netherlands

M. D. de Smet
Montchoisi Clinic
Lausanne
Switzerland

and

Amsterdam Medical Center
University of Amsterdam
Amsterdam
The Netherlands

Chapter 9

Jason Reynoso, Avishai Meyer, Jayaraj Unnirevi and Dmitry Oleynikov*
Center for Advanced Surgical Technology
University of Nebraska Medical Center
985126 Nebraska Medical Center
Omaha
NE 68198-5126
USA

E-mail: doleynik@unmc.edu

Chapter 10

Jenna L Gorlewicz, Robert J. Webster III* and Pietro Valdastri
Department of Mechanical Engineering
Vanderbilt University
VU Station B 351592
2301 Vanderbilt Place
Nashville
TN 37235-1592
USA

E-mail: robert.webster@vanderbilt.edu

Chapter 11

Karim Belharet, David Folio and Antoine Ferreira*
Laboratoire PRISME
Ecole Nationale Supérieure d'Ingénieurs de Bourges
88 boulevard Lahotolle
18020 Bourges
France

E-mail: antoine.ferreira@ensi-bourges.fr

Chapter 12

Noel Sharkey* and Amanda Sharkey
Department of Computer Science
Regent Court
Portobello Rd
University of Sheffield
Sheffield
S1 4DP
UK

E-mail: n.sharkey@dcs.shef.ac.uk; a.sharkey@dcs.shef.ac.uk

Woodhead Publishing Series in Biomaterials

1 **Sterilisation of tissues using ionising radiations**
Edited by J. F. Kennedy, G. O. Phillips and P. A. Williams

2 **Surfaces and interfaces for biomaterials**
Edited by P. Vadgama

3 **Molecular interfacial phenomena of polymers and biopolymers**
Edited by C. Chen

4 **Biomaterials, artificial organs and tissue engineering**
Edited by L. Hench and J. Jones

5 **Medical modelling**
R. Bibb

6 **Artificial cells, cell engineering and therapy**
Edited by S. Prakash

7 **Biomedical polymers**
Edited by M. Jenkins

8 **Tissue engineering using ceramics and polymers**
Edited by A. R. Boccaccini and J. Gough

9 **Bioceramics and their clinical applications**
Edited by T. Kokubo

10 **Dental biomaterials**
Edited by R. V. Curtis and T. F. Watson

11 **Joint replacement technology**
Edited by P. A. Revell

12 **Natural-based polymers for biomedical applications**
Edited by R. L. Reiss et al

13 **Degradation rate of bioresorbable materials**
Edited by F. J. Buchanan

14 **Orthopaedic bone cements**
Edited by S. Deb

15 **Shape memory alloys for biomedical applications**
Edited by T. Yoneyama and S. Miyazaki

16 **Cellular response to biomaterials**
Edited by L. Di Silvio

17 **Biomaterials for treating skin loss**
Edited by D. P. Orgill and C. Blanco

18 **Biomaterials and tissue engineering in urology**
Edited by J. Denstedt and A. Atala

19 **Materials science for dentistry**
B. W. Darvell

20 **Bone repair biomaterials**
Edited by J. A. Planell, S. M. Best, D. Lacroix and A. Merolli

21 **Biomedical composites**
Edited by L. Ambrosio

22 **Drug-device combination products**
Edited by A. Lewis

23 **Biomaterials and regenerative medicine in ophthalmology**
Edited by T. V. Chirila

24 **Regenerative medicine and biomaterials for the repair of connective tissues**
Edited by C. Archer and J. Ralphs

25 **Metals for biomedical devices**
Edited by M. Ninomi

26 **Biointegration of medical implant materials: science and design**
Edited by C. P. Sharma

27 **Biomaterials and devices for the circulatory system**
Edited by T. Gourlay and R. Black

28 **Surface modification of biomaterials: methods analysis and applications**
Edited by R. Williams

29 **Biomaterials for artificial organs**
Edited by M. Lysaght and T. Webster

30 **Injectable biomaterials: science and applications**
Edited by B. Vernon

31 **Biomedical hydrogels: biochemistry, manufacture and medical applications**
Edited by S. Rimmer

32 **Preprosthetic and maxillofacial surgery: biomaterials, bone grafting and tissue engineering**
Edited by J. Ferri and E. Hunziker

33 **Bioactive materials in medicine: design and applications**
Edited by X. Zhao, J. M. Courtney and H. Qian

34 **Advanced wound repair therapies**
Edited by D. Farrar

35 **Electrospinning for tissue regeneration**
Edited by L. Bosworth and S. Downes

36 **Bioactive glasses: materials, properties and applications**
Edited by H. O. Ylänen

37 **Coatings for biomedical applications**
Edited by M. Driver

38 **Progenitor and stem cell technologies and therapies**
Edited by A. Atala

39 **Biomaterials for spinal surgery**
Edited by L. Ambrosio and E. Tanner

40 **Minimized cardiopulmonary bypass techniques and technologies**
Edited by T. Gourlay and S. Gunaydin

41 **Wear of orthopaedic implants and artificial joints**
Edited by S. Affatato

42 **Biomaterials in plastic surgery: breast implants**
Edited by W. Peters, H. Brandon, K. L. Jerina, C. Wolf and V. L. Young

43 **MEMS for biomedical applications**
Edited by S. Bhansali and A. Vasudev

44 **Durability and reliability of medical polymers**
Edited by M. Jenkins and A. Stamboulis

45 **Biosensors for medical applications**
Edited by S. Higson

46 **Sterilisation of biomaterials and medical devices**
Edited by S. Lerouge and A. Simmons

47 **The hip resurfacing handbook: a practical guide for the use and management of modern hip resurfacings**
Edited by K. De Smet, P. Campbell and C. Van Der Straeten

48 **Developments in tissue engineered and regenerative medicine products**
J. Basu and J. W. Ludlow

49 **Nanomedicine: technologies and applications**
Edited by M. Webster

50 **Biocompatibility and performance of medical devices**
Edited by J-P. Boutrand

51 **Medical robotics: minimally invasive surgery**
Edited by P. Gomes

52 **Implantable sensor systems for medical applications**
Edited by A. Inmann and D. Hodgins

53 **Non-metallic biomaterials for tooth repair and replacement**
Edited by P. Vallittu

54 **Joining and assembly of medical materials and devices**
Edited by Y. N. Zhou and M. D. Breyen

55 **Diamond-based materials for biomedical applications**
Edited by R. Narayan

56 **Nanomaterials in tissue engineering: characherization, fabrication and applications**
Edited by A. K. Gaharwar, S. Sant, M. J. Hancock and S. A. Hacking

57 **Biomimetic biomaterials: structure and applications**
Edited by A. Ruys

58 **Standardisation in cell and tissue engineering: methods and protocols**
Edited by V. Salih

59 **Inhaler devices: fundamentals, design and drug delivery**
Edited by P. Prokopovich

60 **Bio-tribocorrosion in biomaterials and medical implants**
Edited by Y. Yan

61 **Microfluidics for biomedical applications**
Edited by X-J. J. Li and Y. Zhou

62 **Decontamination in hospitals and healthcare**
Edited by J. T. Walker

63 **Biomedical imaging: applications and advances**
Edited by P. Morris

64 **Characterization of biomaterials**
Edited by M. Jaffe, W. Hammond, P. Tolias and T. Arinzeh

To Brian Davies, who opened doors to the robotics world for me and many others.
In memory of Wan Sing Ng, an inspirational colleague and surgical robotics pioneer.

Introduction

P. GOMES, Cambridge Consultants, UK

Surgeons continuously push barriers to develop surgical procedures and techniques which result in patient benefits and better clinical outcomes. As the trend towards minimally invasive surgery (MIS) increases, surgery becomes more technically demanding for surgeons and more challenging for medical device technologists. It is clear that robotics has now an established foothold in medicine as an enabling technology for MIS as this book demonstrates. Written by both medical practitioners and engineers, the book covers a wide range of clinical applications: laparoscopy, gastrointestinal, neurology, cardiovascular, otorhinolaryngology, vitreoretinal, urology, orthopaedics. Commercially available and under-development surgical robots are discussed; insights into future directions are provided.

The first recorded robotic surgical procedure took place on 11 April 1985, at the Memorial Medical Center, Long Beach, CA, USA (Kwoh *et al.*, 1988). An industrial robot was used to assist a computerized tomography (CT) guided brain biopsy. The rationale was to use a sturdy mechanical structure to hold a guide steadily in position so that a probe could be inserted to reach a surgical target deep in the brain in a linear trajectory avoiding vital structures of the brain. The straight trajectory was defined by the surgeon using CT guidance such that there was no neurological damage caused by the probe. The gold standard procedure at the time was to use a manually adjustable stereotactic frame and it was intended, with the use of the robot, to achieve improved accuracy and a faster procedure. Although the robot used was capable of autonomous motion, it was locked in position, with power removed for safety once aligned with the trajectory, while the surgeon inserted the biopsy needles, through the guide, into the patient's brain.

There was a long gap of six years until the next milestone in robotic surgery: the first time a robotic device was used to *autonomously* remove a significant amount of tissue from a patient, in a transurethral resection of the prostate (TURP), a minimally invasive surgical procedure. The device used was the Probot, a special purpose robot developed at Imperial College London, and first used in surgery in April 1991 in London, UK (Davies *et al.*, 1991). John E. A. Wickham was the urologist surgeon who operated with the Probot system. Wickham coined the term MIS and vigorously promoted this type of surgery (Wickham, 1987). MIS refers to any procedure which is less invasive than open surgery for the same purpose.

As was the case with industrial robotics, surgical robotics started under the premise that higher accuracy and speed could be achieved in surgery, particularly when precise targeting (such as that required in neurosurgery) or repetitive tasks (such as resecting a prostate gland with a wire loop resectoscope in a TURP) were required. This is corroborated by first reports of robot-assisted surgeries. Kwoh *et al.* (1988) claim improved accuracy and faster procedures as the rationale for their adoption of robotics in brain biopsy. Davies *et al.* (1991) indicate a dramatic potential reduction of TURP times from 1 h to 5 min.

It was not before 1994 that the US Food and Drug Administration cleared Computer Motion's ZEUS® Robotic Surgical System; this became the first commercial robotic device to assist surgeons in the operating room. ZEUS had three robotic arms, which were controlled remotely by the surgeon. Two robotic arms acted like extensions of the surgeon's arms, following the surgeon's movements while allowing for more precise executions by scaling down movements and eliminating tremors resulting from fatigue. The third arm was a voice-activated endoscope named AESOP® (automated endoscopic system for optimal positioning), the function of which was to manipulate a video camera inside the patient according to voice controls provided by the surgeon. AESOP® eliminated the need for a member of the surgical team to hold the endoscope and allowed the surgeon to directly and precisely control the operative field of view, providing a steady picture during MIS. Following patent legal disputes between Computer Motion and its competitor Intuitive Surgical (Sunnyvale, CA, USA), the two companies merged in 2003 and Computer Motion's products were discontinued in favour of Intuitive's *da Vinci®* robotic system.

Although the quest for increased accuracy seems to have been fulfilled, albeit dependent on factors such as imaging and image processing, registration of imaging to the robotic system, and calibration of instrumentation, the claim of reduced times has not been as successfully met and, despite significant improvements in efficiency and workflow, set-up times often make robotic procedures lengthier than their conventional counterparts. This poses a conflict for surgeons and healthcare providers, as fewer procedures can be carried out by the surgeon, and has made the health economics case for surgical robotics a difficult one to argue. However, despite procedure times remaining important and a fundamental market driver, other reasons are driving the adoption of surgical robotics: patient demand, reduction of surgical errors, augmenting surgical capabilities and enabling MIS.

Adding to the surgical and technical complexities, commercial, regulatory and legal restraints can slow down progress and, sometimes, delay and even block the development of new devices. A device that has a higher price than a current one has to show cost effectiveness and requires development of a reimbursement case to gain acceptance in the market place. The ultimate objective of surgical robotics is to improve surgical outcome but the higher costs need to be offset by significantly greater measurable clinical benefits. The regulatory burden on medical device approval is high; the process is slow and favours incremental development rather than radical advances. Intellectual property protection is a double-edged sword and acts both as a driver and as a restraint in the development of surgical robotics and advanced medical technology in general. Although research and innovation are incentivised, because inventors can fend off competitors for a period of time, manufacturers are also forced to design workarounds to avoid patent litigation and may indeed be discouraged from innovating in a particular field altogether.

The practice of robotic surgery is still largely dominated by the *da Vinci*® system, as manifested by recurrent references throughout this book, but other commercial players have now entered the market with surgical robotic products or are appearing on the horizon with medium and long-term propositions. Surgical robotics is currently a vibrant research topic and new research directions may lead to the development of very different robotic surgical devices in the future: small, special purpose, procedure-specific, lower cost, possibly disposable robots rather than the current large, versatile and capital expensive systems. This is a departure from current multimillion dollar, multifunction 'platform' robotic systems, towards low-cost, specific-function, even single-use, micro- or nano-devices. It is too early to predict the winning propositions. Several are reviewed in this book and illustrate what the future may bring.

Chapter 1, by Valentina Vitiello, Ka-Wai Kwok and Guang-Zhong Yang, provides an overview of robot-assisted minimally invasive surgery, including flexible robots for interventional procedures, and introduces recent developments in the integration of synergistic controls such as virtual fixtures, dynamic active constraints, and perceptual docking.

In MIS, where there is no direct view of the surgical site, surgeons need to know with confidence and in real time where the surgical tools are within the patient's body so therapy is delivered to the correct anatomical location in a safe manner. Moreover, in computer-assisted and robotic surgery, the physical locations of the patient and of the surgical instruments have to be accurately mapped to each other and, in image-based surgery, to a preoperative patient's computer model reconstructed from magnetic resonance (MR) or CT images. This is the focus of Chapter 2, where Neil Glossop discusses technologies enabling localisation and position tracking and reviews general requirements for such sensors. Glossop also surveys the main position sensors currently in use and under development, as well as the advantages and drawbacks of the various technologies available and emerging.

Chapter 3, by Tyler Cossetto, Kourosh Zareinia and Garnette Sutherland, focuses on neurosurgery and reviews the evolution of neurosurgical robots, from the first experiences by Kwoh *et al.* (1988) to robots designed to operate with intraoperative magnetic resonance imaging (MRI) resection control to allow for correction for brain shift. An example of the latter, the neuroArm, an image-guided MR-compatible robot for microsurgery and stereotaxy, first used in May 2008 to carry out the surgical removal of a brain lesion, is presented in detail. The chapter also discusses what the future in robotic neurosurgery may bring.

Marco Zenati and Mohsen Mahvash examine robotic systems for cardiovascular interventions in Chapter 4, including available commercial robots, other robotic concepts at the research stage and a discussion of likely future trends. The chapter contains a review of heart conditions and various interventional approaches for treatment, and a reflection on the evolving roles of cardiac surgeons and cardiologists which are being redefined and shaped by technology.

The following two chapters are dedicated to orthopaedic surgery. Chapter 5, by Antony Hodgson, provides a review of the state-of-the-art in orthopaedic robotics and describes five systems commercially available today, encompassing autonomous, active-constraints/collaborative and passive toolholders. Four of the systems are used in joint replacement arthroplasty, the fifth in spinal pedicle screw placement. Autonomous and collaborative systems pave the way for bone-conserving procedures that fit within the broad definition of MIS.

One of the five systems referred to by Hodgson is the object of an in-depth analysis of robot-assisted total knee replacement (TKR) surgery in Chapter 6, written by Christopher Plaskos, Jan Koenig, and Corey Ponder. The chapter provides background information and an overview of conventional and MIS TKR and reports extensive clinical experience with the Apex Robotic Technology (ART) system. The chapter concludes with developments needed to allow widespread adoption of robotic technology in orthopaedics.

Robotic devices available commercially for laparoscopic, cardiovascular, neurological and orthopaedic indications are discussed in the first six chapters. The remainder of the book addresses new applications of robotic technology in ear, nose and throat (ENT), eye, gastrointestinal and natural orifice transluminal endoscopic surgery (NOTES) surgeries.

In Chapter 7, Brett Bell, Marco Caversaccio and Stefan Weber discuss robotics in ENT surgery, a particularly challenging application owing to the small size and complicated layout of the anatomical structures, especially in the middle ear. For nose surgery, MIS has the additional advantage of reduced aesthetic impact. In the absence of commercially available robotic systems specific to head and neck surgery, the authors evaluate the use of the *da Vinci*® telemanipulator in this specialty and present research efforts directed at procedure-specific devices.

Chapter 8, written by Thijs Meenink, Ron Hendrix, Maarten Beelen,

Henk Nijmeijer, Maarten Steinbuch, Gerrit Naus, Eric van Oosterhout and Marc de Smet, focuses on robot-assisted vitreoretinal surgery. As in ENT, the accuracy required to perform eye surgery is challenging and robotics can overcome human limitations. The chapter describes in detail a proof-of-concept demonstrator of a novel master–slave robotic device and lays out the plans for its development to a clinical system.

Ten years ago, all gall bladder removals were done via open surgery in the US. Today, nearly all of these cholecystectomies are performed laparoscopically through three small incisions. The first single-incision laparoscopic surgery (SILS) for cholecystectomy was reported in 1997. SILS, also known as LESS (laparo-endoscopic single site) surgery, has the potential to reduce postoperative pain and port-site complications and, with careful incision closure, can result in no visible scars. Natural orifice surgery (NOS) and NOTES are the ultimate paradigm as there is no external incision. In Chapter 9, Jason Reynoso, Avishai Meyer, Jayaraj Unnirevi and Dmitry Oleynikov review the MIS, SILS and NOTES approaches, presenting overviews, techniques, advantages, disadvantages and clinical applications for the three approaches. Existing robotic technology and technology in development are described and future trends are indicated and analysed.

Chapter 10, by Jenna Gorlewicz, Robert Webster III and Pietro Valdastri, focuses on untethered mobile robots for gastrointestinal MIS which can enter the body through a natural orifice or a small incision and make their way to a target surgical site. An overview of commercial wireless capsule endoscopes is provided. An analysis of the major modules of robotic capsules, which enhance diagnosis and deliver therapy, and of the current technical progress of each of these modules is presented. Perspectives on the future of mobile surgical devices are put forward.

Chapter 10 reviews the state-of-the-art in mesoscale robots (1–100 mm) for the gastrointestinal tract, while Chapter 11 addresses microrobots (a few tens of micrometres) for the circulatory system. Although the former can move freely through the GI tract using peristalsis and can be relatively large, the latter require active locomotion and have tighter size constraints, because the diameters of blood vessels range from 25 mm for the aorta down to 0.01 mm for the capillaries. In chapter 11, Karim Belharet, David Folio and Antoine Ferreira discuss MRI-based navigation for *in vivo* magnetic microrobots and propose an image-processing technique and control algorithms for path planning, tracking and control using a clinical MRI system.

In the final chapter of this book, Chapter 12, Noel Sharkey and Amanda Sharkey debate ethical issues posed by the use of robotics in healthcare and warn of the difficulties that could arise in the future. Their concerns address the patient's experience of robotic surgery, remote telesurgery, automated hospitals and medical care, the marketing of medical robotic systems, surgical training and issues of cost versus access. They conclude that there is much to suggest that medical robotics technology will be of great benefit over the coming years, but we must not let the promise of revolutionary new technology blind us to the difficulties and ethical issues involved in the early stages of developing such technologies.

The editor would like to express her thanks and gratitude to the authors, technologists and clinicians, industrialists and researchers, for their contributions. Without their expertise, dedication, hard work, generosity with their valuable time and willingness to share their knowledge, insights and research results, this book would not have been realised.

Sincere thanks also to the staff at Woodhead Publishing for their professional support and input into this project. Special thanks to Laura Overend, Commissioning Editor, for her invitation to edit this book, her guidance when needed, her patience with my belated responses and for driving this project to its successful conclusion; to Lucy Beg, Publications Coordinator, for liaising and managing all the communications with the authors; and to Cathryn Freear, Senior Project Editor, for working on the manuscript and preparing it for handover to the production department.

References

Davies, B. L., Hibberd, R. D., Ng, W. S., Timoney, A. G. and Wickham, J. E. A., A surgeon robot for prostatectomies, *Fifth International Conference on Advanced Robotics (ICAR)*, pp. 871–875, 1991

Kwoh, Y. S., Hou, J., Jonckheere, E. A. and Hayati, S., A robot with improved absolute positioning accuracy for CT guided stereotactic brain surgery, *IEEE Trans Biomed Eng* February 1988; **35**(2): 153–160

Wickham, J. E. A. The new surgery. *Br Med J* 1987; **295**(6613): 1581–1582.

1
Introduction to robot-assisted minimally invasive surgery (MIS)

V. VITIELLO, K.-W. KWOK and G.-Z. YANG,
The Hamlyn Centre for Robotic Surgery, Imperial College London, UK

Abstract: It is well recognised that the performance of minimally invasive surgery (MIS) imposes an increasing burden on surgeons' manual dexterity and visuomotor control. Tissue deformation, restricted workspace, and a limited field-of-view make manual operation of the procedure difficult. With the advent of robot assisted MIS, manual dexterity is enhanced by microprocessor controlled mechanical wrists, allowing motion scaling and tremor removal. Further enhancement of three-dimensional (3D) vision and intra-operative image guidance permits improved clinical uptake of the technology, ensuring better operative safety and consistency. This chapter provides a detailed overview of robotic surgical systems and introduces recent developments in the integration of synergistic controls such as virtual fixtures, dynamic active constraints, and perceptual docking.

Key words: minimally invasive surgery, medical robotics, robot-assisted surgery, virtual fixtures, perceptual docking.

1.1 Introduction

In the past few decades, surgical practice has been revolutionised by the introduction of advanced instrumentation enabling a paradigm shift from traditional open surgery to minimally invasive surgery (MIS). The main advantage of MIS is attributed to a reduction in patient trauma, resulting in faster recovery and lower hospitalisation costs. However, the very nature of MIS, laparoscopy for example, which involves the use of long, rigid tools inserted into the patient via small incisions, can introduce a range of ergonomic challenges. The loss of wrist articulation together with the fulcrum effect caused by the inversion of motion direction at the trocar, limits the manual dexterity of the surgeon. In addition, the use of a separate display to convey the visual feedback from a laparoscopic camera separates the visuomotor axes, thus affecting the hand-eye coordination of the surgeon (Howe and Matsuoka, 1999).

Improved control and dexterity is one of the main benefits of robotic technologies for MIS. Mechatronically enhanced surgical instruments have been designed to compensate for the loss of wrist articulation caused by the traditional approach. Together with the introduction of master–slave control, this has contributed to the safety and consistency of MIS (Camarillo *et al.*, 2004). However, even with the current state-of-the-art robotic surgical systems, such as the da Vinci from Intuitive Surgical Inc. (Guthart and Salisbury, 2000), tools are still rigid and require careful port placement to ensure required access and workspace for a given procedure. Safe performance of surgical interventions within the tight confines of the chest or cluttered peritoneal cavity involving large-scale tissue deformation is a significant challenge. Current medical robotics research is therefore focused on the integration of multiple control modalities such as perceptual docking and virtual fixtures together with enhanced visualisation and intraoperative image guidance.

Historically, most initial research in medical robotics has been directed to overcoming known limitations of industrial robots, particularly in terms of adaptability and autonomy. The main perceptual differences between humans and robots lie in the ability of processing qualitative and quantitative information. Robots can integrate a large amount of quantitative data precisely through different sensors, thus being able to perform and repeat repetitive tasks with good stability and positional accuracy. On the other hand, surgeons are superior in combining diverse sources of qualitative information for making difficult decisions. Such skills are critical to the success of any surgical intervention, but existing surgical robots are still limited to simple procedures under the direct control of surgeons. Unlike industrial automation, robotic systems for surgery must be considered as a 'surgeon's extender' rather than a 'surgeon's replacement' (Camarillo *et al.*, 2004; Howe and Matsuoka, 1999).

It is important to note that robotic-assisted surgery is only one of the various specialties falling under the broader category of computer-aided surgery (CAS). In this context, the robot represents a single component of a multifunctional system specifically designed to augment the capabilities of surgeons and to improve the overall outcome of surgical procedures. Through a combined use of automated and manually controlled surgical devices, such a system also incorporates preoperative planning, intraoperative registration, and image-guided navigation and visualisation (Taylor and Stoianovici, 2003). In this regard, medical imaging plays a fundamental role in the development of CAS systems and there is a unique opportunity in combining the two. To better understand the benefits and technical challenges of robot-assisted MIS, this chapter provides a detailed overview of robotic surgical systems and introduces recent developments in the integration of multiple control modalities such as perceptual docking and virtual fixtures.

1.2 Minimally invasive surgery and robotic integration

During MIS, a set of three to five incisions of about 1 cm length is usually required to introduce at least two long-handled tissue manipulators, such as grippers and retractors, and one video endoscope to visualise the operative site, as shown in Fig. 1.1a. The main advantages of MIS are related to reduced tissue scar and surgical trauma, less pain and faster recovery (Howe and Matsuoka, 1999). However, the particular configuration of MIS instrumentation also imposes substantial limitations on manual manipulation and hand–eye coordination (Camarillo *et al.*, 2004). The use of rigid, long hand-held tools can result in a loss of surgeon's wrist articulation, while the fixed access port can constrain the lateral movements of the instrument shaft, acting like a fulcrum or remote centre of motion (RCM). The direction of surgeon's hand motion is therefore reversed at the instrument tip and

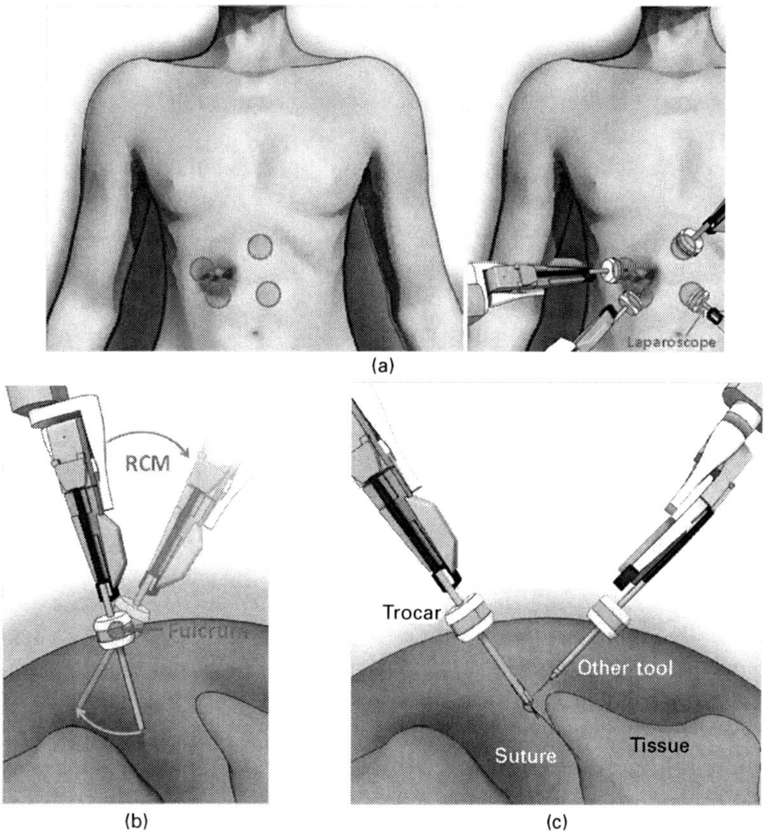

1.1 (a) A typical port arrangement for laparoscopic surgery: (left) four circles indicate the approximate locations of incision points for laparoscopic cholecystectomy; (right) four manipulators holding the instruments and a laparoscope are required to share a small workspace inside the abdominal cavity. (b) An illustration of the fulcrum effect and RCM at the fulcrum point. (c) Possible forces applied by the trocar, suture, tissue and other tool on the laparoscopic instrument on the left.

motion is scaled depending on the relative position of the tool to the trocar, as shown in Fig. 1.1b.

In addition to the fulcrum effect, indirect vision of the operative area through a two-dimensional (2-D) display, often located away from the surgeon, presents an unfamiliar relationship between visual and motor coordinates. Furthermore, the field-of-view is often limited by the use of an endoscopic camera, and the view angle can be unnatural because of the constrained position and orientation of the tool. Finally, the perceptual capabilities of the surgeon are also affected by a lack of tactile sensation and force feedback. During surgery, the instruments are interacting with many objects such as the trocar, tissue or other instruments, as shown in Fig. 1.1c. The use of long, rigid shafts significantly affects force perception at the instrument tip and can lead to undesired damage caused by excessive forces applied on the tissue.

The application of robotic technologies to MIS is aimed at solving many of these drawbacks (Mack, 2001). Recent advances in imaging such as three-dimensional (3-D) wide-angle endoscopic cameras and high-resolution stereoscopic displays have already been incorporated into the current robotic surgical systems (Ballantyne and Moll, 2003). Structural and functional imaging modalities have been integrated for improved tissue characterisation and additional navigational clues (Noonan *et al.*, 2009). The articulated tools incorporate an additional degree of dexterity to allow for improved flexibility and manual dexterity (Low and Phee, 2004; Noonan *et al.*, 2009).

Thus far, much effort has been devoted to the development of teleoperated surgical systems based on one or more robotic slave manipulators at the patient side controlled by the surgeon through a master console that can be remotely located (Low and Phee, 2004). The surgeon can benefit from visual and sometimes haptic feedback at the master console, and highly dexterous slave manipulators. Hand tremor elimination and motion scaling are provided to obtain accurate movements, as well as improved ergonomics and visuomotor integration. Some robotic systems, such as the da Vinci can be used for a range of surgical tasks, whereas others are designed for specific surgical tasks. There are also systems that exploit the stability and geometric accuracy of robots to perform microscopic surgical procedures (Taylor *et al.*, 1999) or for replacing surgical assistants for tasks such as endoscope positioning (Sackier and Wang, 1994) and organ retraction (Osaki *et al.*, 2009). A summary of the drawbacks associated with traditional MIS and the corresponding benefits of robotic integration is presented in Table 1.1

1.3 Definitions and development of surgical robotic systems

In the literature, several authors have attempted to classify surgical robotic systems developed in the last 25 years into specific categories (Camarillo *et al.*,

Table 1.1 Summary of MIS drawbacks and related benefits of robotic integration

Traditional MIS		Robotic MIS	
• Poor depth perception	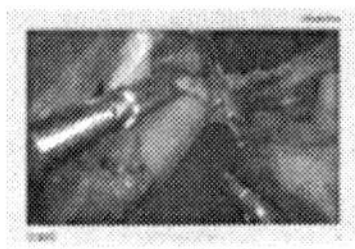	• 3-D endoscopic cameras • High resolution stereoscopic displays	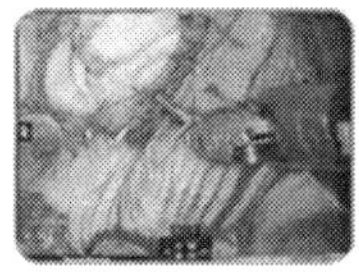
• Poor visual–motor coordination	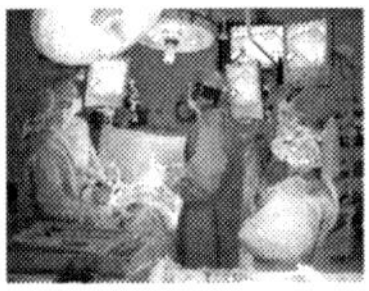	• Immersive visualization • Articulated instruments	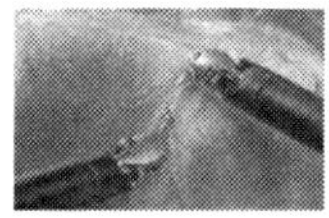 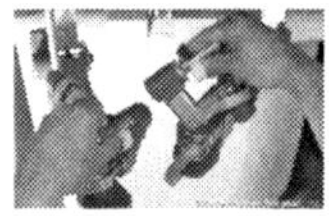
• Fulcrum effect	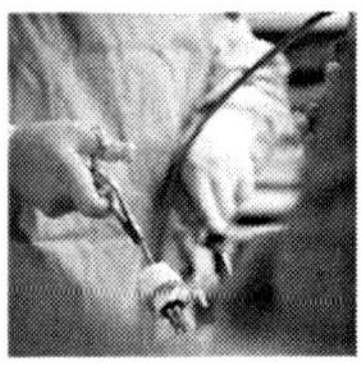	• Articulated instruments • Motion scaling • Tremor filtering	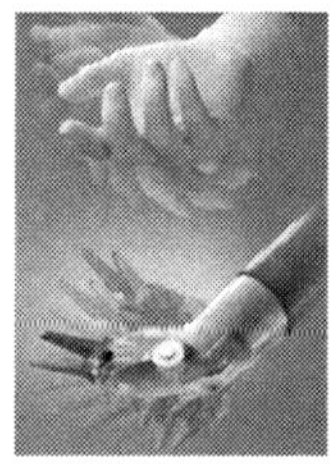
• Tiredness • Physical separation	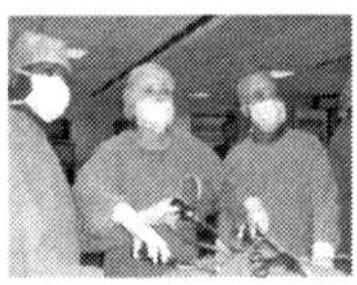	• Ergonomic remote surgical console	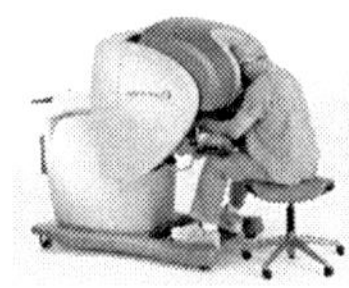
• Hands interaction with tissue	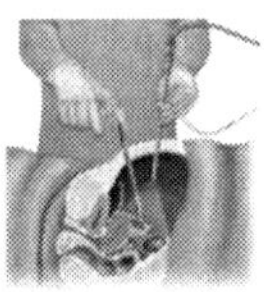	• 'Drive-by-wire' instruments	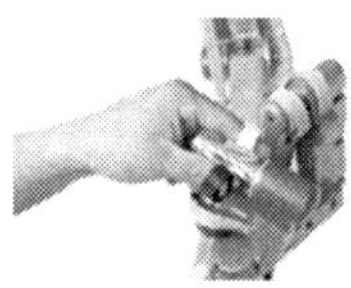

2004; Cleary and Nguyen, 2001; Dario *et al.*, 2003; Davies, 2000; Howe and Matsuoka, 1999; Taylor and Stoianovici, 2003). According to Taylor (Taylor, 1997), these can be based on three main criteria: the interaction mode between the robot and the surgeon, the clinical application, and the role played by the robot during surgical procedures. Systems are defined by the first criterion depending on the level of autonomy of the robot, ranging from autonomous to master-slave systems (Dario *et al.*, 2003; Davies, 2000). Application-based taxonomies focus instead on the clinical area where the robot is used, such as thoracic and orthopaedic surgery (Howe and Matsuoka, 1999; Cleary and Nguyen, 2001). One type of role-based classification divides active and passive robots according to their level of interaction with the patient during the procedure (Camarillo *et al.*, 2004). As a result of the current limitations of robotic technology, active robots are generally associated with a low level of autonomy, being involved in high-risk procedures that require direct supervision of the surgeon. A different role-based categorisation refers to the function of the medical robot within the wider concept of computer-integrated surgical system, distinguishing between surgical computer-assisted design/computer-assisted machining (CAD/CAM) systems and surgical assistants (Taylor and Stoianovici, 2003).

However, given the strong interdisciplinary nature of research and development in surgical robots, it is challenging to define a unique taxonomy that incorporates both technical features and clinical applications. Therefore, the most representative systems for robotic-assisted MIS, as listed in Table 1.2, are presented in the following sections according to their historical order of appearance.

1.3.1 CAD/CAM and assistive systems

One of the most immediate applications of surgical robotics is coupled with surgical CAD/CAM systems based on a matching between preoperative plans and intraoperative execution. This is particularly desirable for orthopaedic surgery or neurosurgery, where the successful outcome of the procedure depends on the surgeon's ability to follow optimal surgical pathways with extreme precision. The benefits of robotic execution in this context include:

- reliability and high accuracy in registration to medical images;
- capability of operating in restrictive environments (*e.g.* radiation from a computerised tomography (CT) scanner);
- ability to precisely and rapidly relocate surgical tools.

A detailed review of the most relevant CAD/CAM systems for surgery is presented in Taylor and Stoianovici (2003). Among these, the surgical robot Minerva was one of the first robotic systems developed for neurosurgery (Burckhardt *et al.*, 1995). It was designed to perform all the stages of a stereotactic brain biopsy completely autonomously inside a CT scanner, so that the surgeon was able to supervise the entire procedure remotely. The robot was mounted on a railed carrier rigidly coupled with the stereotactic frame on the patient's head. The serial kinematic structure of the mechanism has five degrees-of-freedom (DoFs): two linear axes (vertical and lateral), two rotary axes (in a horizontal and a vertical plane) and a linear axis that allows the motion of surgical instruments to and from the patient brain (Glauser *et al.*, 1993). Although two procedures were successfully executed

Table 1.2 Representative robotic systems for MIS

Application	System	Human use	University/company	Reference
Arthroscopy	Semiautomatic endoscope	No	ISSA, Italy	(Dario *et al.*, 2000)
Cardiac	HARP/CardioArm	No	Carnegie Mellon University, USA	(Degani *et al.*, 2006)
Cardiac	HeartLander	No	Carnegie Mellon University, USA	(Patronik *et al.*, 2005)
Cardiac	PADyC	No	Joseph Fourier University, France	(Schneider and Troccaz, 2001)
Cardiac	Sensei RNS	Yes	Hansen Medical, USA	(Kanagaratnam *et al.*, 2008)
Colonoscopy	Inchworm robot	No	CALTECH, USA	(Slatkin *et al.*, 1995)
Colonoscopy	Inchworm robot	Yes	ISSA, Italy	(Dario *et al.*, 1997)
Endoscopy	Legged capsule	No	ISSA, Italy	(Quirini *et al.*, 2008a, 2008b)
Endoscopy	SMA robot	No	Tokyo Institute of Technology, Japan	(Ikuta *et al.*, 1988)
Laparoscopy	AESOP	Yes	Computer Motion Inc., USA	(Sackier and Wang, 1994)
Laparoscopy	CoBRASurge	No	Nebraska University, USA	(Zhang *et al.*, 2009)
Laparoscopy	Da Vinci	Yes	Intuitive Surgical Inc., USA	(Guthart and Salisbury, 2000)
Laparoscopy	Endoassist/FreeHand	Yes/yes	Freehand 2010, UK	(Aiono *et al.*, 2002; Rane *et al.*, 2008)
Laparoscopy	i-Snake	No	Imperial College London, UK	(Shang *et al.*, 2011)
Laparoscopy	MiroSurge	No	DLR, Germany	(Hagn *et al.*, 2010)
Laparoscopy	Modular telesurgery system	No	University of Hawaii, USA	(Berkelman and Ma, 2009)
Laparoscopy	Pneumatic telesurgery system	No	Tokyo Institute of Technology, Japan	(Tadano and Kawashima, 2010)
Laparoscopy	RAVEN	No	University of Washington, USA	(Lum *et al.*, 2009)
Laparoscopy	ZEUS	Yes	Computer Motion Inc., USA	(Low and Phee, 2004)
Microsurgery	neuroArm	Yes	University of Calgary, Canada	(Sutherland *et al.*, 2003)
Microsurgery	RAMS	No	NASA JPL, USA	(Kozlowski *et al.*, 1997)
Neurosurgery	CyberKnife	Yes	Accuray Inc., USA	(Adler Jr *et al.*, 1997)
Neurosurgery	Minerva	Yes	Lausanne University, Switzerland	(Burckhardt *et al.*, 1995)
Neurosurgery	NeuRobot	Yes	Shinshu University, Japan	(Hongo *et al.*, 2002)
Neurosurgery	NeuroMate	Yes	Renishaw Plc, UK	(Benabid *et al.*, 1987)
Neurosurgery	SpineAssist	Yes	Mazor Surgical Technologies, Israel	(Shoham *et al.*, 2007)
Ophthalmic	Micron	No	Carnegie Mellon University, USA	(Ang *et al.*, 2000)
Ophthalmic	Steady-Hand Eye Robot	No	Johns Hopkins University, USA	(Taylor *et al.*, 1999)

(Continued)

Table 1.2 Continued

Application	System	Human use	University/company	Reference
Orthopaedic	Acrobot	Yes	Imperial College London, UK	(Davies *et al.*, 1997)
Orthopaedic	RIO	Yes	MAKO Surgical, USA	(Hagag *et al.*, 2011)
Orthopaedic	ROBODOC	Yes	Curexo Technology Corp., USA	(Kazanzides *et al.*, 1992)
Urology	MrBot	No	Johns Hopkins University, USA	(Muntener *et al.*, 2006)
Urology	Probot	Yes	Imperial College London and Guy's Hospital, UK	(Harris *et al.*, 1997)

by the system in 1993 (Glauser *et al.*, 1995), safety issues related to the amount of radiation exposure for the patient within the CT scanner forced the discontinuation of the device. Nonetheless, the concept of precise tool positioning using a 5-DoF robotic arm was then successfully exploited by Benabid *et al.* (1987) at the Grenoble University Hospital (La Tronche, France), who developed the NeuroMate (Fig. 1.2a), the first robotic device for neurosurgery approved by the US Food and Drug Administration (FDA). The system has been used in over 1000 clinical cases and features a state-of-the-art navigation and planning system that supports 2-D and 3-D image registration and frame-based or frameless navigation (Li *et al.*, 2002). The technology was first acquired by Integrated Surgical Systems (Sacramento, CA, USA) in 1997 and recently purchased by Renishaw Plc (Gloucestershire, England, UK).

Together with standard tools, focused delivery of radiation beams can also be used to perform neurosurgical interventions. The CyberKnife (Accuray Inc, USA) is a complete robotic radiosurgery system that can be used for both intracranial and spinal applications (Adler *et al.*, 1997). It consists of a linear accelerator mounted on a robotic positioning arm. By using the feedback mechanisms provided, it can adjust the beam trajectory to correct for patient movement. The flush mounted image detectors capture high-resolution anatomical images throughout the treatment, while the synchrony respiratory tracking system continuously synchronises beam delivery to the motion of the tumour, allowing clinicians to significantly reduce margins while eliminating the need for gating or breathholding techniques. A recent addition to the system is the RoboCouch Patient Positioning System, which robotically aligns patients precisely with six DoFs, enabling faster patient setup.

Another surgical robot that was recently awarded FDA approval is the SpineAssist robot (Mazor Surgical Technologies, Israel) for spinal surgery (Shoham *et al.*, 2007). The system features a miniature parallel manipulator designed to attach directly to the patient's spine and sophisticated software for image-guidance. It can be used as a guide for tool positioning and implant placement and is no larger than a soda can. Motion of the robotic arm is defined preoperatively and is supervised by the surgeon during the procedure.

As previously noticed, CAD/CAM robotic systems are clinically attractive when applied to orthopaedic surgery. The ROBODOC (first developed by Integrated Surgical Systems, USA and recently acquired by Curexo Technology Corporation, USA) (Kazanzides *et al.*, 1992) was one of the first autonomous robots designed for such application. It is an image-guided system that utilises an industrial SCARA robot with five DoFs to execute autonomously high-precision bone cutting for implant placement. Implant selection, preoperative planning and registration are performed using the integrated ORTHODOC workstation (Taylor *et al.*, 1994). The system is

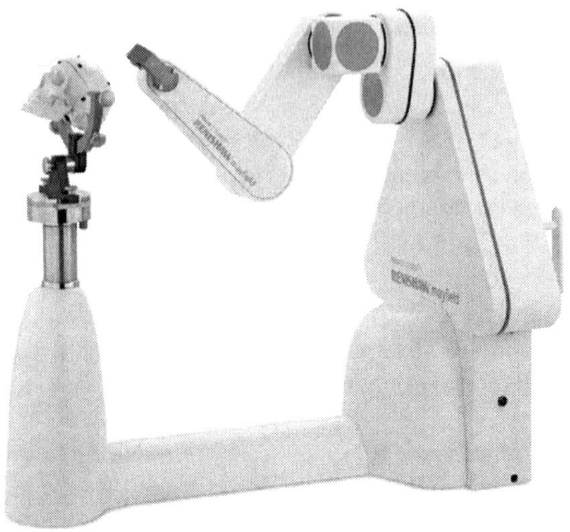

(a)

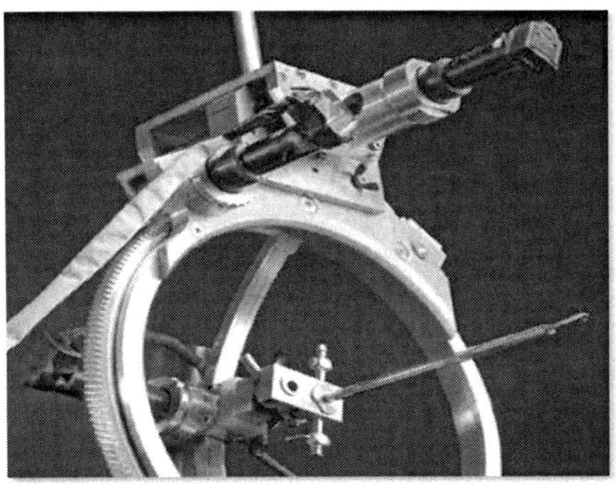

(b)

1.2 CAD/CAM systems for surgery: (a) the NeuroMate accurate tool positioning system for stereotactic brain surgery (Benabid *et al.*, 1987) (© Renishaw plc); (b) the Probot system developed at Imperial College London and especially designed to perform precise cutting of soft tissue within a constrained workspace as required for prostatectomy (Harris *et al.*, 1997) (courtesy of Professor Brian Davies, Imperial College London).

used clinically for total hip replacement (THR) since 1992 (Mittelstadt *et al.*, 1996). Despite the significant precision improvement obtained, the related benefits for patient outcome still have to be demonstrated. Also, the surgical time becomes longer owing to learning curves associated with the initial use of the system and the slow error recovery process. Another drawback of the system is the need for an additional surgery before CT scanning to place aluminium pins on the bone for registration. To overcome this problem, a new non-fiducial based surface registration technique (DigiMatch) has recently been integrated into the system (Nakamura *et al.*, 2009).

Another system for orthopaedic surgery which is currently undergoing human tests for FDA approval is the ARTHROBOT robot for total hip arthroplasty developed by Kwon *et al.* (2001). The manipulator has a 4-DoF parallel structure and is mounted directly on the bone using a simplified gauge-based registration technique. This reduces the preoperative set-up time and guarantees over 90% accurate surface conformity with efficient workspace.

Finally, automatic CAD/CAM systems have also been used in urology, particularly for prostate resection. The Probot system developed at Imperial College London, for example, is especially designed to perform precise cutting of soft tissue within a constrained workspace (Harris *et al.*, 1997). In particular, the resectoscope is placed at the tip of a robotic frame that centres its angular motion around a point, thus allowing resection of a conical cavity. The dimension of the resected part can be adjusted by translating the centre of rotation, as shown in Fig. 1.2b. The desired prostatectomy area is defined pre-operatively through a dedicated surgeon–computer interface featuring both 3-D prostate model construction and on-line imaging capabilities, through which the surgeon can supervise the whole procedure.

In the field of urological interventions, Stoianovici and coworkers at Johns Hopkins University (JHU) are currently developing a magnetic resonance imaging (MRI) compatible robotic system for fully automated brachytherapy seed placement called MRBot (Muntener *et al.*, 2006). The robot has five DoFs to control the position and orientation of an end-effector and can be placed directly inside the 50 cm bore of a standard closed MRI scanner. Four additional DoFs at the end-effector allow the depth of needle insertion to be modified and brachytherapy seeds to be deployed automatically by manipulating a titanium needle. The entire robot is built of non-magnetic and dielectric materials and a new type of pneumatic actuator is used to achieve full MRI compatibility.

Together with CAD/CAM systems, endoscopic camera holders represent one of the first and most widespread applications of robotics to MIS. Traditionally, an assistant has to understand surgeons' needs and move the endoscope accordingly. This becomes a demanding task because of the confined manoeuvring space, uncomfortable body position and difficulty in seamless communication in a busy and often stressful operating environment. In this regard, the introduction of a robotic assistant directly under the command of the operating surgeon makes perfect sense. The main design feature of endoscopic camera holders is the incorporation of a RCM to move the endoscope about the pivoting insertion point on the patient's skin. Although the workspace of the robot must be as large as possible to ensure adequate positional versatility and large field-of-view during surgery, a small footprint is desirable to allow for free motion of the instrument. To achieve these goals, different RCM designs have been proposed.

The automated endoscopic system for optimal positioning (AESOP) from Computer Motion Inc. was the first camera positioning robot to gain FDA approval in 1994 (Sackier and Wang, 1994). It features two revolute joints with intersecting axes creating a passive RCM that constrains the orientation of the instrument inside the patient's body but not between the access point and the robot (Fig. 1.3a). This allows for safe endoscope repositioning in case of accidental patient motion. The first generation of the system featured a foot or hand controller to move the endoscope in six DoFs (in, out, left, right, up and down), while the second generation robot was voice-controlled (Sackier *et al.*, 1997). Although more intuitive, the use of voice commands implied long set-up times for calibration and possible positioning errors.

Two generations of endoscopic camera positioning systems based on infra-red (IR) sensors and head motion have been developed by Prosurgics (previously Armstrong Healthcare, London, UK). Both feature a five-axis SCARA arm for endoscope positioning. The manipulator is mounted on a freestanding, wheeled cart in EndoAssist (Aiono *et al.*, 2002) or directly clamped onto the patient table in FreeHand (Rane *et al.*, 2008), as shown in Fig. 1.3b.

In addition to the above commercial systems, one interesting device currently under development is the compact bevel-geared robot for advanced surgery (CoBRASurge), which features a bevel-gear wrist with three rotational joints defining a mechanically locked RCM at the intersection of their axes (Zhang *et al.*, 2009). The compact and lightweight mechanism has an optimised workspace accounting for collision avoidance between the robot's links and between the patient and the robot, as described in (Zhang and Nelson, 2008). The system is remotely controlled using a joystick and demonstrated good performance as laparoscope holder in recent animal tests (Nelson *et al.*, 2009).

1.3.2 Master–slave surgical systems

Master–slave systems incorporate the lowest level of autonomy because the motion of the surgeon's hands is replicated by the surgical robot. The two parts of the system are physically separated so that this control modality is considered as teleoperation and has the potential for treating patients from afar. The most common teleoperated MIS system currently available on the market is the da Vinci surgical system by Intuitive Surgical Inc. (Sunnyvale, CA) (Guthart and Salisbury, 2000). Although it was initially developed to

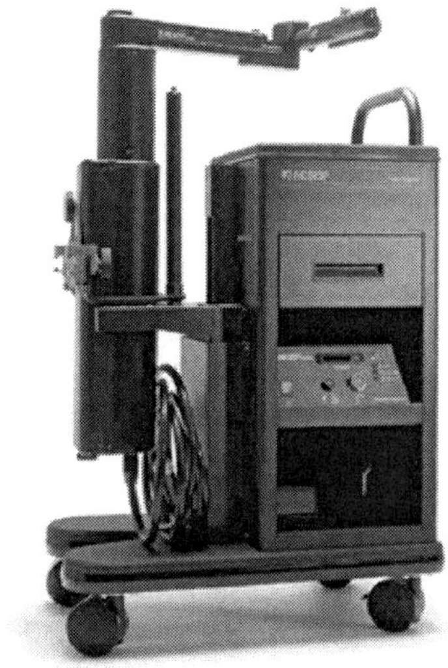

(a)

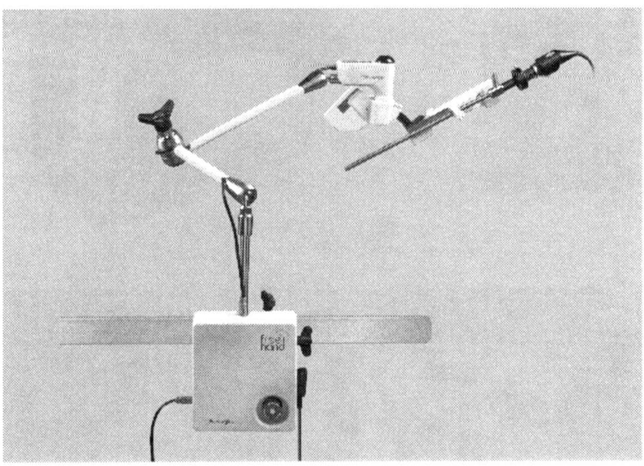

(b)

1.3 Endoscopic camera positioning systems: (a) the AESOP voice-controlled camera positioning robot (Sackier and Wang, 1994) (© Computer Motion Inc.); (b) the FreeHand robotic camera holder controlled through head motion using IR sensors (Rane *et al.*, 2008) (© 2010 FreeHand Ltd).

perform cardiothoracic surgery, currently its main application is laparoscopic radical prostatectomy. The system consists of a master console and a slave, patient-side cart placed in the same operating room, which houses an endoscopic camera and up to three surgical tools, as shown in Fig. 1.4a.

The most important feature of the da Vinci surgical tools is the EndoWrist™ with three-axis articulation mimicking the DoFs of the human wrist. Cable

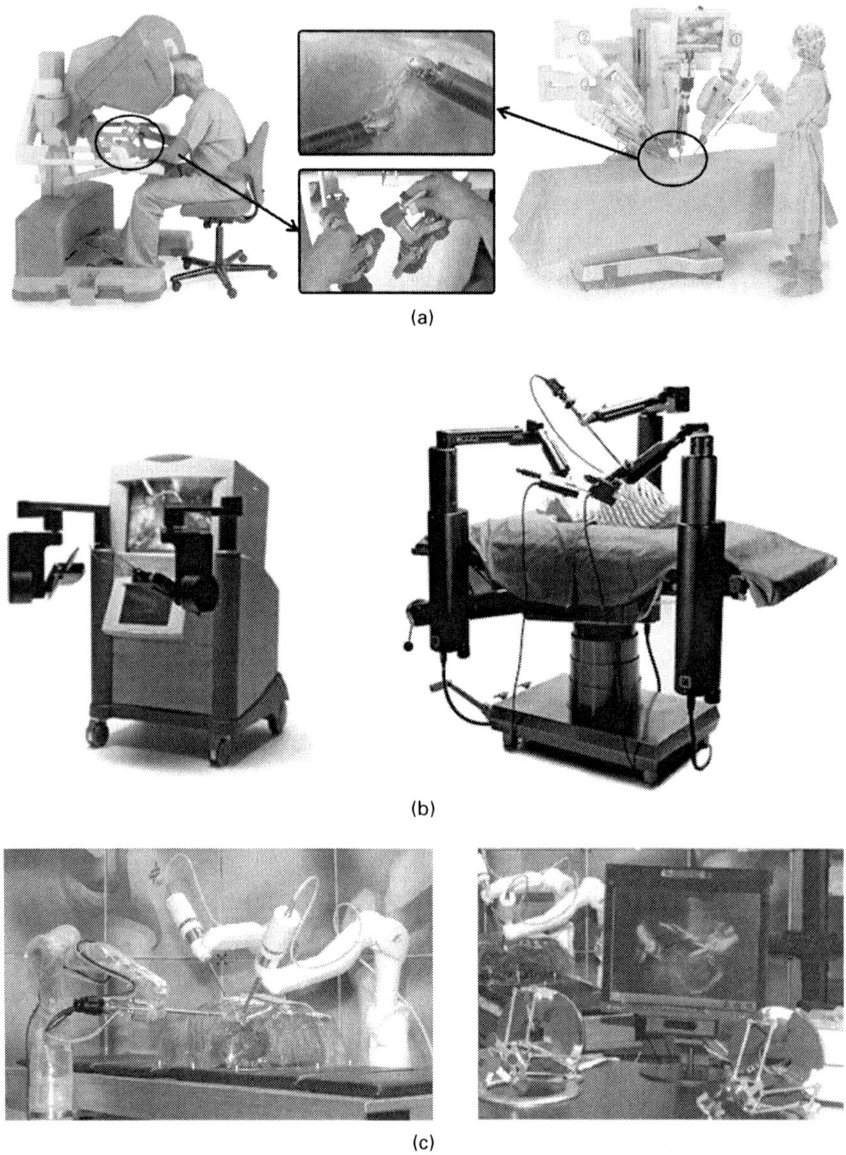

1.4 Master–slave robotic surgical systems: (a) the da Vinci Si surgical system comprising master console with ergonomic handles (middle insert) and slave manipulators (Guthart and Salisbury, 2000) (© 2009 Intuitive Surgical Inc.); (b) the Zeus master–slave robot for MIS (Low and Phee, 2004) (© Computer Motion Inc.); (c) the DLR MiroSurge teleoperated robot for surgical applications (© 2009 IEEE. Reprinted, with permission, from Konietschke *et al.* (2009)).

drives located in the 10 mm shaft of the EndoWrist™ are used to remotely control the tool through actuators placed at the proximal extremity of the holding module. These cables also drive the grasper oriented by the wrist. Finally, the external positioning mechanism controls the roll axis of the wrist.

The master console of the da Vinci system houses a 3-D display receiving the visual information from the operating field through the stereoscopic cameras at the tip of the endoscope. The surgeon docks the head in the console and places the hands inside the master's handles, which are registered to the coordinate frame of the 3-D monitor. The reversion of motion direction typical of MIS tools is avoided, tremor is filtered at 6 Hz, and motion scaling is applied to ensure the global accuracy of surgeon's movements. The main benefits of the system are enhanced dexterity and improved ergonomics as compared with conventional laparoscopy. However, limitations of the system include high cost and a lack of haptic and tactile feedback.

The Zeus teleoperated surgical robot (Low and Phee, 2004) was developed by Computer Motion Inc. (Goleta, CA) in parallel to the da Vinci system. It also features a patient-side slave manipulator with three arms and a master console, as shown in Fig. 1.4b, but the main difference between the two is that the Zeus instruments only have five DoFs. Albeit the system was used in the first transatlantic telesurgery, performed between Manhattan, New York, USA and Strasbourg, France (Marescaux *et al.*, 2001), it is no longer in production since its acquisition by Intuitive Surgical Inc. in 2003.

Although the da Vinci is currently the only master–slave robotic surgical system commercially available, Hongo *et al.* (2002) have developed the NeuRobot telecontrolled system to enable neurosurgery at a micro-scale, which is currently undergoing clinical tests. Together with the slave micro-manipulator and the master device, the system comprises a 6-DoF manipulator-supporting device and a stereo display monitor. The slave manipulator features three 1 mm forceps and a 3-D 4 mm endoscope. The initial position and spatial configuration of the slave arm is defined using the supporting device according to presurgical planning. Each micro-manipulator is then remotely controlled during the procedure by three 3-DoF (rotation, swinging, and translation) levers. Surgical simulations were first performed on a human cadaveric head to validate the system and the NeuRobot was subsequently successfully used to remove a portion of a tumour from a patient with a recurrent, atypical meningioma (Goto *et al.*, 2003).

Another promising system already tested on human patients is the neuroArm, a teleoperated robot for micro- and neurosurgery developed by Sutherland *et al.* (2003) at the University of Calgary, Canada. The design of the magnetic resonance (MR) compatible slave manipulator is based on a SCARA configuration and features seven DoFs plus tool actuation. A 3-DoF optical force sensor to provide haptic feedback is embedded in the end-effector, which can be interfaced with standard neurosurgical tools. The slave part of the system can be mounted on a mobile base for microsurgery or directly clamped onto the patient table for stereotaxis (Sutherland *et al.*, 2008). The master workstation recreates the sound and touch of surgery to enhance the user experience. The user interface comprises four monitors to display visual information from the operative room (OR) and the surgical site, as well as the position of the neuroArm and intra-operative MR images. Binoculars are integrated to convey the images from the surgical microscope and two PHANTOM Omni haptic input devices (SensAble Technologies, Woburn, MA) equipped with a stylus to mimic standard neurosurgical tools are used for manipulation. The first phase of clinical testing has been successfully completed by the system (Pandya *et al.*, 2009).

In addition to the aforementioned clinically applied robots, a number of teleoperated systems are currently under development. Among these, the one by Berkelman and Ma (2009) has the unique feature of combining simple, modular and lightweight components which can be easily integrated in the operating room. The slave part of the system consists of three manipulators less than 2 kg in weight, which can be clamped to a rigid frame fixed on the rails on either side of the patient table. Two of the manipulators are used to position endoscopic instruments while the third one is voice controlled and determines the pose of the endoscope. Also in this case, two PHANTOM Omni haptic devices are used to control the instrument manipulators, but they are customised with a mouse scroll-wheel and encoder to control the gripper opening and closing in a quasicontinuous fashion. The design of each slave manipulator is based on the light endoscope robot (LER) (Berkelman *et al.*, 2003), which consists of a ring-shaped base to be placed on the patient abdomen at the level of the instrument entry point, a clamp to hold the endoscope trocar and two joints guiding the motion of the endoscope about the incision point. The insertion depth of the endoscope can also be remotely controlled. The instrument manipulators feature an additional DoF to control the rotation of the tool shaft. Hitherto, the system performance has only been assessed in a laboratory environment.

Tadano and Kawashima (2010) recently investigated the use of pneumatic actuators to integrate force-sensing abilities in a teleoperated surgical system. The slave manipulator consists of a pneumatically actuated forceps with four DoFs arranged as rotation around its axis, two joints and a gripper (Tadano and Kawashima, 2006), which is positioned using a 3-DoF supporting manipulator (translation and rotation around the pivot point at the trocar insertion). The master manipulator features a total of six DoFs and is constituted by a delta mechanism for 3-DoF translation and a serial gimbal mechanism with three intersecting rotational axes to control the orientation of the forceps tip. Bilateral impedance control is implemented to obtain master–slave teleoperation. In particular, a motion-based impedance control is used for the master manipulator, and a force-type impedance control is adopted without a force sensor for the pneumatic slave manipulator. The accuracy of the bilateral control has been evaluated by measuring positions and forces of the manipulators during a suturing task in an *in vitro* experiment and the results indicated that the force at the slave side is felt by the operator with an uncertainty of about 1.5 N.

A robot-assisted microsurgery (RAMS) cable-driven master–slave telerobotic system for eye surgery has been developed at the NASA Jet Propulsion Laboratory (JPL) only for technology test purposes (Kozlowski *et al.*, 1997). The system enables enhanced dexterity and accuracy using tremor filters and motion scaling. Force feedback is also delivered to the operator, and the motion of the instrument can be constrained to minimise the negative effect of the surgery on the eye. The surgical tool is manipulated by a slave robot featuring six positioning DoFs with 15-μm accuracy and 6-DoF tip-force sensing. The master manipulator has the same kinematic structure of the slave robot with six force-sensed DoFs and 25-μm tip-position measurement accuracy. Bimanual operation can also be implemented by combining two systems with a surgical microscope.

The RAVEN robot developed by Hannaford and coworkers at the University of Washington was recently validated for teleoperation of surgical tasks (Lum *et al.*, 2009). It consists of a patient side featuring two identical manipulators mounted on the sides of the surgical table and a master side with two input devices, a monitor and a laptop. Each 7-DoF cable-actuated surgical manipulator consists of three main parts: a static base, which houses all of the motors; a spherical mechanism to position the tool and the tool interface. The spherical 4-DoF mechanism allows rotation of the tool about the pivot point on the patient abdomen and the remaining three DoFs at the tool interface control its rotation, grasp and wrist axes. The input devices at the surgeon site are PHANTOM Omni devices and the monitor displays a video feed of the operative site. A USB foot-pedal is also used to enable and disable the coupling between master and slave manipulators and allow for position indexing.

Finally, the German Aerospace Center (DLR) has recently designed a teleoperated robot for surgical applications called MiroSurge shown in Fig. 1.4c (Konietschke *et al.*, 2009; Hagn *et al.*, 2010). The master console features an autostereoscopic display and two haptic input devices with force feedback (Omega 7 by ForceDimension, Lausanne, Switzerland). The three slave manipulators at the patient side are lightweight MIRO robots (Hagn *et al.*, 2008) with a kinematically redundant structure resembling one of the human arms. The surgeon controls two of the slave robots equipped with specialised MIS instruments with enhanced articulation and force/torque sensing. The third arm is used to position the endoscopic stereo camera.

1.3.3 Hand-held and mechatronically enhanced surgical tools

Although CAD/CAM systems incorporate a relatively high level of automation, the main goal of robotic surgery is to develop new functional tools enhancing the ability of surgeons. Most medical robots are indeed designed to co-operate with surgeons and assist them during the operation. Among these, robotic hand-held surgical instruments are enhanced mechatronic tools with a certain degree of integrated intelligence and autonomy. They are able to assist the surgeons by adjusting movements and constraining the level of interaction with the operative field.

Several manually-driven prototypes have been designed to improve the accuracy of tissue manipulation, mainly for augmenting a surgeon's tactile or haptic sensing ability. Dario *et al.* (2000) proposed a new endoscope for integration in a computer-assisted arthroscopy system. The steerable tip of the device is cable-actuated and sensors for detecting the position of the tip and its contact with tissue are also embedded, as shown in Fig. 1.5a. The main feature of the device is the ability of semiautomatic collision avoidance to prevent the tip from touching critical areas defined before the surgery (D'Attanasio *et al.*, 2000).

The active tremor compensating microsurgical tool for ophthalmology called Micron was developed at Carnegie Mellon University by Riviere and coworkers (Ang *et al.*, 2000). Six inertial sensors are integrated to monitor the motion of the tool tip and estimate the physiological error. Tremor is cancelled using piezoelectric actuators to move the tip in the opposite direction using three DoFs as shown in Fig. 1.5b. The device has been recently improved by adding visual servoing abilities (Becker *et al.*, 2009).

The Steady-Hand Eye Robot developed at JHU (Taylor *et al.*, 1999) is a co-operatively-controlled robot assistant designed for retinal microsurgery. Co-operative control allows the surgeon to have full control of the system, with his hand movements dictating exactly the movements of the robot. The robot can also be a valuable assistant during high-risk procedures, by incorporating virtual fixtures to help protect the patient, and by eliminating physiological tremor in the surgeon's hand during surgery. The last prototype of the manipulator (Uneri *et al.*, 2010) consists of four components: (1) an XYZ linear stage for translation, (2) a rotary stage for rolling, (3) a tilting mechanism with a mechanical RCM, and (4) a tool adapter with a handle force sensor, as shown in Fig. 1.5c. Further details of synergistic control strategies applied to the system will be given in the last part of this chapter.

1.3.4 Semiautonomous robots for surgery

For MIS, the integration of some degrees of automation in soft tissue endoscopy still remains one of the biggest challenges. The development of tools for endoscopic surgery started 40 years ago with the design of active catheters. These long flexible cables are able to penetrate from the patient's veins to the most inaccessible areas of the cardiovascular system for performing diagnostic sensing at the tip. In recent years, some therapeutic actions have

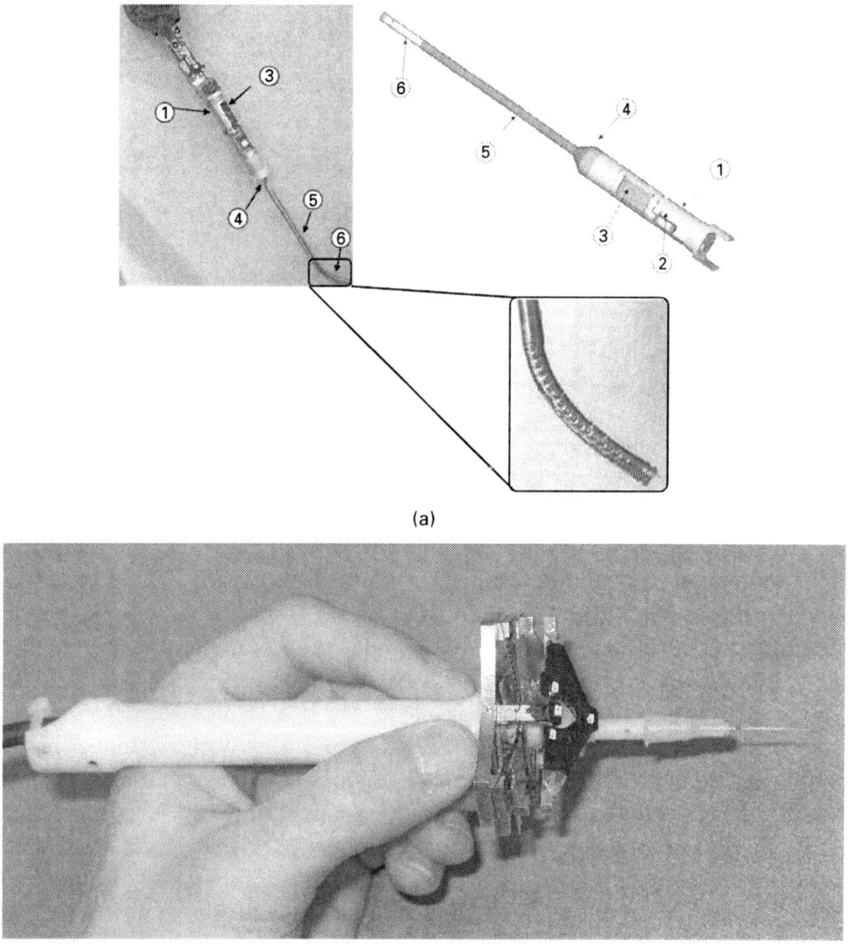

1.5 Robotically enhanced hand-held devices for MIS: (a) collision-avoidance endoscope for computer-assisted arthroscopy: 1 central element, 2 strain gauge sensor, 3 Hall effect sensor, 4 connector, 5 tube, 6 steerable tip (© 2000 IEEE. Reprinted, with permission, from Dario *et al.* (2000)); (b) micron hand-held instrument with active motion and tremor removal for vitroretinal microsurgery (courtesy of Dr Cameron Riviere, Carnegie Mellon University; Ang *et al.*, 2000); (c) schematic of the Steady-Hand Eye Robot and photo of the system set-up for vitroretinal surgery (© 2010 IEEE. Reprinted, with permission, from Uneri *et al.* (2010)).

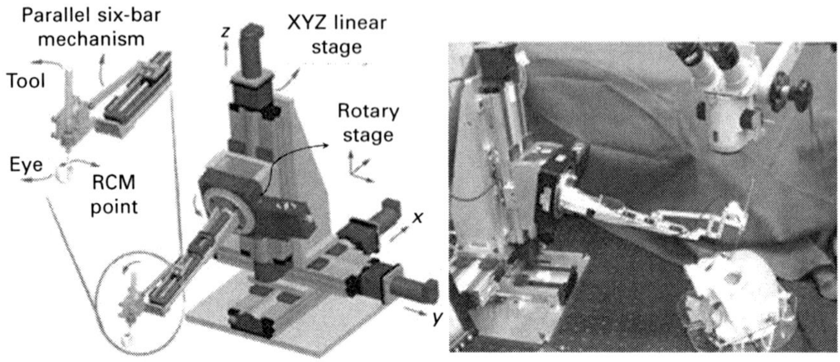

(c)

1.5 Continued.

also been executed using active probes integrating disposable stents to repair aneurysms or superelastic angioplastic balloons (Lim *et al.*, 1996). Although sensorised active catheters possess some degrees of autonomy, they are not considered as real autonomous robots because their advancement is controlled by the surgeon with the aid of external imaging guidance. For example, the Sensei Robotic Navigation System (RNS) (Kanagaratnam *et al.*, 2008) recently introduced clinically by Hansen Medical (Mountain View, CA, USA) is designed to control a steerable catheter under fluoroscopic guidance. The surgeon's workstation features a main display with the fluoroscopic view of the catheter at the surgical site and a 3-D model showing its actual articulation. Local catheter-to-tissue contact information collected using a force sensor at the tip of the catheter is also displayed. Additional screens show intracardiac electrophysiology data and a 3-D reconstruction of the surgical scene, as shown in Fig. 1.6a. The slave part of the system consists of a steerable catheter (Artisan) controlled by a remote catheter manipulator fixed at the patient table. The tendon configuration of the catheter is illustrated in Fig. 1.6a. In particular, the Artisan features two flexible guides controlled by separate remotely located actuation boxes. The combination of outer and inner guide motion allows the catheter to easily conform to any S-shaped curve (Camarillo *et al.*, 2008b). Accurate position control is ensured by detailed modelling of both forward and inverse kinematics of the tendons and real-time vision-based 3-D shape detection and tracking (Camarillo *et al.*, 2008a).

On the other hand, semiautonomous endoscopes integrate intervention and diagnostic ability of the surgeon through autonomous motion and integrated vision. As an example, the tethered epicardial crawling (TEC) robot HeartLander developed by Riviere and coworkers (Patronik *et al.*, 2005) is a miniature mobile robot for cardiac MIS, consisting of two independent components connected by three nitinol wires. Each part can adhere to the

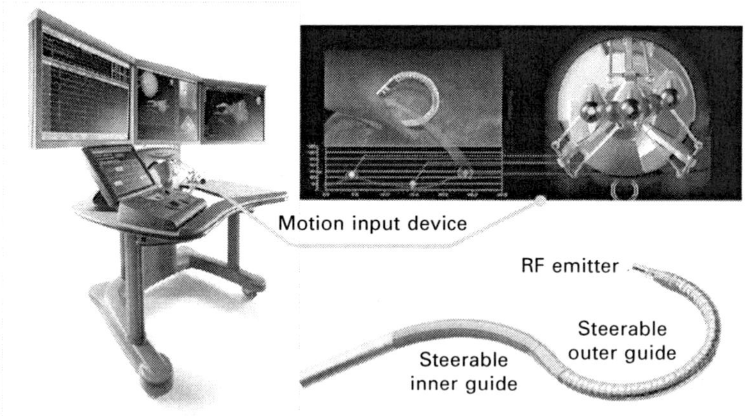

(a)

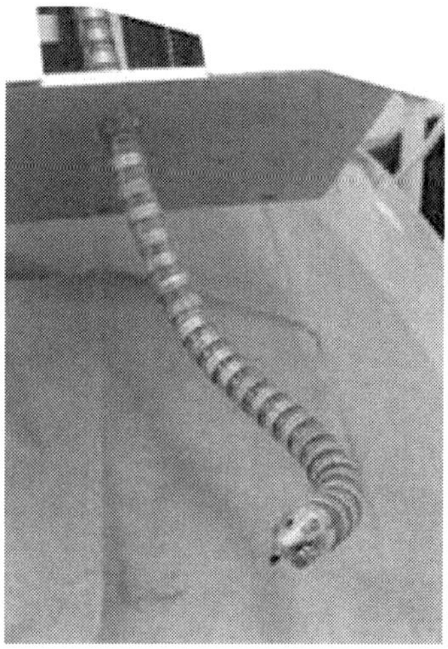

(b)

1.6 Semiautonomous systems for endoscopic surgery: (a) Sensei® X Robotic Catheter System: the parallel manipulator (top right) is a motion input device integrated in the master console (left), featuring tactile vibration feedback corresponding to the contact measure between the tip and the tissue; the Artisan™ Control Catheter (bottom right) allows double-bending flexibility to navigate along the vessels and position the radio-frequency emitter on the vascular wall (Kanagaratnam *et al.*, 2008) (© 2011 Hansen Medical, Inc.); (b) CardioArm highly articulated robotic probe (courtesy of Dr Howie Choset, Carnegie Mellon University and Medrobotics Corporation) (Degani *et al.*, 2006); (c) 12-leg robotic capsule for the exploration of the GI tract (reprinted, with permission, from Quaglia *et al.*, 2009 (© 2009 IOP) and Valdastri *et al.*, 2009 (© 2009 IEEE)).

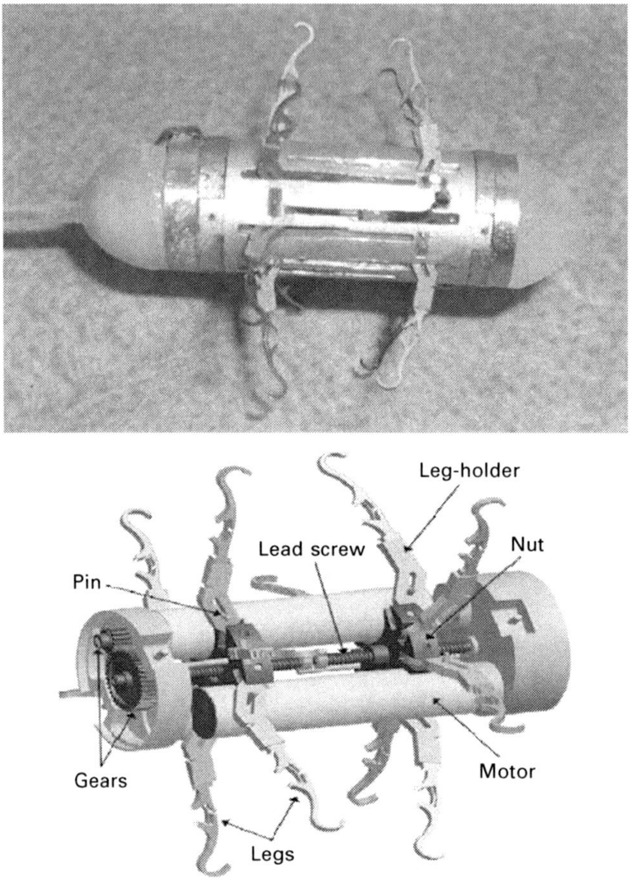

(c)

1.6 Continued.

epicardium using suction pads, thus enabling forward advancement through inchworm-like locomotion. The robot also incorporates an endoscope for visual feedback and an electromagnetic tracking system for real-time 3-D localisation (Patronik *et al.*, 2009). Recently, a new prototype with miniature on-board motors has been proposed for wireless cardiac MIS procedures (Allen *et al.*, 2008).

The highly articulated robotic probe (HARP) developed by Choset and coworkers (Degani *et al.*, 2006) and lately named CardioARM (Ota *et al.*, 2009), is instead designed to perform minimally invasive epicardial interventions through a subxiphoid approach. The flexible part of the device is 300 mm long and has a diameter of 10 mm, and is able to navigate in confined anatomical regions such as the intrapericardial space with minimal interaction with the environment, as shown in Fig. 1.6b. The forward motion is performed by alternating the rigidity of two concentric tubes constituting the probe. Both tubes consist of cylindrical links serially connected by spherical joints. The main advantage of this design is the ability of holding an arbitrary 3-D shape or to become completely flexible if necessary. However, the joints can only bend ±10° and cannot be actuated independently, thus the radius of curvature is limited and the kinematic redundancy is not fully exploited. Furthermore, the forward speed is low and a large external feeding control mechanism is required.

Thus far, most semiautonomous robots are designed for navigation and examination of the gastrointestinal (GI) tract. This is because of both anatomical and safety reasons, given that the GI tract is naturally not sterile, can be accessed through two natural orifices, and its minimum diameter is about 3 cm. Currently, clinically deployable GI robots are limited, apart from endoscopic capsules, which can be considered as passive swallowable imaging tools rather than real robotic devices (Moglia *et al.*, 2007).

Various approaches have recently been proposed to provide wireless endoscopic capsules with active locomotion, either through external (*e.g.* magnetic fields) (Menciassi *et al.*, 2009) or on-board actuation (Tortora *et al.*, 2009). In particular, Dario and coworkers at Instituto Superiore Sant'Anna (ISSA) have used legged locomotion and developed three generations of legged capsular prototypes (Quirini *et al.*, 2008a; 2008b; Valdastri *et al.*, 2009). One of the prototypes is shown in Fig. 1.6c, for which forward motion is performed by cyclic actuation of two identical sets of six legs located, respectively, at the front and rear of the capsule. Each set of legs is driven by a miniature brushless direct current (DC) motor coupled with a slot-follower mechanism. The device has been tested *ex vivo* using excised porcine colon specimens placed inside a GI phantom model. The average speed was 5 cm min^{-1}, which would allow the completion of a colonoscopic procedure in less than 30 min. The device was powered by wired connection to an external source and wireless power delivery and further size miniaturisation still remain a challenge for future designs.

One of the most challenging tasks in the design of an endoscopic robot is the incorporation of an effective locomotion scheme enabling the advance of the robot through the elastic, slippery, peristaltic and collapsed colon without causing tissue damage. Koji Ikuta (Ikuta *et al.*, 1988) was among the first to use shape memory alloy (SMA) actuators to drive an automated snake-like endoscopic robot around obstacles. The device consisted of five flexible segments: four bending in the same direction on a plane, and a tip one which could turn orthogonally. It also featured a fibrescope delivering the vision information. The device was able to navigate smoothly through the sigmoid colon, but the motion was limited to a two dimensional space. One problem related to the use of SMA tendons is that they require high currents for actuation and forward movement is slow.

Burdick and coworkers (Slatkin *et al.*, 1995) designed a robotic endoscope able to perform inchworm-like locomotion in the colon using inflatable balloons and modified bellows as actuators. The balloons located at the robot extremities had the function of grasping the colon walls, while the rubber bellows worked as extensors. The system was moderately efficient *in vitro*, but encountered challenges when tested *in vivo*, as the balloons tended to slip along the intestinal wall owing to insufficient gripping force. Increased dilatation of the colon wall to achieve adequate gripping force carries a risk of producing regional ischemia.

Different generations of semiautonomous inchworm-like robots for colonoscopy have been developed by Paolo Dario and coworkers (Dario *et al.*, 1997; 2004; Menciassi *et al.*, 2002; Phee *et al.*, 2002). Each of them features a steerable distal tip integrating a visualisation system and a locomotion unit comprising two clamping modules and a pneumatically actuated extension module. Each clamping unit houses several small holes to suck the colon tissue and fix the position of the robotic device relative to the intestinal wall. Inchworm-like locomotion is performed by first actuating the rear clamper, then extending the central module and, finally, closing the frontal clamper while the rear clamper is released. After the central module contracts again, the same steps are repeated. The robotic system demonstrated the capability of smoothly adjust its shape in relation to the intestine during locomotion. However, its major drawback was the so called 'accordion effect' which occurs when the colon wall is extending or retracting in accordance with the elongation and contraction phases of locomotion, preventing any advancement of the device.

A flexible access platform for MIS called the i-Snake® has recently been developed at the Hamlyn Centre by Guang-Zhong Yang and his team (Shang *et al.*, 2011). The platform incorporates a hybrid micromotor/tendon design to ensure individually addressable joint articulation and ample space for inner instrument channels (Noonan *et al.*, 2011). As shown in Plate Ia (see Colour Section between pages 136 and 137), the joint design is modular, thus allowing changing the robot configuration according to the specific surgical task. The range of actuation of each DoF is ± 45° and the outer diameter of each joint is 12.5 mm, allowing the integration of two 3 mm diameter internal channels for the passage of camera and instrumentation. The enhanced dexterity of the device allows large area exploration (±90° vertically and ±225° horizontally) from a single incision on the patient skin without the limitations of laparoscopic style external manipulation (Clark *et al.*, 2010; Sodergren *et al.*, 2010; Newton *et al.*, 2012). Plate Ib shows the device in a completely retroflexed configuration during *in vivo* deployment to perform a transvaginal tubal ligation procedure on a porcine model. Gaze-contingent (Noonan *et al.*, 2010) and shape conformance (Vitiello *et al.*, 2011) control strategies have also been implemented with the system.

1.4 Perceptual docking for synergistic control

Although the performance of the surgeon is improved by integrating the aforementioned systems, the human capabilities are not yet fully exploited. A novel concept in robotic surgery is therefore to seamlessly share control between the surgeon and the robot. One example is the active constraint robot known as Acrobot developed at Imperial College London (Davies *et al.*, 1997; Yen and Davies, 2010). The system was first commercialised by the Acrobot Company Ltd and recently re-named 'Acrobot Sculptor Robotic System' after acquisition by Stanmore Implants Worlwide in 2010. It is used in orthopaedic surgery as shown in Fig. 1.7a and features a back-drivable force-controlled bone-milling instrument, which allows 'hands-on' sculpting of the bone. The surgeon is in direct control of the milling tool, but his hand motions are constrained to remain within a permitted region, usually defined preoperatively. Such a system offers the benefits of a CAD/CAM system with enhanced safety, which makes it clinically more acceptable.

Mako Surgical (Fort Lauderdale, FL, USA) has recently developed a second hands-on system for orthopaedic joint replacement called the robotic arm interactive orthopaedic system (RIO) (Hagag *et al.*, 2011). The latest version of RIO derives from the tactile guidance system (TGS), which obtained FDA approval in May 2005 and was originally based on a specialised version of the backdriveable whole arm manipulation (WAM) arm (Barrett Technology Inc., Cambridge, MA, USA), also licensed by Mako. The procedure performed with the RIO has been called MAKOplasty from the company, which is also commercialising the implants. The sculpting ability of robotic devices such as Acrobot Sculptor and RIO allows the execution of complex geometry cuts within the bone, introducing the potential for patient specific, bone conserving, and resurfacing implants, in contrast with the original simple orthopaedic implant design obtainable with conventional instrumentation.

A variation of the same concept has been implemented by Troccaz *et al.* using a 6-DoF passive arm with dynamic constraints (PADyC) (Schneider and Troccaz, 2001). This system can constrain the surgeon's hand motion inside a predefined region or along a desired trajectory and was developed for application in cardiac surgery (pericardial puncture). The system comprises a three-axis SCARA robot with two additional axes (one for rotation and one for translation) and a modular sixth joint for either translation or rotation. Even though the use of a passive robot ensures increased safety, motion accuracy and stiffness are compromised.

A novel approach to synergistic control called 'perceptual docking' has recently been proposed by Yang *et al.* (2008). The fundamental idea is to gain knowledge from subject-specific motor and perceptual behaviour through *in situ* sensing. One example is to integrate eye-tracking as an

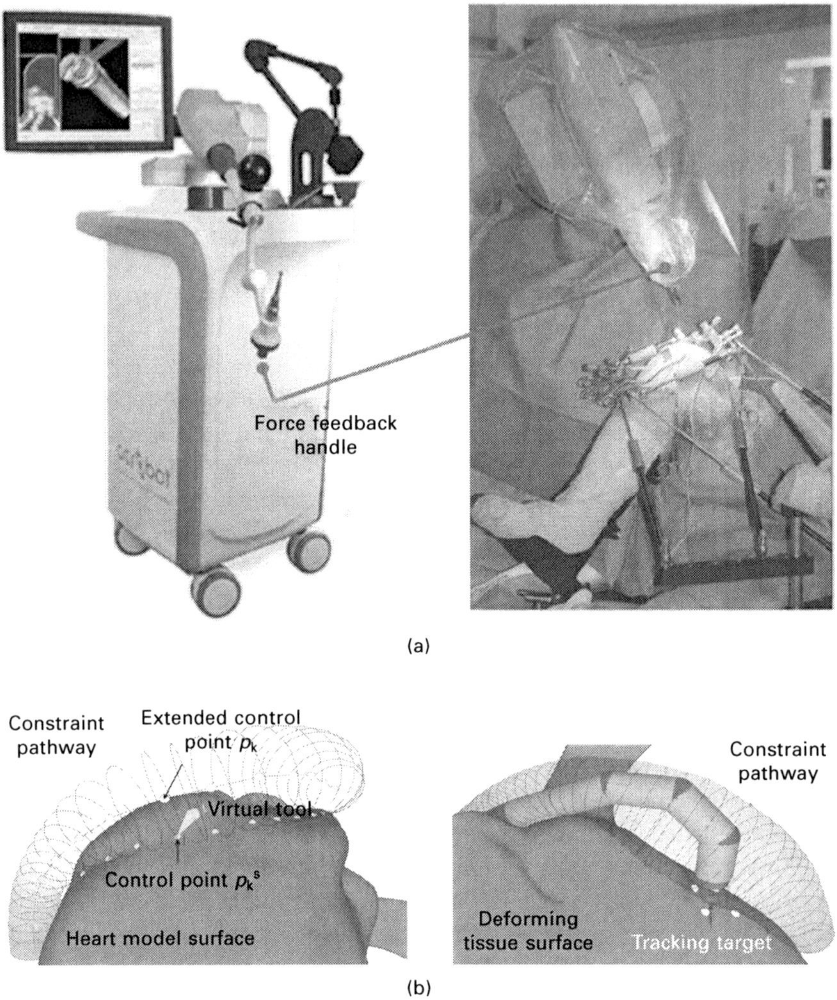

1.7 Synergistic control applications in robot-assisted MIS: (a) the Acrobot system for actively constrained orthopaedic surgery (courtesy of Professor Justin Cobb, Imperial College London) (Yen and Davies, 2010); (b) dynamic active constraint generated on the surface of the beating heart (Kwok *et al.*, 2009a). The superimposed tubular constraint can be used to determine optimal robot configurations for safe visual stabilisation when tracking a target on a deforming tissue surface (Kwok *et al.*, 2010); (c) a schematic illustration of dynamic active constraints defined on the surface of the beating heart as conical pathways carved out from the active constraint boundary and directed towards the ablation targets based on the eye fixation points tracked during the experiment (Mylonas *et al.*, 2008). (Reprinted from (Lee *et al.*, 2010) © 2010, and (Mylonas *et al.*, 2012), © 2012, with permission from Elsevier).

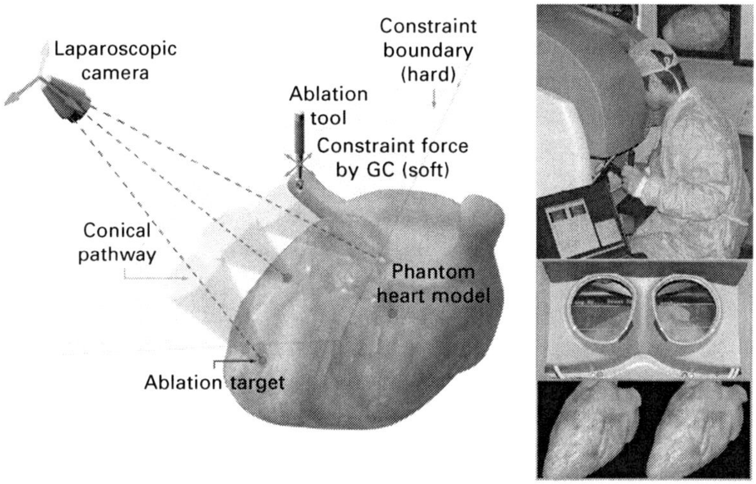

(c)

1.7 Continued.

additional human-robot interface modality and perform gaze-contingent attention selection, 3-D tissue deformation recovery (Mylonas *et al.*, 2004; 2005) or motor channelling with haptic constraints (Mylonas *et al.*, 2008). A perceptually docked control framework for multiple robotic devices operating in the gastric cavity has also been designed and validated (Kwok *et al.*, 2009b).

1.4.1 Virtual fixtures

As already discussed, incorporating haptic feedback can permit a number of safety features to be implemented on the current robotic platforms. Over the past decade, virtual fixtures (VFs) have been widely used in many robotic platforms. The concept was originally proposed by Rosenberg (1993) for telerobotic manipulations. Perceptual overlays are generated so as to reduce the mental burden in performing a remotely manipulated task, and to alleviate the workload of processing certain sensory modalities. The idea behind VFs is simple yet effective, just as using a ruler to guide a pen in drawing a straight line. Such perceptual overlays can be computer-generated haptic signals interacting with operators in order to maintain the consistency and accuracy of the movement.

The original idea of VFs was not limited to haptic interaction; it also included audio signals or other multimodal interaction cues. However, the use of haptic interaction is the most common mode of operation. In general, VFs can be divided into two categories (Ren *et al.*, 2008): forbidden-region VFs (FRVFs) and guidance VFs (GVFs). FRVFs constrain the motion of a robot so as to keep its end-effector away from the defined space. Surface contact and reaction forces are commonly adopted to provide the operator with a strong sensation of the barrier. In contrast, GVFs are used to assist the operator in manoeuvring the robot end-effector along a virtually defined pathway. The design of GVFs is specific to the task objectives such as targeting at specific anatomical objects. Soft attractive forces are usually generated as guidance to hand motion. However, the operator is always in full control of the robot and his/her hand would not be overpowered by the haptic interface.

Although the term VFs was rarely used for several years after its inception, the control concept was applied to many remote manipulation tasks. Joly and Andriot (1995) proposed a mathematical model of VF control that incorporated different force profiles such as spring and damping forces, into the controller. The VFs were modelled by generating tangential forces along a complex curve or orthogonal forces to the outer surface of a cylinder. The control stability and the manipulator singularity in VF tasks were considered by Micaelli *et al.* (1998), who also enhanced a VF remote manipulation system with the synergistic use of different master–slave controllers. Provided with the adjustable parameters of these controllers, different behaviours could be achieved depending on the manipulation tasks. The dynamics of both master and slave manipulators, including their Coriolis force during motion, was studied by Itoh *et al.* (2000). They proposed a control algorithm capable of scaling the motion and force generated by both manipulators.

The introduced VFs represent an interaction mode where the motion or force exerted by the robot is a subset or limited version of those requested by the operator (Mylonas *et al.*, 2012). This control concept is well-suited to some of the challenges faced by robot assisted MIS. For instance, as a result of the sensory deprivation and confined workspace as discussed earlier, the implementation of VFs for the human–robot interface can help the surgeon locate particular tissue structures or dissect near a structure with a defined safety margin to prevent inadvertent tissue damage. In this way, the robot is prevented from moving outside of a safe region, ensuring the preservation of critical features.

One clinical application for which VFs are critical is microsurgery. As discussed earlier, the JHU Steady-Hand Eye Robot with admittance VF control (Bettini *et al.*, 2004) provides the operator with 7-DoF manipulation and force sensing at the handle. With the motion constrained by anisotropic stiffness, this hand-held robot is used to enhance the dexterity of manipulating delicate tissue membranes. One of the objectives is to deliver a safe retinal vein cannulation, which involves epiretinal membrane peeling and needle insertion into the lumen of a retinal vein. Experimental validations were conducted on a phantom eye model, which demonstrated promising results in minimising the lateral forces applied on the trocar by the instrument shaft.

These undesirable forces can deteriorate the tool positioning accuracy by distorting the required force transferring from sclera to the tissue inside the eye. By evaluating the performance in terms of completion time and the magnitude of the forces required for the task, improved performance can be achieved by augmenting the VF interaction force with audio feedback (Balicki *et al.*, 2010).

By integrating an endoscopic instrument into the same mechanical framework of the JHU Steady-Hand Eye Robot, Li *et al.* (2007) proposed a constrained optimisation approach which enabled surgical navigation to be conducted deep inside the nasal and sinus cavity. To consider the instrument as an entity, rather than only its tip, it was the first work that attempted to generate constrained motion based on the configuration of the instrument body. During the task, the tip is guided along a reference target using the admittance control; meanwhile, the instrument manipulation is also subject to the interaction between the instrument body and the bone cavity. The static anatomical model of the cavity is obtained by CT scan and the reference target for path-following is preoperatively defined. The robot configuration in joint space is optimised in order to avoid collision and excessive force on the target anatomy. In addition to hands-on manipulation by using the Steady-Hand robot, remotely controlled manipulation is also implemented by using a master interface capable of force sensing. The improvement of targeting accuracy and task efficiency was experimentally demonstrated for both modes of manipulation.

Finally, the extension of the control concept to procedures involving soft tissue, cardiac surgery, for example, had been suggested in the very early stage of robotic assisted MIS. By using the ZEUS surgical robot, Park *et al.* (2001) proposed to perform blunt dissections adjacent to the artery with the aid of VFs. Borelli *et al.* (2004) also attempted to apply active constraints to minimally invasive cardiac surgery with 2-DoF master control. More significant work was proposed by Ren *et al.* (2008) who first introduced dynamic VFs capable of adapting the rapid morphological changes of epicardial surface according to the intraoperative ultrasound images. The method requires accurate registration of ultrasound images to the MR/CT model of the entire cardiac surface. The experiment was conducted in a simulation environment. The operator can slide the virtual tool on hard FRVFs which are generated based on a potential field along the surface using generalised sigmoid function (Ren *et al.*, 2007). Soft GVFs based on generalised Gaussian functions have also been used to attract the tool tip to the ablation target. The penetration depth is also constrained by the VF force model while performing a simulated cutting task for ablation. For tracking deforming epicardial surfaces, Gibo *et al.* (2009) also studied the effectiveness of using moving FRVFs for remote manipulation. The motion, however, only involved translation. Nevertheless, the work demonstrated the clinical value of using predictive filters (Ginhoux *et al.*, 2005) to estimate a proper translation of FRVFs in response to the physiological motion.

1.4.2 Dynamic active constraints

As mentioned earlier, the basic concept of active constraints was introduced by Davies *et al.* (1997) to enhance surgical safety during robot-assisted orthopaedic surgery using the Acrobot system. In fact, the concept of active constraints can be deduced from VFs because the idea is based on gradually increasing the haptic stiffness when the cutter approaches the predefined forbidden region. Sensing the guidance forces directing the hand-held instrument either perpendicularly or tangentially away from the virtual boundaries of the prosthesis, the surgeon can sculpture the knee bone precisely. However, the clinical application of VFs and active constraints is, thus far, mainly limited to orthopaedic procedures, which are conducted under a static frame-of-reference because of the relatively rigid anatomical structures involved. With recent advances in intraoperative real-time tissue deformation recovery based on accurate feature tracking and fusion of multiple visual cues, the field of VFs and active constraints is finding its way for more complex procedures involving large-scale soft-tissue deformation. The use of articulated flexible robotic devices augmented by enhanced ergonomics under the framework of active constraints can further improve the perceptual-motor capabilities of the surgeon, thus allowing surgical procedures to be carried out with greater accuracy and efficiency. To this end, Kwok *et al.* (2009a) recently developed a scheme for real-time modelling of dynamic active constraints for an articulated robot adapting to both cardiac deformation and local changes of tissue morphology. In contrast to existing methods, the manipulation boundaries of the forbidden region are defined for the entire length of an articulated surgical tool. Constraining the motion of a single point (*e.g.* the tip) of the instrument is not enough, especially when manoeuvring within the tight confines of chest cavity and pericardium. Moreover, accurate path following is critical for many procedures, such as epicardial ablation. For example, the maze procedure currently needs to be performed during open heart surgery or through multiple small incisions on both sides of the chest to ensure accurate vessel encirclement. In the minimally invasive case, a catheter is passed along the posterior of the heart through two narrow spaces strictly confined by the great vessels and the surrounding pericardium. The lack of visual feedback strongly affects the hand–eye coordination of the surgeon. The development of more flexible devices for safe access and navigation, combined with the application of active constraints, can enhance both the speed and the accuracy of such procedures.

Within the active constraint framework, a haptic interface is used to input 3-D coordinates, so that the operator can place a series of points precisely along the surface of the preoperative anatomical model with the sensation of contact force feedback, as shown in Fig. 1.7b (left). Together with the specification of adjustable radius values that determine the cross-sectional area along the obstacle-free centreline, dynamic active constraints are constructed as a predetermined constraining pathway comprising a series of circular contours. Note that the contours are not restricted to circles only, but also they can be represented by any polygon in polar coordinates on a 3-D plane. This prescribed pathway, as well as the preoperative model, can be co-registered with intraoperative images. To provide a smooth 3-D constraint pathway without having to define too many control points along the anatomical structures, a rescaled domain is applied to parameterise the constraint into numerous segments. Such smoothing effect becomes particularly obvious in the case of high-curvature surfaces with large radius variation.

When considering the spatial constraints applied on the robot motion, such a constraint model is not only a 3-D tessellation boundary for facilitating visual guidance during navigation, but it is also important to provide proximity queries (PQs) between the robot and the constraint pathway. These queries can be included as optimisation conditions for controlling the robot without exceeding the safety margin. To this end, Kwok *et al.* (2010) have also proposed an analytical approach to compute the robot deviation from the constraint pathway. In contrast to the existing PQ algorithms (Gilbert *et al.*, 1988; Lin and Canny, 1991; Mirtich, 1998), the proposed algorithm is more efficient as it does not require any complex data structure and preprocessing because the spatial constraint model has to adapt to tissue deformation rapidly. It is also general for any robot objects even in non-convex complex shapes. The programming architecture of the approach is intrinsically parallel and the computational time can be significantly reduced when using the currently advanced parallel architectures such as graphics processing unit (GPU) or field-programmable gate array (FPGA), thus fulfilling the requirements for real-time haptic interaction and optimal kinematic control of the robot.

One example of kinematic control under dynamic active constraints is motion stabilisation of a redundant snake robot, as shown in Fig. 1.7b (right). The main objective of the control algorithm is to enable the robot to track the visual target accurately and steadily on deforming tissue. The optimal kinematic configuration that conforms to predefined anatomical constraints is first determined. The proposed motion tracking can also be augmented with manual control. The importance of visual–motor synchronisation for performing accurate smooth pursuit movements has also been demonstrated by considering the physical limits in terms of maximum frequency response of the system (manifested as a delay between the input of the manipulator and the movement of the end-effector) (Kwok *et al.*, 2010).

1.4.3 Gaze-contingent motor channelling

A more intuitive way to update the active constraint intraoperatively is to incorporate human interaction within the framework of gaze contingent perceptual docking control (Yang *et al.*, 2008). As mentioned before, this is defined as a novel method of knowledge acquisition for robotic systems that utilises *in situ* learning of operator specific motor and perceptual/cognitive behaviour, such as gaze direction. Firstly, the 3-D position of the fixation point on the tissue can be calculated by tracking the binocular eye movement and computing ocular vergence. Subsequently, the distance between the laparoscopic instrument and the gaze fixation point can be determined on the basis of the known intrinsic and extrinsic parameters of the calibrated stereo laparoscopic camera.

Based on the perceptual docking framework, Mylonas *et al.* (2008) have introduced gaze-contingent haptic constraints. Through the use of motor channelling, real-time binocular eye tracking can be exploited to improve the performance and accuracy of robotic manipulation. This is achieved by generating a haptic force with intensity proportional to the relative separation between the fixation point and the instrument tip. Figure 1.7c illustrates how dynamic active constraints are defined as conical pathways guiding the instrument tip towards the target determined by the fixation point. This effectively bridges the visual and motor modalities using a perceptually enabled channel and alleviates the burden of the instrument control as well as the cognitive demand on the surgeon.

1.5 Conclusions and future trends

In this chapter, the robotic surgical systems currently available on the market and under research development demonstrate how the technology is still in its infancy, especially for application to more complex procedures involving soft tissue manipulation. Indeed, the systems that have been successfully integrated in the operative theatre and have effectively improved the procedure in terms of either surgeon performance or patient outcome, only offer advantages related to the capabilities of traditional industrial robots. Their role is therefore limited to a minimum number of low-level tasks such as precision cutting or endoscope holding and positioning. Although some CAD/CAM systems are used for both preoperative planning and intraoperative tasks, long preoperative procedures, high cost and large footprint are major issues, together with the questionable improvement in patient outcome that has yet to be demonstrated.

As robot-assisted MIS evolves, it is expected that a new generation of smaller and lighter surgical robots with stronger and more flexible manipulator will emerge. With miniaturised robotic instruments, the robot actuation can take place inside the body without being driven by external mechanisms with a large footprint inside the operating room. This will also facilitate the development of VFs and active constraints for more complex surgical procedures using manipulators of higher DoFs. This will bring the surgeons back to the operating table, thus permitting a more natural surgical workflow as we did before. In this case, the surgery will truly become robot-assisted, rather than robot-dominated, MIS.

Although some instruments are incorporated with a number of DoFs close to the tip, such as the EndoWrist™ instruments used in da Vinci, it is difficult to perform smooth pursuit movement on complex anatomical pathways. This is particularly important for many targeted-therapy or tissue-ablation procedures. As mentioned earlier, the main problem is that the use of long and rigid instruments through a fixed entry port restricts the robot workspace and the accessibility to the surgical site inside a confined anatomical cavity. To facilitate adequate surgical exploration, there has been a rising demand on developing snake-like articulated robotic devices that allow flexible access inside the human body, thus relaxing the requirement on accurate port placement. These have motivated the recent development of natural orifice transluminal endoscopic surgery (NOTES) and single incision laparoscopic surgery (SILS). Although the clinical justification for these procedures is still under continuing debate, the need for improved articulation to allow for seamless navigation along a curved anatomical pathway represents a major step in the future development of MIS robots.

The recent advances in pre- and intraoperative imaging have permitted detailed guidance for procedures involving soft tissue deformation. In order to follow the general trend of flexible articulated devices, it is necessary to consider the interaction of the entire body of the robot with the surrounding anatomical structures. This is because relying only on the buttressing of anatomical structures to constrain and guide the robot is unsafe as this can easily cause perforation particularly of delicate or diseased tissue. Constraining the navigation with effective guidance to avoid excessive forces and collisions by the robot body is a key criterion in introducing VFs or active constraints. Additionally, consideration of the actual robot actuation limits is also important in remote manipulation tasks. Scaled-down hand motion with tremor removal has been achieved by using master–slave control interfaces; however, the input motion can still be relatively fast compared with the actual actuation limit of the device. This can cause mis-synchronisation and instability of the control loop. In order to enhance smooth manipulation matched to the dynamic response of the robot, impedance forces based on its actuation capabilities have to be incorporated as a new control feature of VFs or active constraints. Furthermore, in soft-tissue surgery, the safety manipulation margin interacting with the entire snake-like robot body can change continuously owing to tissue deformation. The active constraints therefore need to be updated accordingly to ensure dynamic shape conformance. All these represent significant technical challenges and unmet surgical requirements that need to be addressed by future research.

1.6 References

Adler Jr J R, Chang S D, Murphy M J, Doty J, Geis P and Hancock S L (1997), The cyberknife: a frameless robotic system for radiosurgery, *Stereotact Funct Neurosurg*, **69**, 124–128.

Aiono S, Gilbert J M and Soin B (2002), Controlled trial of the introduction of a robotic camera assistant (Endo Assist) for laparoscopic cholecystectomy, *Surg Endosc*, **16**, 1267–1270.

Allen P, Patronik N and Zenati M A (2008), A mobile robot driven by miniature onboard motors for cardiac intervention, *34th Annual Northeast Bioengineering Conference*, 9–10.

Ang W, Riviere C and Khosla P (2000). 'An active hand-held instrument for enhanced microsurgical accuracy', in Delp S L, DiGoia A M and Jaramaz B, *Medical image computing and computer-assisted intervention – MICCAI 2000*, Berlin, Springer, 878–886.

Balicki M, Uneri A, Iordachita I, Handa J, Gehlbach P and Taylor R (2010). 'Micro-force sensing in robot assisted membrane peeling for vitreoretinal surgery', in Jiang T, Navab N, Pluim J and Viergever M, *Medical image computing and computer-assisted intervention – MICCAI 2010*, Springer Berlin/Heidelberg, 303–310.

Ballantyne G H and Moll F (2003), The da Vinci telerobotic surgical system: the virtual operative field and telepresence surgery, *Surg Clin North Am*, **83**, 1293–1304.

Becker B C, Voros S, MacLachlan R A, Hager G D and Riviere C N (2009), Active guidance of a handheld micromanipulator using visual servoing, *IEEE International Conference on Robotics and Automation*, 339–344.

Benabid A L, Cinquin P, Lavalle S, Le Bas J F, Demongeot J and de Rougemont J (1987), Computer-driven robot for stereotactic surgery connected to CT scan and magnetic resonance imaging, *Stereotact Funct Neurosurg*, **50**, 153–154.

Berkelman P, Boidard E, Cinquin P and Troccaz J (2003), LER: the light endoscope robot, *IEEE/RSJ International Conference on Intelligent Robots and Systems*, 2835–2840.

Berkelman P and Ma J (2009), A compact modular teleoperated robotic system for laparoscopic surgery, *Int J Robot Res*, **28**, 1198–1215.

Bettini A, Marayong P, Lang S, Okamura A M and Hager G D (2004), Vision-assisted control for manipulation using virtual fixtures, *IEEE Trans Robot*, **20**, 953–966.

Borelli J, Bello F, Rodriguez Y Baena F and Davies B (2004), An active constraint environment for minimally invasive heart surgery: early experience of a cutting operation, *Stud Health Technol Inform*, **98**, 31–33.

Burckhardt C W, Flury P and Glauser D (1995), Stereotactic brain surgery, *IEEE Eng Med Biol Mag*, **14**, 314–317.

Camarillo D B, Krummel T M and Salisbury J K J (2004), Robotic technology in surgery: past, present, and future, *Am J Surg*, **188**, 2–15.

Camarillo D B, Loewke K E, Carlson C R and Salisbury J K (2008a), Vision based 3-D shape sensing of flexible manipulators, *IEEE International Conference on Robotics and Automation*, 2940–2947.

Camarillo D B, Milne C F, Carlson C R, Zinn M R and Salisbury J K (2008b), Mechanics modeling of tendon-driven continuum manipulators, *IEEE Trans Robot*, **24**, 1262–1273.

Clark J, Sodergren M, Noonan D P, Shang J, Payne C J, James D R C, Teare J, Athanasiou T, Darzi A and Yang G-Z (2010), A novel articulated robotic laparoscope for single incision and natural orifice surgical applications; preliminary usability trials in a live porcine model, *Surg Endosc*, **24**, 314–701.

Cleary K and Nguyen C (2001), State of the art in surgical robotics: clinical applications and technology challenges, *Comput Aided Surg*, **6**, 312–328.

D'Attanasio S, Tonet O, Megali G, Carrozza M C and Dario P (2000), A semi-automatic handheld mechatronic endoscope with collision-avoidance capabilities, *IEEE International Conference on Robotics and Automation*, 1586–1591.

Dario P, Carrozza M C, Lencioni L, Magnani B and D'Attanasio S (1997), A microrobotic system for colonoscopy, *IEEE International Conference on Robotics and Automation*, 1567–1572.

Dario P, Carrozza M C and Marcacci M (2000), A novel mechatronic tool for computer-assisted arthroscopy, *IEEE Trans Inform Technol Biomed*, **4**, 15–29.

Dario P, Ciarletta P, Menciassi A and Kim B (2004), Modeling and experimental validation of the locomotion of endoscopic robots in the colon, *Int J Robot Res*, **23**, 549–556.

Dario P, Hannaford H and Menciassi A (2003), Smart surgical tools and augmenting devices, *IEEE J Robot Autom*, **19**, 782–792.

Davies B (2000), A review of robotics in surgery, *Proc Inst Mech Eng H J Eng Med*, **214**, 129–140.

Davies B L, Lin W J and Hibberd R D (1997), Active compliance in robotic surgery – the use of force control as a dynamic constraint, *Proc Inst Mech Eng H J Eng Med*, **211**, 285–292.

Degani A, Choset H, Wolf A, Ota T and Zenati M A (2006), Percutaneous intrapericardial interventions using a highly articulated robotic probe, *1st IEEE/RAS-EMBS International Conference on Biomedical Robotics and Biomechatronics*, 7–12.

Gibo T L, Verner L N, Yuh D D and Okamura A M (2009), Design considerations and human-machine performance of moving virtual fixtures, *IEEE International Conference on Robotics and Automation*, 671–676.

Gilbert E G, Johnson D W and Keerthi S S (1988), A fast procedure for computing the distance between complex objects in three-dimensional space, *IEEE J Robot Autom*, **4**, 193–203.

Ginhoux R, Gangloff J, de Mathelin M, Soler L, Sanchez M M A and Marescaux J (2005), Active filtering of physiological motion in robotized surgery using predictive control, *IEEE Trans Robot*, **21**, 67–79.

Glauser D, Fankhauser H and Epitauz M (1995), Neurosurgical robot Minerva: first results and current developments, *J Image Guid Surg*, **1**, 266–272.

Glauser D, Flury P and Epitauz M (1993), Mechanical concept of the neurosurgical robot Minerva, *Robotica*, **11**, 567–575.

Goto T, Hongo K, Kakizawa Y, Muraoka H, Miyairi Y, Tanaka Y and Kobayashi S (2003), Clinical application of robotic telemanipulation system in neurosurgery, *J Neurosurg*, **99**, 1082–1084.

Guthart G S and Salisbury J K, Jr. (2000), The Intuitive™ telesurgery system: overview and application, *IEEE International Conference on Robotics and Automation*, 618–621.

Hagag B, Abovitz R, Kang H, Schmitz B and Conditt M (2011). RIO: Robotic-Arm Interactive Orthopedic System MAKOplasty: User Interactive Haptic Orthopedic

Robotics, in Rosen J, Hannaford B and Satava R M, *Surgical robotics – systems applications and visions*, New York, Springer, 219–246.

Hagn U, Konietschke R, Tobergte A, Nickl M, Jörg S, Kübler B, Passig G, Gröger M, Fröhlich F, Seibold U, Le-Tien L, Albu-Schäffer A, Nothhelfer A, Hacker F, Grebenstein M and Hirzinger G (2010), DLR MiroSurge: a versatile system for research in endoscopic telesurgery, *Int J Comput Assist Radiol Surg*, **5**, 183–193.

Hagn U, Nickl M and Jorg S (2008), The DLR MIRO: a versatile lightweight robot for surgical applications, *Ind Robot*, **35**, 324–336.

Harris S J, Arambula-Cosio F, Mei Q, Hibberd R D, Davies B L, Wickham J E A, Nathan M S and Kundu B (1997), The Probot – an active robot for prostate resection, *Proc Inst Mech Eng H: J Eng Med*, **211**, 317–325.

Hongo K, Kobayashi S and Kakizawa Y (2002), NeuRobot: telecontrolled micromanipulator system for minimally invasive microneurosurgery – preliminary results, *Neurosurgery*, **51**, 985–988.

Howe R D and Matsuoka Y (1999), Robotics for surgery, *Annu Rev Biomed Eng*, **1**, 211–240.

Ikuta K, Tsukamoto M and Hirose S (1988), Shape memory alloy servo actuator system with electric resistance feedback and application for active endoscope, *IEEE International Conference on Robotics and Automation*, 427–430.

Itoh T, Kosuge K and Fukuda T (2000), Human–machine cooperative telemanipulation with motion and force scaling using task-oriented virtual tool dynamics, *IEEE Trans Robot Autom*, **16**, 505–516.

Joly L D and Andriot C (1995), Imposing motion constraints to a force reflecting telerobot through real-time simulation of a virtual mechanism, *IEEE International Conference on Robotics and Automation*, 357–362.

Kanagaratnam P, Koa-Wing M and Wallace D T (2008), Experience of robotic catheter ablation in humans using a novel remotely steerable catheter sheath, *J Interv Card Electrophysiol*, **21**, 19–26.

Kazanzides P, Zuhars J, Mittelstadt B, Williamson B, Cain P, Smith F, Rose L and Musits B (1992), Architecture of a surgical robot, *IEEE International Conference on Systems, Man and Cybernetics*, 1624–1629.

Konietschke R, Hagn U, Nickl M, Jorg S, Tobergte A, Passig G, Seibold U, Le-Tien L, Kubler B, Groger M, Frohlich F, Rink C, Albu-Schaffer A, Grebenstein M, Ortmaier T and Hirzinger G (2009), The DLR MiroSurge – a robotic system for surgery, *IEEE International Conference on Robotics and Automation*, 1589–1590.

Kozlowski D M, Morimoto A K and Charles S T (1997), Micro-telerobotic surgical system for microsurgery, *Stud Health Technol Inform*, **39**, 216–223.

Kwok K-W, Mylonas G, Sun L, Lerotic M, Clark J, Athanasiou T, Darzi A and Yang G-Z (2009a), Dynamic active constraints for hyper-redundant flexible robots, in Yang G-Z, Hawkes D J, Rueckert D, Noble A and Taylor C, *Medical image computing and computer-assisted intervention – MICCAI 2009*, Berlin, Springer, 410–417.

Kwok K-W, Sun L W, Vitiello V, James D R C, Mylonas G P, Darzi A and Yang G-Z (2009b), Perceptually docked control environment for multiple microbots: application to the gastric wall biopsy, *IEEE/RSJ International Conference on Intelligent Robots and Systems*, 2783–2788.

Kwok K-W, Vitiello V and Yang G-Z (2010), Control of articulated snake robot under dynamic active constraints, in Jiang T, Navab N, Pluim J and Viergever M, *Medical image computing and computer-assisted intervention – MICCAI 2010*, Springer Berlin/Heidelberg, 229–236.

Kwon D-S, Yoon Y-S, Lee J-J, Ko S-Y, Huh K-H, Chung J-H, Park Y-B and Won C-H (2001), ARTHROBOT: a new surgical robot system for total hip arthroplasty, *IEEE/RSJ International Conference on Intelligent Robots and Systems*, 1123–1128.

Lee S-L, Lerotic M, Vitiello V, Giannarou S, Kwok KW, Visentini-Scarzanella M and Yang G-Z (2010), From medical images to minimally invasive intervention: computer assistance for robotic surgery, *Comput Med Imaging Graph*, **34**(1), 33–45.

Li M, Ishii M and Taylor R (2007), Spatial motion constraints using virtual fixtures generated by anatomy, *IEEE Trans Robot*, **23**, 4–19.

Li Q H, Zamorano L, Pandya A, Perez R, Gong J and Diaz F (2002), The application accuracy of the NeuroMate robot – a quantitative comparison with frameless and frame-based surgical localization systems, *Comput Aided Surg*, **7**, 90–98.

Lim G, Park K and Sugihara M (1996), Future of active catheters, *Sens Actuator A*, **56**, 113–121.

Lin M C and Canny J F (1991), A fast algorithm for incremental distance calculation, *IEEE International Conference on Robotics and Automation*, 1008–1014.

Low S C and Phee L (2004), A review of master–slave robotic systems for surgery, *IEEE Conference on Robotic Automation and Mechatronics*, 37–42.

Lum M J H, Friedman D C W, Sankaranarayanan G, King H, Fodero K, Leuschke R, Hannaford B, Rosen J and Sinanan M N (2009), The RAVEN: design and validation of a telesurgery system, *Int J Robot Res*, **28**, 1183–1197.

Mack M J (2001), Minimally invasive and robotic surgery, *J Am Med Assoc*, **285**, 568–572.

Marescaux J, Leroy J, Gagner M, Rubino F, Mutter D, Vix M, Butner S E and Smith M K (2001), Transatlantic robot-assisted telesurgery, *Nature*, **413**, 379–380.

Menciassi A, Park J H, Lee S, Gorini S, Dario P and Jong-Oh P (2002), Robotic solutions and mechanisms for a semi-autonomous endoscope, *IEEE/RSJ International Conference on Intelligent Robots and Systems*, 1379–1384.

Menciassi A, Valdastri P, Quaglia C, Buselli E and Dario P (2009), Wireless steering mechanism with magnetic actuation for an endoscopic capsule, *Annual International Conference of the IEEE Engineering in Medicine and Biology Society*, 1204–1207.

Micaelli A, Bidard C and Andriot C (1998), Decoupling control based on virtual mechanisms for telemanipulation, *IEEE International Conference on Robotics and Automation*, 1924–1931.

Mirtich B (1998), V-Clip: fast and robust polyhedral collision detection, *ACM Trans Graph*, **17**, 177–208.

Mittelstadt B, Kazanzides P and Zuhars J (1996), The evolution of a surgical robot from prototype to clinical human use, in Taylor R H, *Computer-integrated surgery*, Cambridge, MA, MIT Press, 397–407.

Moglia A, Menciassi A, Schurr M O and Dario P (2007), Wireless capsule endoscopy: from diagnostic devices to multipurpose robotic systems, *Biomed Microdev*, **9**, 235–243.

Muntener M, Patriciu A, Petrisor D, Mazilu D, Bagga H, Kavoussi L, Cleary K and Stoianovici D (2006), Magnetic resonance imaging compatible robotic system for fully automated brachytherapy seed placement, *Urology*, **68**, 1313–1317.

Mylonas G, Kwok K-W, Darzi A and Yang G-Z (2008), Gaze-contingent motor channelling and haptic constraints for minimally invasive robotic surgery, in Metaxas D, Axel L, Fichtinger G and Szekely G, *Medical image computing and computer-assisted intervention – MICCAI 2008*, Berlin, Springer, 676–683.

Mylonas G P, Darzi A and Yang G-Z (2004), Gaze contingent depth recovery and motion stabilisation for minimally invasive robotic surgery, in Yang G-Z and Jiang T, *Medical imaging and augmented reality*, Berlin, Springer, 311–319.

Mylonas G P, Kwok K-W, James D R C, Leff D, Orihuela-Espina F, Darzi A and Yang G-Z (2012), Gaze-contingent motor channelling, haptic constraints and associated cognitive demand for robotic MIS, *Med Image Anal*, **16**, 612–631.

Mylonas G P, Stoyanov D and Deligianni F (2005), Gaze-contingent soft tissue deformation tracking for minimally invasive robotic surgery', in Duncan J, *Medical image computing and computer-assisted intervention – MICCAI 2005*, Berlin, Springer, 843–850.

Nakamura N, Sugano N, Nishii T, Miki H, Kakimoto A and Yamamura M (2009), Robot-assisted primary cementless total hip arthroplasty using surface registration techniques: a short-term clinical report, *Int J Comput Assist Radiol Surg*, **4**, 157–162.

Nelson C, Zhang X and Shah B C (2009), Tool guidance using a compact robotic assistant, *J Robot Surg*, **3**, 171–173.

Newton R, Noonan D, Vitiello V, Clark J, Payne C, Shang J, Sodergren M, Darzi A and Yang G-Z (2012), Robot-assisted transvaginal peritoneoscopy using confocal endomicroscopy: a feasibility study in a porcine model, *Surg Endosc*, DOI 1007/s00464-012-2228-1.

Noonan D, Elson D, Mylonas G, Darzi A and Yang G-Z (2009), Laser-induced fluorescence and reflected white light imaging for robot-assisted MIS, *IEEE Trans Biomed Eng*, **56**, 889–892.

Noonan D P, Mylonas G P, Shang J, Payne C J, Darzi A and Yang G-Z (2010), Gaze contingent control for an articulated mechatronic laparoscope, *3rd IEEE/RAS-EMBS International Conference on Biomedical Robotics and Biomechatronics*, 759–764.

Noonan D P, Vitiello V, Shang J, Payne C J and Yang G-Z (2011), A modular, mechatronic joint design for a flexible access platform for MIS, *IEEE/RSJ International Conference on Intelligent Robots and Systems*, 949–954.

Osaki M, Takayama T, Omata T, Ohya T, Kojima K, Takase K and Tanaka N (2009), Single-trocar assemblable retractor-hand for laparoscopic surgery, *IEEE International Conference on Robotics and Automation*, 3490–3495.

Ota T, Degani A and Schwartzman D (2009), A highly articulated robotic surgical system for minimally invasive surgery, *Ann Thorac Surg*, **87**, 1253–1256.

Pandya S, Motkoski J W, Serrano-Almeida C, Greer A D, Latour I and Sutherland G R (2009), Advancing neurosurgery with image-guided robotics, *J Neurosurg*, **111**, 1141–1149.

Park S, Howe R and Torchiana D (2001), Virtual fixtures for robotic cardiac surgery, in Niessen W and Viergever M, *Medical image computing and computer-assisted intervention – MICCAI 2001*, Springer Berlin/Heidelberg, 1419–1420.

Patronik N A, Ota T, Zenati M A and Riviere C N (2009), A miniature mobile robot for navigation and positioning on the beating heart, *IEEE Trans Robot*, **25**, 1109–1124.

Patronik N A, Riviere C N and El Qarra S (2005), The HeartLander: a novel epicardial crawling robot for myocardial injections, *Int Congr Ser*, **1281**, 735–739.

Phee L, Accoto D and Menciassi A (2002), Analysis and development of locomotion devices for the gastrointestinal tract, *IEEE Trans Biomed Eng*, **49**, 613–616.

Quaglia C, Buselli E, Webster III R J, Valdastri P, Menciassi A and Dario P (2009), An endoscopic capsule robot: a meso-scale engineering case study, *J Micromech Microeng*, **19**(10), 105007 (11pp.).

Quirini M, Menciassi A and Scapellato S (2008a), Design and fabrication of a motor legged capsule for the active exploration of the gastrointestinal tract, *IEEE/ASME Trans Mechatron*, **13**, 169–179.

Quirini M, Menciassi A, Scapellato S, Dario P, Rieber F, Ho C-N, Schostek S and Schurr M O (2008b), Feasibility proof of a legged locomotion capsule for the GI tract, *Gastrointest Endosc*, **67**, 1153–1158.

Rane A, Kommu S S, Grange P, Anderson C and Rimington P (2008), Initial laboratory experience with the freehand camera holding robotic arm in laparoscopic urological surgery, *J Endourol*, **22**, 129.

Ren I, Patel R V, McIsaac K A, Guiraudon G and Peters T M (2008), Dynamic 3-D virtual fixtures for minimally invasive beating heart procedures, *IEEE Trans Med Imaging*, **27**, 1061–1070.

Ren J, McIsaac K A, Patel R V and Peters T M (2007), A potential field model using generalized sigmoid functions, *IEEE Trans syst, man, and cyber, Part B: cyber*, **37**, 477–484.

Rosenberg L B (1993), Virtual fixtures: perceptual tools for telerobotic manipulation, *IEEE Virtual Reality Annual International Symposium*, 76–82.

Sackier J M and Wang Y (1994), Robotically assisted laparoscopic surgery, *Surg Endosc*, **8**, 63–66.

Sackier J M, Wooters C and Jacobs L (1997), Voice activation of a surgical robotic assistant, *Am J Surg*, *174*, 406–409.

Schneider O and Troccaz J (2001), A six-degree-of-freedom passive arm with dynamic constraints (PADyC) for cardiac surgery application: preliminary experiments, *Comput Aided Surg*, **6**, 340–351.

Shang J, Noonan D P, Payne C, Clark J, Sodergren M H, Darzi A and Yang G Z (2011), An articulated universal joint based flexible access robot for minimally invasive surgery, *IEEE International Conference on Robotics and Automation*, 1147–1152.

Shoham M, Lieberman I H, Benzel E C, Togawa D, Zehavi E, Zilberstein B, Roffman M, Bruskin A, Fridlander A, Joskowicz L, Brink-Danan S and Knoller N (2007), Robotic assisted spinal surgery – from concept to clinical practice, *Comput Aided Surg*, **12**, 105–115.

Slatkin A B, Burdick J and Grundfest W (1995), The development of a robotic endoscope, *IEEE/RSJ International Conference on Intelligent Robots and Systems*, 162–171.

Sodergren M, Clark J, Noonan D P, Shang J, Payne C J, James D R C, Athanasiou T, Teare J, Darzi A and Yang G-Z (2010), Feasibility of transvaginal peritoneoscopy using novel articulated stereo-laparoscope robot, *Surg Endosc*, **24**, 314–701.

Sutherland G R, Latour I and Greer A D (2008), Integrating an image-guided robot with intraoperative MRI, *IEEE Eng Med Biol Mag*, **27**, 59–65.

Sutherland G R, McBeth P B and Louw D F (2003), neuroArm: an MR compatible robot for microsurgery, *Int Congr Ser*, **1256**, 504–508.

Tadano K and Kawashima K (2006), Development of 4-DOFs forceps with force sensing using pneumatic servo system, *IEEE International Conference on Robotics and Automation*, 2250–2255.

Tadano K and Kawashima K (2010), Development of a masterslave system with force-sensing abilities using pneumatic actuators for laparoscopic surgery, *Adv Robot*, **24**, 1763–1783.

Taylor R, Jensen P and Whitcomb L (1999), A steady-hand robotic system for microsurgical augmentation, *Int J Robot Res*, **18**, 1201–1210.

Taylor R H (1997), Robots as surgical assistants: where we are, wither we are tending, and how to get there', in Keravnou E, Garbay C, Baud R and Wyatt J, *Proceedings of the 6th Conference on Artificial Intelligence in Medicine in Europe*, London, Springer–Verlag, 3–11.

Taylor R H, Mittelstadt B D, Paul H A, Hanson W, Kazanzides P, Zuhars J F, Williamson B, Musits B L, Glassman E and Bargar W L (1994), An image-directed robotic system for precise orthopaedic surgery, *IEEE Trans Robot Autom*, **10**, 261–275.

Taylor R H and Stoianovici D (2003), Medical robotics in computer-integrated surgery, *IEEE J Robot Autom*, **19**, 765–781.

Tortora G, Valdastri P, Susilo E, Menciassi A, Dario P, Rieber F and Schurr M O (2009), Propeller-based wireless device for active capsular endoscopy in the gastric district, *Minim Invasive Ther Allied Technol*, **18**, 280–290.

Uneri A, Balicki M A, Handa J, Gehlbach P, Taylor R H and Iordachita I (2010), New steady-hand Eye Robot with micro-force sensing for vitreoretinal surgery, *3rd IEEE RAS and EMBS International Conference on Biomedical Robotics and Biomechatronics (BioRob)*, 814–819.

Valdastri P, Webster R J I and Quaglia C (2009), A new mechanism for mesoscale legged locomotion in compliant tubular environments, *IEEE Trans Robot*, **25**, 1047–1057.

Vitiello V, Kwok K-W, Payne C and Yang G-Z (2011), DOF minimization for optimized shape control under active constraints for a hyper-redundant flexible robot, in Taylor R and Yang G-Z, *Information processing in computer-assisted interventions – IPCAI 2011*, Springer Berlin/Heidelberg, 67–78.

Yang G-Z, Mylonas G P and Kwok K-W (2008), Perceptual docking for robotic control, in Dohi T, Sakuma I and Liao H, *Medical imaging and augmented reality*, Berlin, Springer, 21–30.

Yen P-L and Davies B L (2010), Active constraint control for image-guided robotic surgery, *Proc Inst Mech Eng, Part H: J Eng Med*, **224**, 623–631.

Zhang X, Lehman A, Nelson C A, Farritor S M and Oleynikov D (2009), Cooperative robotic assistant for laparoscopic surgery: CoBRASurge, *IEEE/RSJ International Conference on Intelligent Robots and Systems*, 5540–5545.

Zhang X and Nelson C A (2008), Kinematic analysis and optimization of a novel robot for surgical tool manipulation, *ASME J Med Devices*, **2**, 021003.1-021003.8.

2
Localization and tracking technologies for medical robotics

N. GLOSSOP, Queen's University, Canada

Abstract: The general requirements for medical position sensors for use in robotic surgical navigation systems are reviewed, including accuracy, form factors, update rate, degrees of freedom, working envelope and patient safety. Position sensors are described that are currently in use to accurately and unobtrusively track the location and potentially the orientation of several targets affixed to the robot's end-effector or to a surgical instrument; systems under development are also mentioned. Technologies described comprise external mechanical linkages, optical sensors, electromagnetic systems, fiber-optic based systems, global positioning system (GPS) based systems, impedance based sensors, infra-red emitting diodes, and in-bore magnetic resonance imaging (MRI) tracking systems. Applications of the sensors are discussed and their advantages and disadvantages are compared.

Key words: position sensor, GPS tracking, fibre optic sensor, robotic surgical navigation, surgical safety, infra-red emitting diodes.

2.1 Introduction

One of the fundamental requirements of all surgical systems is the requirement to know the location and trajectory of the end effector. Conventional non-robotic image-guided intervention (IGI) systems use external position sensors applied to a hand-held instrument such as a probe, needle or drill. In surgical robotic systems, this information can be provided by encoders on the joints of the robot itself or through an external measurement device. Position sensors have had a long history in non-robotic image-guided intervention with even the earliest IGI systems incorporating some form of location sensor. Several technologies have been used including mechanical linkages, various types of optical sensors, electromagnetic sensors, ultrasonic sensors and global positioning system (GPS) based technology. Many of the systems have been used extensively in the field of metrology, biomechanics, navigation and image-guided intervention. Several systems have been specifically adapted to the medical market and are commercially available from multiple vendors and sold as discrete building blocks for integrated systems. Some position sensors are proprietary devices, developed and owned by individual medical device manufacturers. For the most part, these are substantially similar to those developed by the commercial suppliers often using almost identical technology.

This chapter reviews some of the general requirements for medical position sensors including accuracy, form factors, update rate, degrees of freedom (DOF), working envelope and patient safety. It also surveys the main position sensors currently in use along with some of the systems currently under development. Advantages, disadvantages and examples of the systems are also discussed.

2.2 Requirements for position sensors

Requirements of surgical position sensors include position and orientation accuracy, update frequency, and number of targets simultaneously trackable. The size and shape of the working volume of the position sensor is also critical. Depending on the precise application, the dimensions and weight of the system components, particularly the 'tracking targets' that are attached to the end effector, may also be critical in the selection of a particular technology. Several technologies also have fundamental weaknesses such as metal interference or line-of-sight problems that may influence the selection. Electrical and biocompatibility issues have to be to addressed.

It is usually necessary to determine the position of the tracked device in either three, five or six degrees of freedom, i.e. the (x,y,z) spatial location together with the roll–pitch–yaw orientations relative to a reference. At the very least the system should be capable of 3 DOF but in some applications five (x,y,z plus pitch and yaw) or all six DOF may be required. Fortunately it is possible to resolve the missing rotational parameters if required, by using multiple tracked devices.

Position sensors are usually required to measure the tip of a surgical device in the range of 1–2 mm and orientation ranging from 0.5 to 2 degrees, but this is highly application dependent.[1] In some specialized applications such as electrophysiological mapping, raw errors of several millimeters may be acceptable. There can be a tendency to overspecify the accuracy requirement of the position sensor, but extensive experience has shown that, in most applications to date, 1–2 mm is sufficient. This is because accuracy in computer and robotically assisted surgical systems is a combination of several cumulative errors that arise from the resolution of scans used to plan the procedure, anatomical changes such as tumor changes or organ motion from the time of the scan, patient movement during the procedure, registration errors (arising from the process used to match the physical patient with the scan) as well as the accuracy of the position sensor.[2] Taken together these errors are often much larger than the 1–2 mm of the position sensor so improvements to the position sensor would have little effect on overall accuracy of the intervention.

Depending on the type of system, the update frequency is typically 5–20 Hz, although some systems do have special high-frequency requirements, particularly when powered end-effectors are involved. The update frequency of some commercial position sensors falls as the number of tracked targets increases. This can be a problem in some applications where the maximum sampling speed is required.

Working volumes vary with application, with 500 mm × 500 mm × 500 mm generally regarded as a minimum useful volume, but again this is application dependent – some applications can make do with smaller or some may require larger volumes. Some position sensors now offer odd shaped volumes such as pyramids or 'silos' that have been developed over the years to facilitate the needs of customers. Some can also be custom calibrated to specific shaped sampling volumes.

Most modern position sensors consist of two parts, namely the 'tracked targets', 'tracker', or 'applied component' and, secondly, the fixed component. Applied components can either be emitters (that send out or relay some kind of signal) or sensors (that receive the signal). Which of these parts is the applied component and which is the fixed component depends on the system being used, as one part tends to be fairly bulky whereas the other can be miniaturized and attached to instruments or end effectors. For example, in electromagnetic tracking systems, the EM sensor coils are the applied component, as they can be made extremely compact. The emitter (field generator) on the other hand is comparatively bulky and constitutes the fixed component. Conversely, in optical tracking systems, the emitters – infrared emitting diodes (IREDs) – are the applied component as they are small compared with the receiver (in this case the camera).

Location and orientation of the applied components are determined by the position sensor system, and are usually expressed relative to a coordinate system attached to the fixed component. For example, optical position sensors report the location of the tracked IREDs relative to the camera system, and magnetic position sensors report the location of the coils relative to the field generator as shown in Fig. 2.1. This is occasionally used to eliminate the necessity for the tracking part of the system by attaching the fixed component directly to part of the system such as a robot, microscope, gantry or table, thus obviating the need for tracking the object and reducing the number of applied components that must be tracked.

Information regarding the tracked targets is transferred from the position sensor to a computer application by a high-speed wired or wireless method. The data is used to drive a display of the instrument's location or to otherwise facilitate the intervention by for example controlling a robotic actuator. The logical form of the data transfer can be 4 × 4 rotation–translation matrices or as quaternions that can be readily converted to other standard formats. The translation matrix is denoted as T in Fig. 2.1 and is the matrix required to transform the position of the applied component from the origin of the fixed component. A stream of these matrices (or the quaternion representation) for

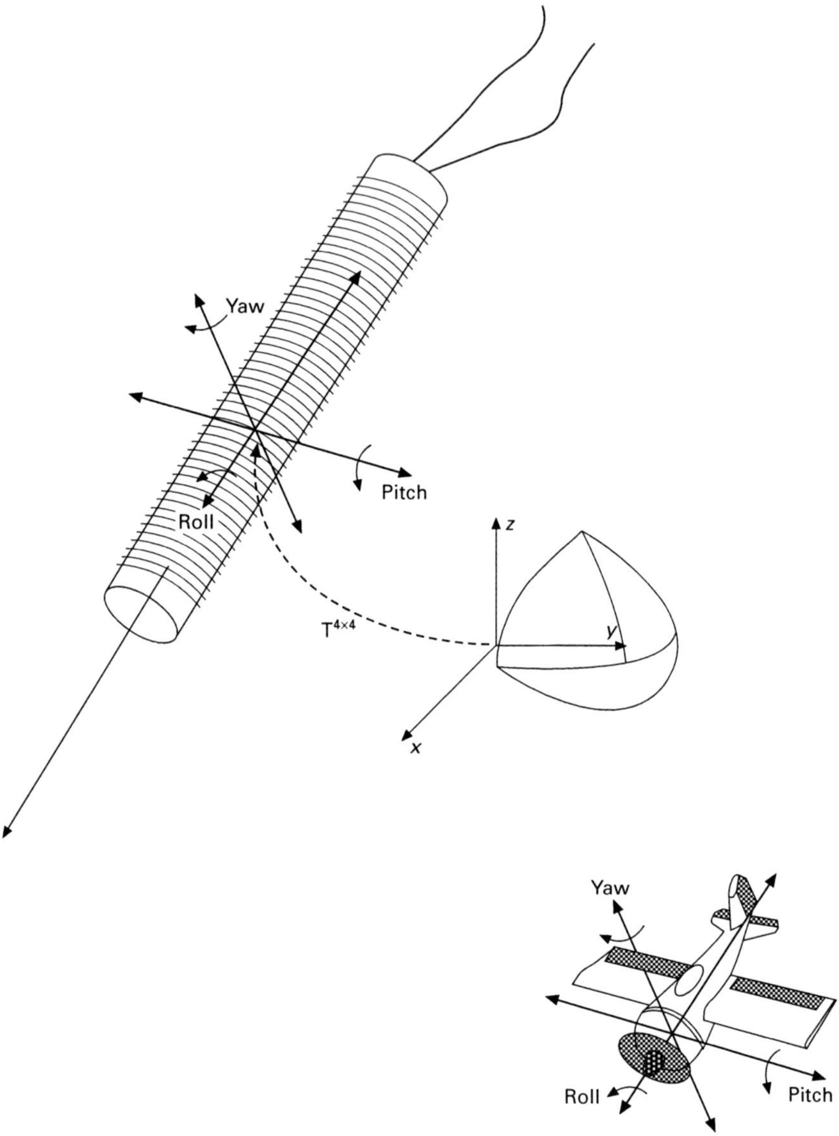

2.1 Co-ordinate system for tracking system. The location and orientation of the tracked coil is expressed in the co-ordinate system of the fixed component, here the field generator.

each target is typically transferred from the position sensor at high speed over a serial, USB, network or other connection. The matrix is often augmented with status information and time stamps.

Although at least a single target must be tracked, it is preferable to simultaneously track multiple targets, with a minimum of three probably the most useful. Current position sensors are capable of tracking multiple trackers simultaneously or virtually simultaneously. When dealing with medical applications, at least one applied component is usually attached to or near the anatomy of interest to 'dynamically reference' the motion, compensating at least in part for patient motion. A second tracker is attached to the instrumentation. If the procedure is being observed by an external device such as a microscope, video camera, endoscope, interventional X-ray or ultrasound, to provide real-time imaging feedback, a third applied component can be used to track the location of that device. This can be used to provide an 'augmented reality' view showing a virtual overlay of the instrument, anatomy or plan. Multiple instruments are also sometimes tracked, especially when two devices are targeting the same location from different approaches (e.g. 'rendezvous procedures'). Tracking systems may also need to accommodate multiple instrument types with appropriate adaptors, and the ability to change tools on the fly with some sort of 'plug-and-play' capability.

In most cases, it is necessary to minimize the size of the applied part so that it does not affect the instrument or anatomy to which it is attached. Typically, the smaller and less obtrusive these are, the more useful the overall system. Some systems that provide only three DOF for each tracked component (such as optical systems) may require several of these applied components to be used to uniquely specify the position and orientation of the end effector in six DOF. In these instances, at least three non-collinear targets must be formed into a tracker or 'rigid body'. The orientation can be determined by combining the position information from the three markers. The overall dimension of the applied part can therefore be much larger than that of the subcomponents.

Wireless tracking is a feature that can either be a convenience or vital depending on the application. Wireless dynamic referencing can be used in radiation therapy systems for example to account for organ motion during treatment. These implanted markers are essential for the application, which could otherwise not be easily accomplished. Other examples of wireless tools include the retroreflective spheres used in many optical instruments. Trackers may be integrated into the end effector or instrument or be attached to it at the time of the procedure. This means that they will be exposed to the surgical environment and must be sterilized. They should be able to withstand the sterilization process without degrading in accuracy or functionality. This is sometimes a difficult requirement, as the processes of cleaning and sterilization, particularly for reusable devices, can be onerous. If the applied part is disposable, it must be inexpensive enough to be consumed. Applied parts if exposed must also be biocompatible and not cause any adverse biological reaction when in contact with the patient tissue. Finally, the appropriate electrical components must be electrically isolated from one another so the patient does not experience a harmful voltage.

2.3 Dynamic referencing

Dynamic references are applied to the anatomy to account for tissue and patient motion. These consist of either tracking components attached directly to the anatomy or external measurement devices such as ultrasound systems, laser scanners, x rays or magnetic resonance imaging (MRI) systems used to image the tissue directly. Dynamic referencing increases the accuracy of minimally invasive robotic procedures. In the simplest case, the tissue is treated as a rigid structure, but scanners and imaging systems or the use of multiple tracking elements distributed over the tissue enable higher order motion correction. Complex motion correction is not always required but most procedures benefit significantly from the use of some dynamic referencing.

2.4 Types of position sensors

Several technologies have been used for position sensors. They include mechanical, optical, electromagnetic, GPS, fiber optic, MRI-based, impedance-based and hybrid systems. Each system has strengths and weaknesses of its own and selection of a position sensor is very application dependent as system requirements for one type of procedure may be missing in another. Several technologies are available 'off-the-shelf' and are designed to be incorporated into customized end user applications. These systems often have at least partial medical approvals (e.g. electrically compliant to medical device standards) or may be designed specifically for medical use.

2.4.1 Mechanical linkages

Passive instrumented spatial mechanical linkages have been used in biomechanical measurement of joint position and in some of the earliest IGI systems. They have also been extensively used in metrology in particular for three-dimensional (3D) co-ordinate measurement and digitization tasks such as reverse engineering or mechanical quality control. They are essentially mechanical arms without actuators but with encoders at the joints of a mechanism that connects the end effector to the base or origin. Each joint records a rotation or a translation which are superimposed to determine the location and orientation of the end. These devices are simple, well understood and can be very accurate. They can also be sampled at high rates. When used in computer-assisted image-guided intervention, a physician can attach an instrument or device to the end of the arm and manually position the arm to help identify anatomy or trajectories for screws or blades. Encoders are often incorporated into conventional mechanical robot arms. In this case, they are invisible to the system and function extremely well.

The most famous mechanical IGI system was the 'ISG Viewing Wand' which was commercially sold in the early 1990s (ISG Technologies, now Merge Healthcare, Mississauga, ON Canada). It was used in cranial neurosurgery, and consisted of a customized Faro (Lake Mary, FL, USA) digitizing arm that was attached to a Mayfield skull clamp in which the patient's head was immobilized. This ensured that the arm remained referenced to the patient's skull in the event that the headclamp was moved. The system featured a pointer inserted by the surgeon, into the patient's brain during the intervention and the position of the pointer was displayed as a live virtual object on dynamically reformatted two-dimensional (2D) and 3D computed tomography (CT) or MRI scans, helping to spatially locate the target anatomy or tumor. Manual mechanical systems such as the viewing wand can be clumsy and bulky to use, because the physician must manipulate the device by hand, and joint limitations can cause the linkage to become tangled or locked up. They are also not suited to tracking more than a single instrument and dynamic referencing can only be accomplished by the use of a second arm or by attaching the base of the unit directly to the anatomy. This is not possible except in rare occasions such as the neurosurgical application. Newer technologies have displaced mechanical linkages as the method of choice for computer-assisted IGI systems, but they remain an important method of position sensing for rigid robotic systems.

2.4.2 Optical systems

Optical position sensors have evolved over the last forty or more years. Based on the long standing principles of photogrammetry, optical position sensors use multiple cameras to determine the location of one or more targets. Originally applied to topographic mapping measurement, architecture and engineering, the technique was later applied medically in the study of human gait and in radiostereometric analysis (RSA) for precise quantitative measurements within X-rays. Systems initially made use of reflective markers placed onto the patient that were digitized either manually or automatically in multiple camera views. These were not in real time because the digitization could not be performed quickly enough but post-processing of film or video frames was used to obtain the marker locations in space. Applications to image-guided intervention began with the arrival of real-time systems in the 1980s and 1990s such as the 'Watsmart' manufactured by Northern Digital Inc. (NDI, Waterloo ON, Canada), Image Guided Technologies 'Flashpoint' (IGT, now Boulder Innovation Group, Inc., Boulder CO) and by Qualysis (Gothenburg, Sweden). These systems enabled automatic optical tracking of devices for the first time. Gait analysis systems also became available with near-real-time performance around this time.

The commercial systems developed by NDI and IGT initially made use of active infrared-emitting diodes (IREDs). These infrared-emitting diodes were designed to emit small spots of light in the near infrared, approximately (850–950 nm wavelength). The systems 'strobed' the IREDs so that only a single marker was visible to the camera system for a brief period of time, generally well under a millisecond, the 'frame rate' of the cameras. When multiple IREDs were used, they would be sequentially illuminated so that they could be uniquely identified by the tracking system. Because the position sensor system controlled the time and sequence that each was illuminated, it was able to uniquely identify each marker. IREDs were grouped into rigid bodies consisting of three or more markers that were affixed to the handle of rigid instruments or standardized 'trackers' that were attached to anatomy, instruments or devices.

This type of camera system used three linear 1D arrays of detectors in the camera heads instead of conventional 2D charge coupled device (CCD) arrays used in most systems today. These arrays were separated by several tens of centimeters from one another mounted on a long boom pointed at fixed angles relative to one another. They were more accurate than the 2D arrays available at that time, but necessitated the cameras assemblies to be quite large and the systems contained complex and costly electronics. They also came 'precalibrated' because the orientation and location of each of the cameras was precisely known at the time of manufacture. The NDI Optotrak 3020, for example, was over 1 m long and weighed 40 kg. Accuracy of the Optotrak was in the range of 0.1 to 0.2 mm, which was more than that required for surgical applications, where registration and other errors could easily be 1–2 mm. The price of these systems was also high, approximately US$60 000 at the time. Current versions of three camera systems include the Certus (NDI) and Atracsys (Lausanne, Switzerland) cameras. They are better suited to surgical applications than the original systems, but the Certus is certainly more accurate than required for most medical applications.

The Qualysis system was developed originally for biomechanics but was employed in the original Brainlab (Feldkirchen, Germany) IGI system. The device made use of a pair of 2D cameras that were mounted on a rigid boom. The system was field-calibrated using the concepts of the direct linear transform (DLT) used in biomechanics to determine the location of markers mounted on the instrument. Most modern camera systems such as the Polaris (NDI) use 2D cameras like this but they are precalibrated.

These cameras made use of a pair of high-resolution 2D CCD arrays that are filtered to allow only bright infrared light in a certain narrow frequency range to be viewed by the cameras. The original Polaris camera that was introduced by NDI in 1996 used continuously illuminated IRED markers instead of strobed markers. By using unique marker geometries, the position and orientation of several rigid bodies could be simultaneously simultaneously determined by lower cost 2D CCD arrays. A few years later, a 'hybrid' Polaris was introduced, which included accommodation of passive markers as well as the traditional IREDs. The passive systems used an annular arrangement of 'illuminator' IREDs that surrounded the camera lenses. Instruments were fitted with retroreflective spheres or discs that made up the rigid body. The wireless convenience of passive systems made them attractive to physicians, especially for hand-held instruments.

The hybrid Polaris system proved to be a turning point in the use of this technology for image-guided surgical application, and the descendants of the Polaris still form the vast majority of all image-guided systems available. The price point of these was less than a third of the Optotrak systems and prices are continuing to fall and performance rise as competitors enter the market and the manufacturing processes become more efficient. Passive optical systems of a different variety are also available from some manufacturers such as Claron Technologies (Toronto, ON Canada). These systems use a pair of inexpensive 2D ambient light cameras together with special 'checkerboard' targets attached to instruments. The transition points between the light and dark checker patterns are identified by the cameras and used as virtual markers. Tracking targets are extremely simple and inexpensive and can be simply printed onto a material and attached to an instrument.

Current optical systems are relatively affordable and offer acceptable accuracy for many surgical, diagnostic and therapeutic applications. The overall position sensor accuracy is in fact a combination of the design of the rigid body and the camera system, with larger rigid bodies offering enhanced accuracy, but less convenience to the physician. The latest generation of passive systems using retroreflective targets are also far more convenient than wired systems, but have higher running costs owing to the recommended one-time use of the passive spheres.

Optical systems have also had a long history of use in robotic surgical interventions.[3,4] They are straightforward to incorporate into the setup and can offer advantages over encoder-only based position tracking. All optical systems suffer from line-of-sight issues, meaning that a continuous unobstructed line must be maintained between the cameras and the targets on the instrument. This can sometimes be challenging and inconvenient in surgical environments, but is less of a problem with the smaller cameras in use today. The setup of the room is one of the most challenging aspects of this technology, but after some experimentation, the room setup can usually accommodate the system.

Optical systems also require that the portion of the instrument being tracked is completely rigid from the point of tracking target fixation to the instrument tip because the tip location is extrapolated from the location of the tracking targets. Even small orientation errors caused by instrument bending can magnify into large errors in tip position (Fig. 2.2), thus limiting the type of instrument being tracked and also interfering with the instrument's form and function. These errors do not occur in instruments where the sensor is located at the tip of the instrument, as can be accomplished using electromagnetic technology.

The size of the rigid bodies can be limiting in some cases. Clearly, the larger the rigid body, the more accurate the instrument. This means that certain small rigid bodies may not accurately track the instrument. Practically, it is difficult to create a trackable rigid body that is under about 3–5 cm in diameter, unless certain close-range cameras are used that restrict the sampling volume. Dynamic referencing of anatomy is therefore limited to rigid objects such as bone, because most soft tissue cannot support the tracker. It is possible to apply IREDs directly to skin surfaces.

Infrared light from sources such as operating room lights can affect optical tracking systems. Modern optical systems use bandpass filters tuned to the IRED or illuminator wavelength, and contain sophisticated algorithms that attempt to distinguish between stray light. It is still possible, however, to lose a target by flooding the environment with infrared. Modern surgical lamps emit less infrared and this problem can usually be addressed by careful room setup.

Optical systems are robust and rarely report incorrect information. They are designed to report no data rather than the potential of an error. Because some of the systems do use predictive algorithms and internal averaging to determine the future location of the instrument it is not advisable to use rapid instrument motions that exceed the specifications of the systems. As with all precision equipment, it is also important to ensure both targets and rigid bodies are properly calibrated regularly. Rigid bodies in particular can degrade through improper handling or after multiple cleaning and sterilization cycles.

Optical technology has been widely used in spine, cranial neurosurgical and orthopaedic procedures, particularly trauma. It has also been used in ear, nose and throat (ENT) applications, but is generally not appropriate for

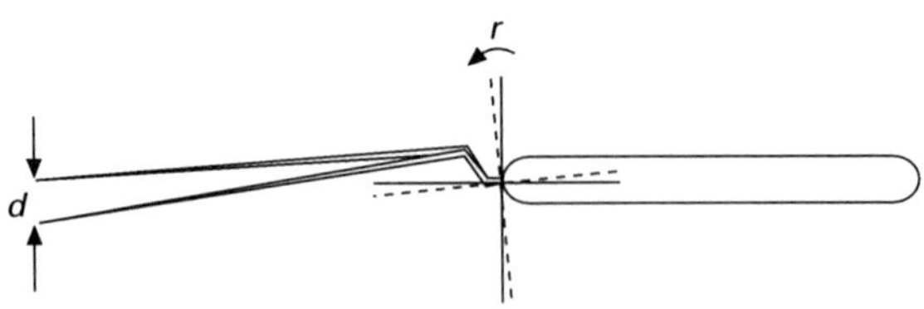

2.2 Effect of tip bending on tip displacement accuracy. Even a small bend in the tip near the base of the instrument can lead to a large tip inaccuracy.

internal tracking of flexible endoscopes, fine needles or deformable anatomy. Optical systems have been used in therapeutic radiation therapy devices such as the Cyberknife (Accuray, Sunnyvale, CA) to track patient motion so that sensitive structures are not inadvertently irradiated. Ultrasound devices have also been tracked optically when performing image fusion between pre-procedure CT or MRI with live ultrasound (e.g. Ultraguide, Haifa, IL – no longer in business)

2.4.3 Sound-based systems

A few early systems used time of flight from sound pulses to triangulate on instruments. Small emitters or spark gaps applied to instruments emitted bursts of sound that were received by three or more sensitive microphones fixed to a frame. One IGI system (first generation Picker ViStar system, Picker Inc., Cleveland OH) was released that used a sonic position sensor from Science Accessories Corporation (SAC).[5] The accuracy suffered from speed of sound variations in the environment owing to temperature fluctuations along the paths to each of the three receivers. As distances were short, even small temperature fluctuations could lead to errors in the perceived locations of the emitters. Sonic systems also had line-of-sight issues and could be affected by ambient high-frequency sounds present in the environment for example from suction devices. These were later replaced by optical systems and sonic devices are no longer used in medical IGI applications.

2.4.4 Electromagnetic tracking systems

Electromagnetic (EM) tracking systems have a long history beginning in the 1970s. There have been several generations of these systems, each substantially improved over previous versions. They have become particularly interesting in recent years as they offer the possibility of addressing soft-tissue IGI for the first time.

EM tracking systems consist of a fixed unit known as a transmitter or field generator. The field generator contains several emitter coils that set up a transient or constant electromagnetic field that is detected by one or more applied sensors that typically take the form of coils or occasionally Hall-effect sensors. The field generated by modern systems is generally very weak, generally less than 100 μT. This field induces a current in the receiver coil that can be detected by the position sensor. Depending on the characteristics such as intensity or phase of the receiver current, the position of the sensor can be calculated.

Most EM systems offer at least five DOF from a single sensor coil. This means that both the (x,y,z) position and pitch–yaw orientation of the end effector or surgical instrument can be determined. The axial symmetry makes it difficult to determine the 'roll' of the sensor accurately, but the 'pitch' and 'yaw' can be obtained (Fig. 2.1). Using more than one sensor coil or using more complicated 'dual wound' six DOF coils (in which two coils are wound onto the same core) enables all six DOF to be obtained from a single coil. The use of multiple coils can have other advantages: the additional information can be used by the tracking system to enhance the accuracy of the end effector, because the system for solving the location of the instrument tip is overdetermined and it can also be used to detect environmentally induced errors. For example, if the sensors are arranged in a known spatial relationship to one another, this relationship can be continually tested to ensure that the generated field is uniform in the region around the additional sensors.

The earliest systems by Polhemus (Colchester, VT) and Ascension (Burlington, VT) and others were developed in the 1970s and 1980s and were extremely susceptible to ambient EM and noise and not very accurate. They used large sensors, up to 3–5 cm in diameter, and were used for gross measurement, particularly in applications in the entertainment industry for motion capture for live animation of actors. Some were also used in military applications such as head tracking for pilots for weapons targeting (e.g. Elscint, Tel Aviv, Israel), and in general digitizing applications for reverse engineering. Sensor coils (Fig. 2.3) have become much smaller as this technology has evolved and are now available less than 0.5 mm in diameter and 7 mm long. Multiple different technologies are used by various vendors for locating the sensor, including intensity and phase measurements of the electromagnetic field at the coil. These technologies are capable of determining the coil position to around 1–2 mm.

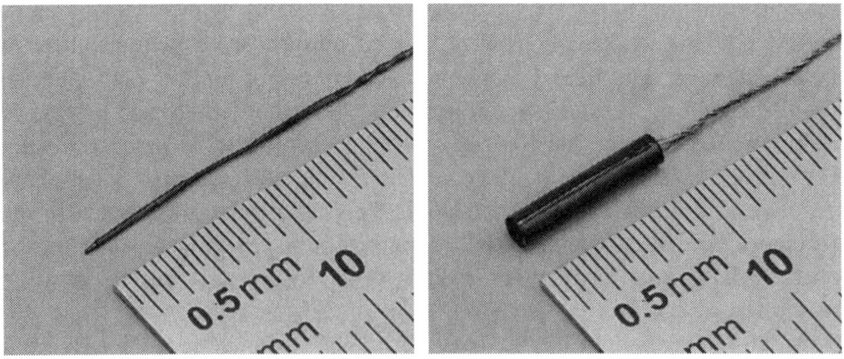

2.3 Sensor coils for electromagnetic tracking system.

In the late 1990s, Biosense-Webster (Diamond Bar, CA) developed the first widely used EM tracking system for cardiac mapping that used small coil technology, and this is still in use today. In this system, the sensing coil was small enough to be directly embedded in a catheter for the first time. Wires are strung along the catheter to a plug on the proximal end of the catheter. Similar small sensors were developed by NDI for their Aurora system and Ascension for their Instatrak system. Spin-offs from the military supplier Elscint are now incorporated in products by Mediguide-St Jude and Superdimension/Covidien (Minneapolis MN). The NDI system can track at around 40 Hz, but this decreases as multiple sensors are added.

EM systems are generally susceptible to metal, particularly ferromagnetic materials and conductors, which distort the magnetic field that is set up by the field generator. In systems that use alternating or pulsed magnetic fields, conductors such as metal plates are susceptible to eddy currents that are induced by fluctuating fields. Although advances have been made in the systems to make them less susceptible to metal compared with the early systems, it is always best to promote an 'electromagnetically clean' environment. Although original systems tended to show errors of several centimeters upon introduction of electronic devices (the 'cellphone test', where a working cellphone is placed in the measurement volume) or even small metal objects, this is no longer the case. Most systems are remarkably tolerant to the introduction of surgical instruments and probes of the appropriate material with very small distortions.[6] Manufacturers are working diligently to minimize the number of distortion artifacts caused by metal.

Other advantages of EM systems are the small size, and the lack of line-of-site issues inherent in the competing optical technology. Sensors as small as those supported by the current generation of EM systems can be embedded into a variety of instruments including needles as small as 22G, catheters, and even vascular guidewires. The size and ability of EM systems to track devices inserted into the patient make them ideally suited to soft-tissue interventions that cannot be addressed by optical technology. These include cardiac electrophysiology (EP) mapping and ablation, and oncological applications such as radiofrequency, microwave and cryoablation, targeted biopsy. EM sensors are less well suited than optical systems to orthopaedics[7] although they have been used experimentally for certain specialty applications such as pain management in the spine.

The Philips PercuNav (formerly Traxtal, Toronto ON, Canada) makes extensive use of EM tracking technology. This system employs an array of needles and trackers with tracking sensors embedded in the tip in order to facilitate interventional radiology procedures, particularly interventional oncology[8] and urology.[9] The tracked needles enable tumors pinpointed by use of ultrasound, CT, MRI or positron emission tomography (PET) to be precisely targeted and biopsy probes or ablation devices delivered to the location. The PercuNav system also employs dynamic referencing in the form of tracked skin patches and needles that are used for tissue tracking. A similar system is available from Esaote (Genova, Italy) called the 'Virtual Navigator' and from General Electric ('Logiq E9', GE, Wauwatosa, WI).

The Calypso-Varian (Seattle WA, USA) system makes use of a wireless EM tracking system. This system is unique in that it uses radiofrequency identification (RFID) trackers that are powered using an external magnetic field. They then transmit information regarding their location wirelessly to the receiver. The 'beacons' are embedded in glass and are suitable for implant to assist with dynamic motion tracking of organs such as the prostate or breast during radiation therapy. Amedo GmbH (Bochum, Germany) is also investigating RFID technology for position sensing.

2.4.5 Impedance-based tracking systems

Impedance systems are in routine use in the field of electrophysiological mapping and ablation. The system marketed by St Jude Medical, the Ensite-NavX (St Jude Medical, St Paul, MN) uses impedance measurements in an electronic field of 5.6 kHz alternating in the *x*, *y*, and *z*-axis between fixed 'patches' attached to the body surface of the patient. This system is only appropriate for intracorporal measurement, with the measurements being made by the same catheters used for the cardiac electrical measurements. The systems are also non-line-of-site and are not affected by ambient metal in the environment. This technology can be somewhat inaccurate, with errors varying with location within the patient from a few millimeters to almost 7 mm.[10] This is owing to the non-uniformity of the systems, which are dependent on placement of patches and body parameters. The nature of the task and the correction procedures employed enables them to be used effectively for the specific purpose of relative positional mapping and to measure the electrical potential in the heart as it beats. In the NavX system, the spatial data is subsequently morphed onto a geometrically correct model derived from CT or MRI scans. The primary advantage is that there is no requirement for specialized trackers – the EP electrodes on the catheter themselves can be used as tracking elements. Biosense Webster also uses an impedance-based system in its latest release, Carto-3, but it is used in conjunction with their EM system to calibrate the space *in situ*, thus increasing the accuracy. Furthermore, the manufacture of the catheter does not need to incorporate sensors into their devices. This system is used to steer robotically driven catheters such as the Stereotaxis ('Epoch', St Louis, MO) and Hansen ('Sensei', Mountain View CA, USA) systems, but has not been used outside of the specific application of EP mapping. Although mature, this technology appears to have hit a limit on attainable accuracy. Newer versions of the

St Jude system appear to be incorporating EM technology at least for some applications, possibly in a mode similar to the Biosense-Webster system.

2.4.6 In-bore MRI tracking

Robin Medical (Baltimore, MD, USA) manufactures a system that is used within MRI systems to track the position and orientation of a device, making use of specialized MR pulse sequences to track special coils placed on the tips of instruments within the magnet.[11] During a scan, it uses the gradient command signals and signals from a tracking sensor that consists of three orthogonal pick up coils. Several form factors for the sensor are available including a cube sensor for a hand-held guided tool, a 1.5 mm diameter coil for catheters, needles and flexible endoscopes. The accuracy of the Robin Medical system is 2 mm spatial and 1.5 degrees, with a sampling rate of up to 16 Hz. The system is ideal for in-gantry procedures because live anatomy can be imaged with the sensor being able to direct the scan plane. This technology is appropriate for procedures that are performed within the magnet bore including certain biopsies and catheter procedures.

2.4.7 Video matching

The use of mutual information to match surface features has been demonstrated by Higgins *et al.*,[12] and is in use in image-guided bronchoscopic applications by Broncus Medical (Broncus Lungpoint, Mountain View CA, USA). The system uses optical images of internal anatomical features (such as branch points within an airway) that are visualized by a flexible bronchoscope and used to determine the location of the scope by comparing the viewed scene to a surface model of the airways generated from a segmented CT scan. This type of system requires high resolution optical and CT images to obtain adequate matching, in addition to a sufficient number of distinct features to properly register the images with the pre-procedure map. It also requires extensive computer processing power and is subject to distortions between the time of the CT and the intervention. Video matching is a very specific technology that is appropriate for certain niche applications and has the advantage of being a ‘software only’ solution, with no requirement for field generators or special camera systems. No modifications to instruments are needed to incorporate tracking elements. Attempts have been made to use vessel tracking in a modified version of this approach that uses ultrasound.

2.4.8 Fiber optic tracking systems

There are two different types of fiber optic tracking systems. A microbend-based system from Measureand Inc. (Fredericton, NB, Canada), and a system based on Bragg gratings that is in development by Luna Technologies (Blacksburg, VA, USA), Hansen Medical (CA, USA), and Philips (Eindhoven, Netherlands).[13,14] Neither system has yet been used commercially within the medical field but the potential, in particular for the Bragg grating-based sensor, is large.

Fiber optic systems are capable of resolving location information along the entire length of the optical fiber, enabling 'shape' sensing in addition to tip location sensing. The main advantages are in elongated devices such as flexible catheters or flexible endoscopes. In some applications, continuous knowledge of the shape of the device or a portion of the device potentially enables advanced registration or motion compensation techniques to be used. In addition, some procedures such as EP mapping may be accelerated by using shape sensing. No doubt these technologies will also enable other procedure types. Fiber optics is also MRI compatible and not affected by strong electric or magnetic fields. The sensors from Luna are also thin, typically 125 μm in diameter and can potentially be embedded into needles and catheters.

Fiber optic sensors based on interferometry such as the Luna device have been well known for many years but remain very expensive and complicated. Because of the processes used to etch the gratings on the fibers and the complexity of the fibers themselves, it is difficult to make such devices affordable. Interferometry-based fiber optics sensors are also notoriously susceptible to temperature and applied strain. These problems will likely be addressed as the technology evolves.

2.4.9 GPS-based systems

GPS systems use local transmitters to track targets much in the same way that conventional GPS is used. These systems have been proposed using local transmitters in an effort to increase the accuracy of satellite-based GPS, but at this time they are still not sufficiently accurate for surgical interventions.

2.4.10 Hybrid systems

Some systems that have been developed are composed of one or more technologies. Notably the Calypso–Varian system, which contains a combination of optical and EM tracking. These systems are rare because of the increased cost but have the potential to benefit from aspects of both of the technologies used. The Calypso system requires the beacons to be close to the field generator and it has a restricted field of view. To compensate for this, the system uses the optical system to determine the location of the field generator which also assists in determining the relative gantry position.

2.5 Future trends

Surgical navigation systems for the near future will continue to use the most popular position-sensing systems including optical, electromagnetic and encoders for traditional robots. As the need to perform less invasive surgical procedures becomes the gold standard, robots that include bendable actuators such as the long arms of the DaVinci and Hansen robots will require secondary position sensors (e.g. EM trackers) to be placed close to the tips of the instruments. This will help to more accurately locate the instruments as they begin to deflect.

Tracking technology will continue to advance with an emphasis on smaller, less invasive sensors. The technology will show incremental increases in accuracy over the next few years. Shape sensors such as the new fiber optic devices may begin to be adopted if the cost can be reduced and the systems can be made robust and reliable. GPS systems hold promise but they have so far been slow to develop and it is not yet clear if these will ever have the accuracy needed for surgical intervention. In constrained natural orifices, such as the airways of the lung, it is likely that video matching algorithms will become dominant as the image quality improves and the computer power required for these tasks becomes sufficient.

Much algorithmic work remains to be done in the area of tissue deformation, especially in soft tissue. Once good models of tissue behavior are available, it will be possible to more accurately understand tissue interaction with the robot potentially leading to improved technical outcomes. As these concepts are refined, the need for small sensors that can detect and measure tissue deformations may become more important. Minimally invasive measurement devices such as laser scanners, ultrasound and MRI scanners that are already used in some procedures as well as small implantable devices will become more prevalent and are likely to be used in conjunction with position sensors placed solely on the robots.

2.6 Conclusion

As technology advances, position sensors are continually changing. Currently, optical and EM systems are preferred for handheld instruments and for certain robotic applications such as semiconstrained robots. Traditional robot encoders tend to be the most cost effective for conventional robotic uses.

2.7 References

1. Birkfellner, W., Hummel, J, Wilson, E, and Cleary, K, Chapter 2: Tracking devices, in Peters, T, and Cleary, K, eds., *Image guided interventions: technology and applications*, Springer 2008.
2. Widmann G, Stoffner R and Bale R, Errors and error management in image-guided

craniomaxillofacial surgery. *Oral Surg Oral Med Oral Pathol Oral Radiol Endod*, 2009 May; **107**(5): 701–15.

3. Korb W, Engel D, Boesecke R, Eggers G, Kotrikova B, Marmulla R, Raczkowsky J, Wörn H, Mühling J and Hassfeld S, Development and first patient trial of a surgical robot for complex trajectory milling. *Comput Aided Surg*, 2003; **8**(5): 247–56.
4. Matthäus L, Giese A, Wertheimer D and Schweikard A., Planning and analyzing robotized TMS using virtual reality. *Stud Health Technol Inform*, 2006; **119**: 373–8.
5. Barnett, GH, Kormos, DW, Steiner, CP and Weisenberger, J, Use of a frameless, armless stereotactic wand for brain tumor localization with two-dimensional and three-dimensional neuroimaging. *Neurosurgery*, 1993; **33**: 674–8.
6. Birkfellner, W, Watzinger, F, Wanschitz, F, Enislidis G, Kollman C, Rafolt, D, Nowotony, R, Ewars, R and Bergmann, H, Systemic distortion in magnetic position digitizers, *Med Phys*, 1998; **25**(11): 2242–8.
7. Glossop, N, Advantages of optical compared with electromagnetic tracking, *J Bone Joint Surg (Am)*, 2009; **91**: 23–8.
8. Kruecker J, Xu S, Venkatesan A, Locklin J, Amalou H, Glossop N and Wood BJ, Clinical utility of real-time fusion guidance for biopsy and ablation. *J Vasc Interv Radiol*, 2011; **22**: 515–24.
9. Rastinehad A, Baccala A, Chung P, Proano J, Kruecker J, Xu S, Locklin J, Turkbey B, Shih J, Bratslavsky G., Linehan WM, Glossop N, Yan P, Kadoury S, Choyke, P, Wood, B and Pinto P, D'Amico risk stratification correlates with degree of suspicion of prostate cancer on multiparametric magnetic resonance imaging. *J Urol*, 2011; **185**: 815–20.
10. Brooks AG, Wilson L, Kuklik P, Stiles MK, John B, Shashidhar, Dimitri H, Lav DH, Roberts-Thomson RL, Wong CX, Young GD and Sanders P, Image integration using NavXFusion: initial experience and validation, *Heart Rhythm*, 2008 Apr; **5**(4): 526–35.
11. Atalar E, Kraitchman DL, Carkhuff B, Lesho J, Ocali O, Solaiyappan M, Guttman MA and Charles HK Jr, Catheter-tracking FOV MR fluoroscopy. *Magn Reson Med*, 1998 Dec; **40**(6): 865–72.
12. Higgins WE, Helferty JP, Lu K, Merritt SA, Rai L and Yu KC, 3D CT-video fusion for image-guided bronchoscopy. *Comput Med Imaging Graph*, 2008 Apr; **32**(3): 159–73.
13. Moore, JP and Rogge, MD, Shape sensing using multi-core fiber optic cable and parametric curve solutions, *Opt Express*, 2012; **20**: 2967–73.
14. Duncan, RG, Froggatt, ME, Kreger, ST, Seeley, RJ, Gifford, DK, Sang, AK, and Wolfe, MS, High-accuracy fiber-optic shape sensing, Proc. SPIE6530, 65301S, 65301S-11, 2007.

3
Robotics for neurosurgery

T. L. COSSETTO, K. ZAREINIA and
G. R. SUTHERLAND, University of Calgary, Canada

Abstract: The integration of robotic technologies into neurosurgery is reviewed and the latest technological advances to improve the precision and accuracy of surgery are described. Applications such as neuroArm are described that enable surgeons to access a variety of imaging data without interrupting surgery. The use of increasingly sophisticated audio, visual, and haptic technologies for the quick and effective manipulation of information during surgery is examined.

Key words: neurosurgery, robotics, haptics, neuroArm.

3.1 Introduction to neurosurgical progression

The proliferation of computer technology throughout the information age has revolutionized neurosurgical practice. Preoperative computerized tomography (CT) and magnetic resonance imaging (MRI) coupled to surgical navigation and microsurgical techniques have dramatically improved lesion localization and surgical dissection. The recent introduction of image-guided robotics has begun to enhance surgical precision and accuracy beyond innate human ability. Although patient outcome, surgical safety and efficiency have all improved, the neurosurgical team is reaching their functional capacity owing to the knowledge required to effectively utilize these various technologies. Although both training neurosurgeons and experienced physicians attempt to stay current with the latest technology, they must also remain aware of advances in the field of medicine relevant to their practice. The world of knowledge is too large for any individual to master; the demands of merging technology with medicine can be met through collaboration.

Progress in neurosurgical technology and instrumentation has been influenced by the need for more precisely targeted approaches to brain and spine lesions (Fig. 3.1). During the development of modern neurosurgery in the late 19th century, neurosurgeons operated with poorly adapted tools designed for general surgery, guided only by clinical diagnosis. The advent of neuroimaging began in the early 1900s with radiographic visualization of the cerebral ventricles and subarachnoid space via pneumoencephalography (Dandy, 1919). Pneumocephalography required the invasive replacement of cerebral spinal fluid with air. Ultrasonography was introduced after World

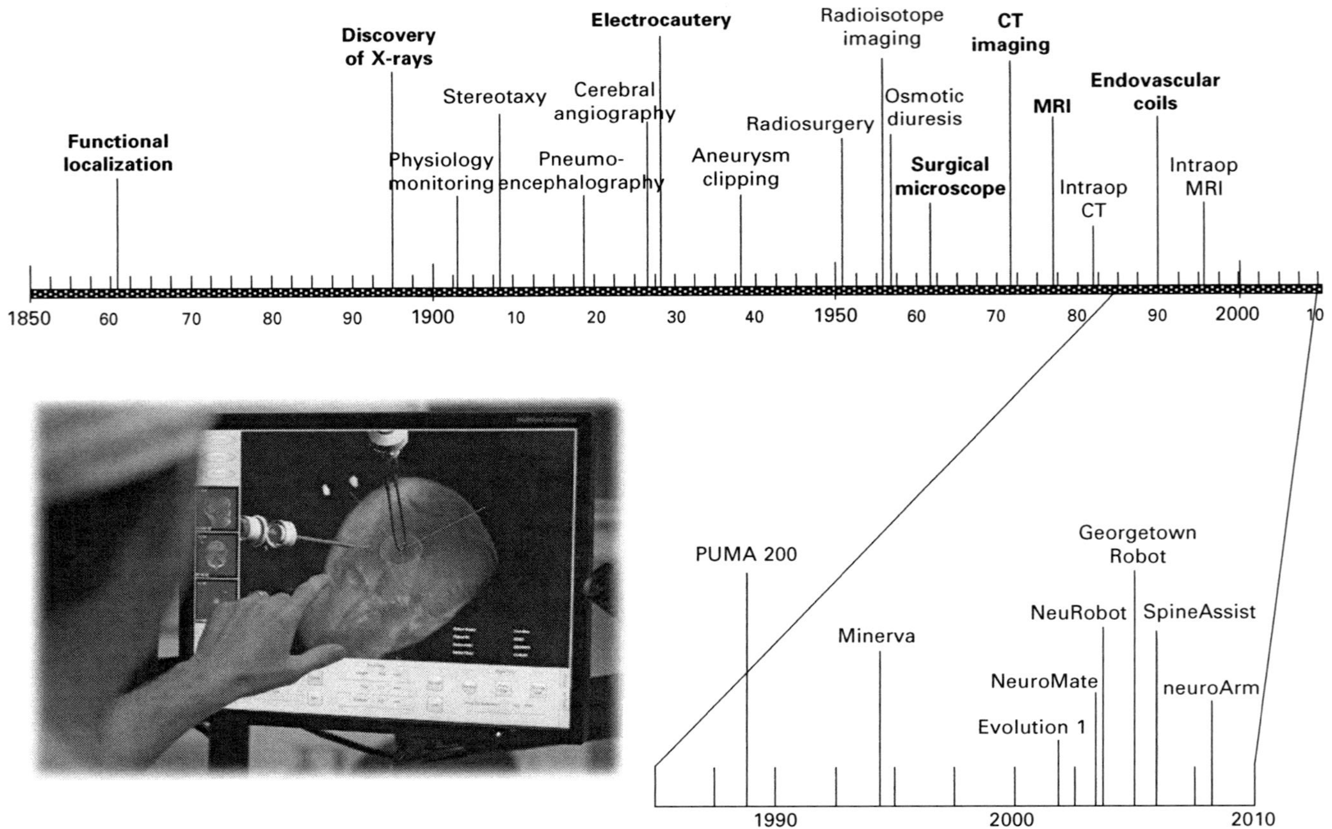

3.1 A timeline showing the historical progress of neurosurgery. The bolded events represent the major developments that significantly altered the field. Over the past two decades, robotics has established a presence in neurosurgery (expanded timeline, bottom right). The insert (bottom left) shows the MR image display of neuroArm.

War II, but found limited utilization in adults because of sound wave obstruction by the thick cranium (Baumgartner, 1997). By the 1980s, computed tomography, positron emission tomography, and MRI were established for accurate localization of central nervous system (CNS) pathology (Lee and Newberg, 2005). Today, intraoperative MRI (iMRI) resection control provides the ability to correct for brain shift, an inevitable consequence of surgical intervention. This allows surgeons to know where they are working relative to the position of the brain during operation.

Minimally invasive techniques have developed in tandem with neuroimaging technologies. The introduction of the microscope for neurosurgery in the 1960s enabled clearer visualization of the surgical field by improving magnification and illumination. Surgeons developed new techniques to operate on a finer scale. As a result, neurosurgeons began to operate in narrower surgical corridors, which necessitated superior dexterity, accuracy and precision.

These improvements in imaging and technique led to the consideration of robotics for neurosurgery. Robots could not only enhance surgical accuracy and precision, but could also accommodate the increasing number of machines in the operating room (OR) by moving the surgeon to a central control area. Neurosurgical robotic design can be classified into three broad categories: supervisory-controlled systems, telesurgical systems, and shared-control systems (Nathoo, 2005). These systems differ with respect to human–machine interaction (Fig. 3.2). In supervisory-controlled systems, the specified motions of the robot are preplanned by the surgeon and carried out autonomously by the robot. The surgeon overlooks the procedure to ensure that there are no errors. The main risk of a supervisory-controlled system is uncontrolled motion; if the operating robot experiences an error, it can take up to a few seconds for that error to be relayed to the computer. The best system designs ensure that errors are reported to the control system. This problem can be minimized if the supervisory surgeon has an emergency switch that bypasses the computer to immediately halt the machine. In telesurgical systems, the surgeon indirectly controls the robot through a master–slave configuration, in which a hand controller acts as a master control and a surgical manipulator acts as a slave. In shared-control systems, the surgeon directly performs the entire procedure while the robot augments hand-steadiness.

3.2 The evolution of neurosurgical robots

Early neurosurgical robots were generally supervisory-controlled systems. They required preoperative images to determine stereotactic co-ordinates and could execute simple, well-defined tasks such as probe placement. Some examples of these pioneering achievements include the first neurosurgical robot – the Programmable Universal Machine for Assembly (PUMA; Advance

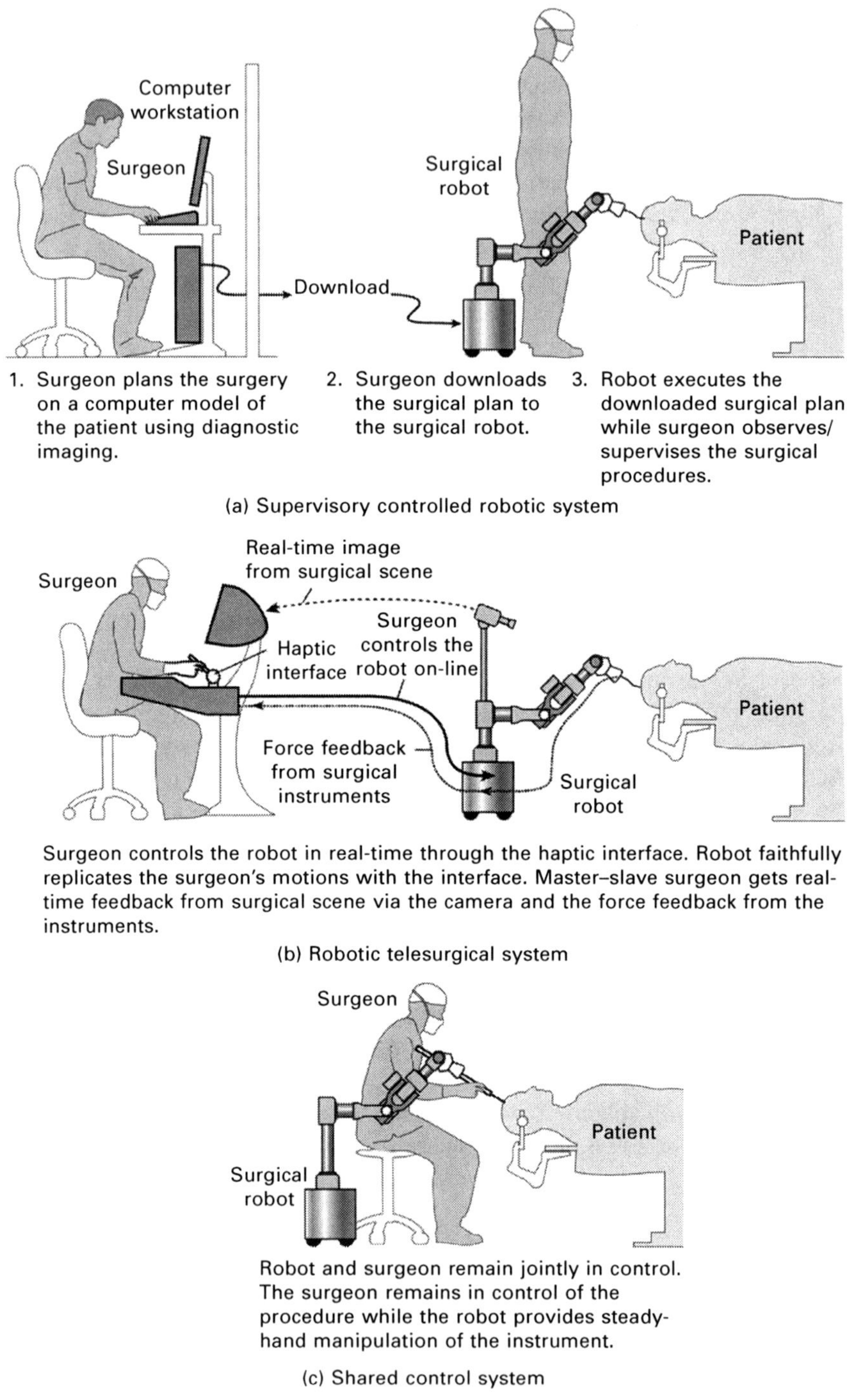

3.2 The three robotic system designs proposed by Nathoo (2005).

Research and Robotics, Oxford, Connecticut), an industrial robot adapted for neurosurgery (Kwoh *et al.*, 1988), and NeuroMate (Integrated Surgical Systems, Davis, California), a robot designed specifically for neurosurgery (Li *et al.*, 2002). Although these systems were instrumental in indicating the potential value of robotics in neurosurgery, they were large, lacked sensory feedback, and also did not include image-guidance capabilities. Consequently, surgeons were unable to correct for brain shift.

In order to develop more reliable systems, real-time, image-guided robots were developed. Minerva was designed to operate within a CT scanner (University of Lausanne, Switzerland), and numerous other robots were designed to operate with MRI (Fankhauser *et al.*, 1994). The Brigham and Women's Hospital (Boston, Massachusetts) and the Surgical Assist Technology Group of the Agency of Industrial Science and Technology (Tsukuba, Japan) developed a MR-compatible robot for stereotactic procedures mounted outside the magnet (Chenzei and Miller, 2001). The Mechatronics Laboratory at the University of Tokyo, Japan, developed a robotic system with a manipulator arm that operates within the aperture of the magnet also for stereotactic surgery (Masamune *et al.*, 1995). The field of neurosurgery is constantly striving for better imaging, which explains the drive to integrate robotics with the superior display of soft-tissue contrast in MRI (Sutherland *et al.*, 1999). As technology advances, decreases in component size will accommodate this integration. With the first neuroArm, only one robotic arm could fit inside the magnet (Sutherland *et al.*, 2008). By the second generation of neuroArm, the components were small enough for two arms to fit into the MRI, greatly increasing functionality.

For micromanipulation, robots with better tool manipulation and actuation capabilities are being developed. The end effector holds the tool, and must be able to move in multiple ways as well as actuate the tool – open and close scissors, for instance. Dexterity is one of the fundamental challenges in robot development, but advances in technology are meeting this challenge with a growing rate of success. Shared-control and telesurgical systems are ideal for microsurgery. These systems keep the human in the control loop, which combines human decision-making capabilities with the precision and accuracy of the robot. Several robotic systems have been developed for micromanipulation. The robot-assisted microsurgery system (RAMS; National Aeronautic and Space Administration's Jet Propulsion Laboratory, Pasadena, California, and MicroDexterity Systems Inc., Memphis, Tennessee) is a telesurgical system that enhances surgical performance by including features such as motion scaling, force scaling, and tremor filtering in the design (Le Roux *et al.*, 2001). The Steady-Hand robotics system is a shared-control system (Johns Hopkins University, Baltimore, Maryland) that is similar to RAMS, and also features force feedback (Taylor *et al.*, 1999). The NeuRobot (Shinshu University School of Medicine, Matsumoto, Japan) is a telesurgical system with a manipulator arm that houses a rigid three-dimensional (3D) endoscope and three manipulators (Takakura, 2002).

These robotic systems, however, operate through a simple human–machine interface (HMI) and have limited versatility. One problem with the NeuRobot was that its tools could only pick up a very small amount of tissue. Payload (the amount a robot can lift), the speed at which the payload can be moved, and accuracy are essential factors to consider in the development of any robot because they determine the practicality of use. With the forward march of technology, surgical robots will become more dexterous, expediting their global adoption.

neuroArm is a contemporary robot that takes advantage of recent trends in technology to provide the operating surgeon with sight, sound, and touch. One of neuroArm's most exciting features is its sophisticated HMI (Greer *et al.*, 2008) Currently, neuroArm is the only MR-compatible telesurgical system designed for both stereotaxy and microsurgery. It was developed through collaboration between the University of Calgary (Calgary, Alberta, Canada) and MacDonald Dettwilder and Associates (Brampton, Ontario, Canada), who created the Space Arm for NASA's shuttle program and the Special Purpose Dexterous Manipulator for the International Space Station. Following development of the prototype the intellectual property was transferred to IMRIS Inc. (Winnipeg, Manitoba, Canada), a company that markets image-guided therapeutic solutions, for commercialization. IMRIS and MacDonald Dettwiler and Associates are now manufacturing and obtaining international regulatory approval for the second generation neuroArm.

The neuroArm HMI acts as a control center for the neurosurgical operating system. Although surgeons have always been like conductors co-ordinating orchestra members through complex performances, the neuroArm workstation provides a surgeon with the ability to efficiently connect with surgical team members, patient information and high-resolution images during a procedure. Although the engineering behind neuroArm's HMI is complex, it may serve as a model of how an intuitive HMI may solve the issue of functional capacity by providing surgeons with immediate access to a vast collection of knowledge. In additiona, a digital workstation can also record all interactions that a surgeon makes with the HMI during an operation, preserving the procedure for both review and educational purposes.

3.3 Maintaining operator control

Patient care and safety are always the first priority in the development of neurosurgical robotics. Regulatory agencies require that surgical robots be manufactured to a high level of safety standards. Whether performed by human or machine the act of surgery always has risk, but regulatory agencies have determined an acceptable margin of safety for surgical robots. During non-robotic surgery, the surgeon's hand motions provide tool force and actuation. The instruments are under direct control of the surgeon and thus the surgeon is immediately aware of tool or equipment failure. During robotic surgery, on the other hand, uncontrolled motions can cause potential injuries regardless of the surgeon's experience or skill. With the use of a computer-controlled system, a human-operated emergency stop with direct manipulator interface greatly mitigates this well-recognized risk.

To reduce harm to the patient, operator training requirements, safety design features, risk management strategies, and quality assurance are fundamental to the use of robotics in neurosurgery. The neuroArm robot, for example, uses numerous safety features to minimize hazards including inadvertent motion, loss of function, electric shock or burn, and contamination (Fig. 3.3). neuroArm was built to aerospace as well as medical standards and, when it comes to robotics, aerospace regulations are in some manners stricter than those of medicine. Coupling regulatory approval to aerospace ensured that neuroArm was built to a very high standard that facilitated other regulatory approvals. The operator is responsible for tool manipulation during surgery, and an assistant is required at the surgical site to ensure that no accidental collisions occur when the tool is out of microscopic view. If an unintended movement is observed by anybody in the operating room, they can immediately communicate to the surgeon via headset, allowing the surgeon to activate the emergency stop footswitch. In the event of a power loss, a built-in braking system is used to stop the actuators and the manipulators can be manually extracted from the surgical site. neuroArm also incorporates additional safety features such as patient position monitoring, no-go zones, and MR visible markers within the tools for verification imaging to assess the accuracy of tool overlay.

3.4 Human–machine interface (HMI)

The interposition of machine between surgeon and patient has created a new approach to surgery. Remotely executed surgeries require the re-establishment of connectivity between the surgeon and the surgical environment. Headsets can be utilized to facilitate communication between a surgeon at a HMI workstation and the operating team, which enables a constant two-way flow of information during a procedure. Engineers, neuroscientists and physicians must continue to collaborate on ways to restore the sight, sound, and touch of surgery to surgeons operating at a remote workstation.

The HMI of a robotic system is the primary site for this exchange of visual, auditory, and tactile information between a user and a device. HMI is the link between the surgeon and the surgical suite. Better sensory information enables superior performance; thus the goal of the HMI should be to enhance,

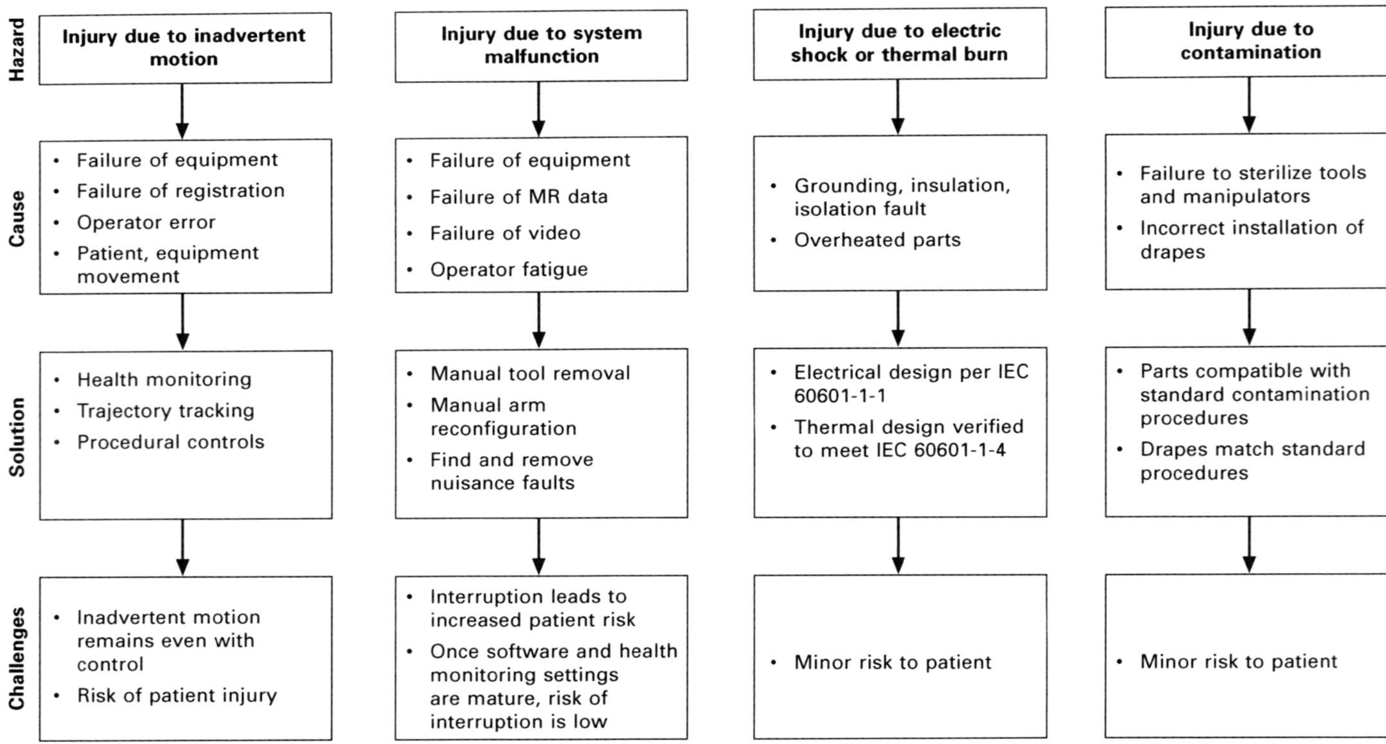

3.3 Hazards related to the introduction of robotics into neurosurgery. Described are the causes of the hazard, the control used to mitigate the risk, and the consequences if not controlled.

rather than replace, sensory input. With the overload of information and technology in neurosurgery, the surgeon also requires the ability to connect the technology that is present in the operating room, as well as digitized knowledge from around the world.

3.4.1 Vision

To operate a telesurgical robot, the neurosurgeon relies on the transmission of visual information from the operating site. The neurosurgeon needs to see both the operating field and the surgical tools in spatial relationship to the surgical pathology and brain. The neuroArm workstation initially contained two visual feedback systems to allow the surgeon to function within both real and virtual environments. The primary system was a binocular stereoscopic unit mounted on the workstation to mimic the OR microscope. Images were transmitted to the binocular display unit by two high-definition cameras (Ikegami Tsushinki Co., Ltd, Tokyo, Japan) mounted on the surgical microscope. The images were displayed on two miniature full-color monitors (Rockwell Collins Inc., Cedar Rapids, Iowa) positioned within the binocular display with extended graphic array (XGA) resolution, or 1024 × 768.

In 2011, the binocular stereoscopic display unit was upgraded to a 24 inch widescreen 3D stereoscopic monitor (provided first by Alienware, The Hammocks, Florida and now Sony, Tokyo, Japan) with 1920 × 1200 resolution, 60 Hz refresh rate, and 3D micro polarizer filter. The primary neurosurgeon wears active 3D glasses to visualize the display (Fig. 3.4). With the movement away from the binocular display, the surgeon regains a field of vision that includes the hand controller, which enables the surgeon to orient hand motion with the surgical corridor visualized on the monitor. Improved monitors provide greater visual clarity, progressing towards an image similar to that seen through the microscope. Surgery is benefiting from competition in the field of television technology. The translation of technology from one field to another is occurring faster than ever before. The 3D monitor has an additional advantage over the binocular display as it allows the surgeon to operate from a more ergonomic posture, thereby increasing comfort and stamina. It also allows residents and observers wearing 3D glasses a stereoscopic view of the operating field, which was limited to the primary neurosurgeon in the case of neuroArm I.

The secondary visual feedback system has retained an original configuration of four LCD displays mounted on the prototype workstation (two video displays and two touchscreens). The first video display shows the view of the field camera, which is mounted on an adjustable base behind the robot's two manipulators. The second video display screen shows single-channel images transmitted from left ocular of the microscope. The first touchscreen is a MRI graphical user interface (GUI) used for surgical navigation. It displays

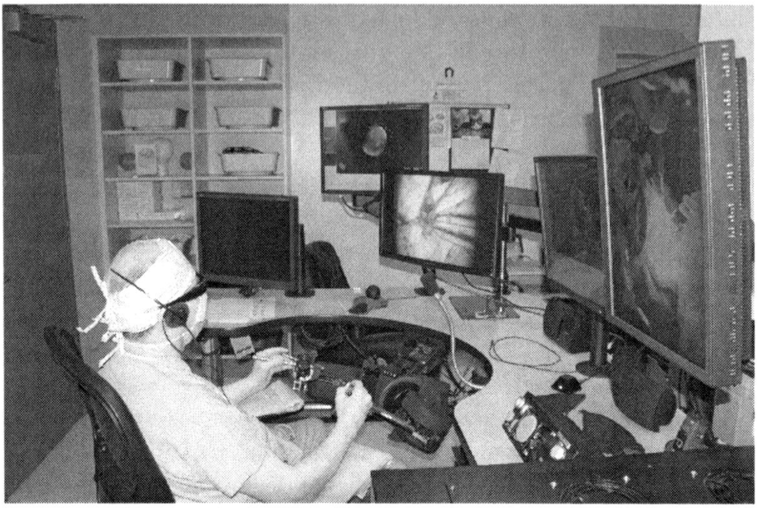

3.4 neuroArm workstation showing the 3D display with the surgeon wearing active 3D glasses. Also shown are the modified PHANToM hand controllers.

precise 3D scenes using open graphics library (OpenGL) and virtual reality modeling language (VRML) models that are rendered through a special volume accelerator card. The MRI display also allows the option of virtual tool overlay to track the motion of the surgical tools through telemetry from the manipulator encoders for a more dynamic view. The images may be manipulated through the touchscreen interface or by a Spaceball 3D motion controller allowing the user to pan, rotate, and zoom. The second touchscreen is a command and status display (CSD) GUI that provides a 3D virtual scene of the robotic manipulators and serves as the main graphical control interface. The second generation neuroArm workstation is a commercial product that is more ergonomic and incorporates advances in technology since the manufacture of the prototype. It has two vertically stacked display monitors: a stereoscopic display on the mid-monitor and an MRI display on the top monitor. The CSD has been decreased in size and been conveniently located between the hand controllers so that the surgeon can operate it without disengaging from the surgical procedure. neuroArm's workstation is made of components that can be upgraded independently as technology advances in different fields.

In comparison to conventional surgery, the integration of visual feedback at the workstation has numerous advantages. To view diagnostic images during a conventional surgery, the surgeon would need to move to a set of monitors, turning attention away from the patient, and then return to the surgical site. If the surgeon needs to change the images, either someone else in the room has to do it, or the surgeon needs to change gloves. The process of leaving the patient to view images is too disengaging for surgeons to do frequently during surgery, which means that surgeons cannot take full advantage of available imaging data. It is common for a neurosurgical patient to undergo various imaging modalities as aids in understanding diagnosis, anatomy, and brain function before surgery. Given the size of this dataset it is difficult for the surgeon to interact with the images during surgery. At a workstation, however, the surgeon has the ability to better interact with various diagnostic imaging sets and can easily transfer between hand controllers and display monitors. The integration of video game motion sensors in the operating room may also provide a solution for quick diagnostic image manipulation, which will eventually allow surgeons hands-free access to images without leaving the sterile field (Wachs *et al.*, 2011).

3.4.2 Audio

In a telesurgical system, high-fidelity two-way audio devices are used to enable communication between staff. In the OR, the surgical team is equipped with wireless headsets, while, in the workstation room, a microphone and speakers are mounted to the HMI table. The neurosurgeon has the option to communicate with an individual or the entire surgical team, and can speak and hear simultaneously. Secure transmission is attained through digital encryption and frequency hopping. The acoustics of surgical dissection are transmitted to the neurosurgeon by microphone mounted to the microscope. Remote audio communication and volume control reduces distracting ambient noises generated by operating room machinery and ventilation systems. Thus, the surgeon is better able to hear and focus on sounds relevant to the surgical dissection.

3.4.3 Tactile

Restoring the tactility of surgery is perhaps the most difficult challenge in engineering a neurosurgical robot. The touch of surgery, the precise mimicking of the surgeon's hand motion by tool manipulators, is vital for technical efficacy. The feel of surgery, or the haptic force feedback to the surgeon's hands by the hand controllers, is essential for spatial awareness. Thus, in order to connect neurosurgeon and machine through a more realistic sensory experience, detailed two-way force data must be exchanged through the HMI.

To recreate the precise touch of the neurosurgeon, neuroArm houses only high-precision components. neuroArm's sensors provide the surgeon with enough tactile data for the performance of microsurgery (Pandya *et al.*, 2009). Linear ultrasonic piezoelectric actuators (Nanomotion, Yokneam, Israel) are used for their 1 nm resolution. Joint input and output is provided by 16-bit sine/cosine rotary electric encoders (Netzer Precision Motion Sensor, Misgav, Israel) allowing for 0.01 degree accuracy. The encoders retain positional information during imaging, even when the actuators are powered off, and provide fault detection in the event that an encoder should fail. All gears have high precision antibacklash mechanics to provide smooth motion even when reversing direction.

The anthropomorphic arms allow for seven degrees of freedom (DOF). The end effector of each arm is designed to hold a variety of tools. Tool roll and tool actuation is controlled by the surgeon, and tool exchange can be automated for uninterrupted rhythm in surgery. All components on the robot are MR-compatible to ensure the robot's performance is not affected by the magnetic field or gradients.

At the workstation, the robot is controlled by two modified PHANToM haptic hand controllers (SensAble Technologies Inc., Woburn, MA) each equipped with a stylus (Quanser, Inc., Markham, Ontario, Canada). The stylus allows six DOF of position and orientation control over the surgical tool to mimic natural hand-tool motion. On the stylus is an index finger-activated lever for the actuation of any tool type including microscissors, bipolar forceps, suction devices, and needle holders.

To recreate the feel of neurosurgery, tooltip forces on each robotic arm are measured by two nano17 six-axis force/torque sensors located between the tool and the end effector (ATI Industrial Automation, Apex, North Carolina) (Fig. 3.5). The force sensors have a diameter of 17 mm and provide a resolution of approximately 1.466 mN (0.15 g) of three translational DOF to the hand controllers. Optimally, future neuroArm hand controllers will have six or seven DOF force generating capability to provide the surgeon with more accurate tactile feedback. At the time of neuroArm's manufacture, haptic hand controllers were only available in three DOF; today there are multiple companies producing seven DOF haptic devices. Although neuroArm's force sensors are in contact with the top of the tool, which provides fairly good force feedback, now there are optical force sensors available that could perhaps be mounted on the tool tip. The current challenge is discovering an efficient way to sterilize the sensors after each use.

Overall, there are roughly four main tactile advantages of a telesurgical operation over conventional procedure: force scaling, motion scaling, tremor filtering, and no-go zones. Force sensors produce real-time quantification of the physical deformation of brain tissue. This quantification could be a major breakthrough in improving the quality of surgery because surgeons will be able to specify the forces of deformation in newtons. In machines, this will allow safety margins to be defined, reducing the risk of inadvertent force on normal structures. The improved understanding of tool–tissue interaction could also expedite surgical training because of the ability to provide specific measurements of acceptable force to new surgeons.

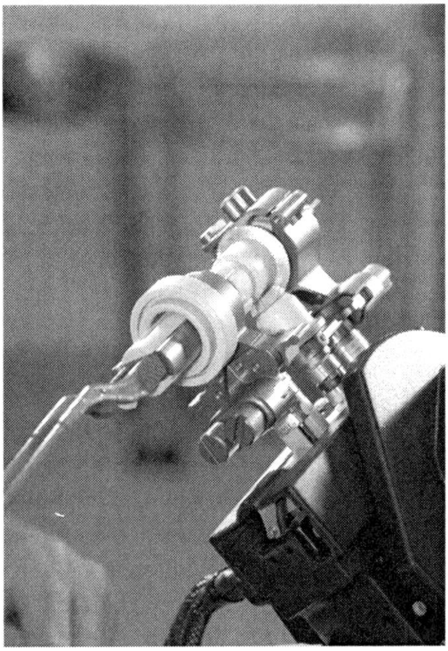

3.5 neuroArm end effector showing bipolar forceps, tool holder, and force sensors. The force sensors are between the tool holder and the wrist.

Force sensors can be adjusted to limit the amount of force applied to tissues; this is known as force scaling. Force scaling is advantageous in the field of neurosurgery, which requires delicate manipulation during surgical dissection. Through force scaling, the neurosurgeon is able to scale up forces beyond innate human ability allowing for more technically challenging surgeries to be performed. For example, when performing a bypass procedure, suturing is difficult owing in part to the imperceptible sensation of tool manipulation. A force feedback system that can scale up these forces to within human perception has the potential to improve surgical performance.

Motion scaling is similar to force scaling, but alters the magnitude of spatial displacement rather than force. It is also advantageous in neurosurgery, in which surgeons often operate in narrow corridors. The scaling down of larger motions made by the surgeon, improves precision and accuracy (Prasad *et al.*, 2004). By using robotic assistance, for example with neuroArm, neurosurgeons can improve spatial resolution from millimeters to less than 50 μm.

In neurosurgery, a robotic system that can filter out tremor is also advantageous for working in narrow corridors. Physiological tremor, which can increase with age, fatigue, and caffeine intake, decreases surgical performance. neuroArm, RAMS, and the Steady-Hands robotic system have the ability to distinguish tremors from intentional gestures and filter them out, thereby increasing precision and reducing errors.

The last feature of a robotic system that enhances a surgeon's movements is the addition of no-go zones. No-go zones are virtual geometrical regions reconstructed from MRIs to outline surgical corridors. The concept of no-go zones comes from aerospace, where engineers building space technology require a high degree of precision. This software feature adds additional safety to the medical robotic system by disallowing the surgeon to come in contact with defined anatomical structures.

3.4.4 Humanizing haptics

Despite the latest improvements in telesurgery, further innovations are needed to fully integrate the surgeon into a sensory reality. The human hand is a naturally engineered biomechanical system with approximately 23 DOF controlled by 40 muscles (Turk, 2004). Designing a slave manipulator with human-like dexterity poses significant design challenges, mainly in software design, which at the present time is rate-limiting. Although in many cases the simplification of human movements does not interfere with accomplishing a surgical procedure, oversimplification can lead to decreased performance. Even for the execution of simple tasks, every motion made by the user must be recorded, processed, and recreated by the machine. This requires substantial computational power, as calculations must be performed in real time resulting in delay. It is possible that as technology progresses, robotics will surpass human dexterity. Many robots are currently designed to mimic the function of the human body; but as new robotic capabilities are imagined, that might cease to be the case, thus allowing robots to accomplish feats that are currently considered impossible.

To enhance the dexterity and smoothness of the robot tool manipulators, technological advancements must occur in two key areas. First, more humanoid-like tool manipulators must be developed for greater tool control. Developments in this area are being made at rapid pace. The Shadow Dexterous Hand is the most advanced commercial robotic hand in the world exhibiting 24 DOF (Walker, 2003) (Fig. 3.6). In comparison with the neuroArm tool manipulator that exhibits six DOF, this is a considerable improvement (Fig. 3.7). Wielding the power that 24 DOF offers requires increased processing power. Real-time modeling and simulation of complex robotic systems requires of the order of thousands of computations per second (Zomaya, 1996). Thus, the second obstacle is to develop computer systems that can process vast amounts of data. Advancements in parallel computing may expand the capabilities of modern computer hardware. Parallel computing is a mode of computation in which multiple calculations are performed simultaneously (Shikhare and Prakash, 2004). This is accomplished by dividing large problems into smaller sets

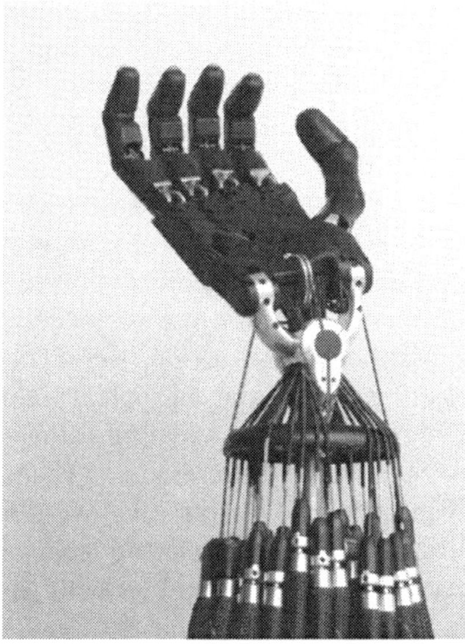

3.6 The Shadow Dexterous Hand.

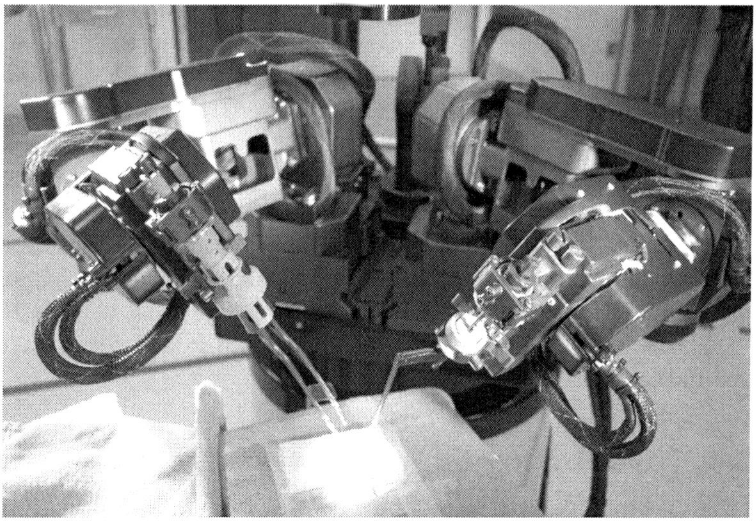

3.7 neuroArm manipulators holding bipolar forceps with right arm and microscissors with left arm.

to be solved concurrently by multiple processors. Computation performed by the human brain is accomplished through parallel processing and forms the basis for the world's most powerful supercomputers and also allows for human dexterity. From 2008 to 2010, the peak speed of the world's fastest supercomputers has more than doubled from 1.105 peta floating operations per second (PFLOPS) to 2.566 PFLOPS (Barker *et al.*, 2008; Stone and Xin, 2010). The processing power of neurosurgical robots will probably parallel global advances in processing capacity and computer technology. In the future, robotic neurosurgery may allow for microdissection at the cellular level.

Recreating the feel of neurosurgery is also an extremely challenging endeavor. The human skin contains a dense population of sensory receptors including cutaneous mechanoceptors, thermoreceptors, nociceptors for supplying the somatosensory cortex with a rich sense of touch, pressure, vibration, temperature, and pain (Vallbo and Johansson, 1984). In fact, the human fingerpad is capable of detecting and locating an applied pressure with a precision <0.2 mm (Loomis, 1979). Thus, when standing at the operating table, the neurosurgeon is able to feel the texture, deformation character, and shape of anatomical structures. Even dampened by surgical gloves, the human hand has a much higher sensory acuity than current haptic technology.

Current hand controllers allow some degree of kinesthetic sense, but more modalities of haptic feedback are needed to accurately mimic the force feedback the neurosurgeon is accustomed to. Haptic technology is lagging behind visual and audio technology largely owing to differences in the commercial market. Electronic image technology has advanced for nearly a century as televisions have become ubiquitous for entertainment. Analog audio recording and reproduction has been perfected over several centuries and digital recording has been mastered over the past several decades for music and telecommunication. Haptic force feedback technology, however, still remains in an infancy stage, as investigators only proposed the field in the mid- to late 1900s (Stone, 2001). The majority of research until now has been reserved for aeronautics and defense applications, but has expanded its scope greatly in the past decade as the mobile consumer technologies and video gaming has created a market for leading-edge haptic devices. Hopefully in the near future, improved sensor technology will lead to precise recording and recreation of telesurgical forces.

3.5 Future trends: informatic surgery

Over the past few decades, the quantity of medical data has increased exponentially, and there is a growing body of research dedicated to managing the myriad of data. The concept of electronic records, for example, has been an evolving attempt to amalgamate a wide range of patient data in order to streamline workflow in healthcare. Efforts are also being made to modernize how physicians interact with the data sets. Advancements in this area, for example, have stimulated the progress of new interactive mediums such as virtual autopsy tables which display high-resolution 3D reconstructed MRIs on a multitouchscreen surface (Dirnhofer, 2006). In the same manner, surgical robotics has the ability to restructure how surgical data is recorded, organized, analyzed, and manipulated.

Teleoperation requires user inputs to be detected, encoded into digital data, and performed by the device. Thus, in telesurgery, each motion of the surgeon is digitized and may be recorded. The implications of recording and digitizing surgical information are profound. Although not built into contemporary neurosurgical robotics, recording in the future may allow surgeons to index challenging and rare procedures for training purposes or surgical planning. Cases from top neurosurgical centers performed by world-leading physicians would be downloaded to serve as a template for preoperative and perioperative decision making of similar cases. Virtual brain renderings could be used for procedural simulation. Recipes of required surgical instruments and procedural instructions built into the GUI could help to streamline preoperative planning and perioperative execution.

Over time, database acquisition for surgical recordings could provide the instructional data for procedure automation. Automation would require a computer with the ability to make educated guesses based on accumulated information, much like humans do. For example, craniotomies would be performed autonomously using thousands of prerecorded case sets completed by surgeons. Such advances, however, will require quantum leaps in expert systems and heuristic planning (Lang and Sutherland, 2010).

3.6 Conclusion

During the industrial revolution, the productivity, accuracy, and reproducibility of manual labor were improved exponentially as the manufacturing industry transitioned towards machine-based production. Similarly, early industrial robots adapted to neurosurgery brought about advantages of precision, accuracy, and reproducibility. The human–machine interface allowed surgeons to control and manipulate surgical robotics remotely through a master–slave configuration. Like a snowball rolling down an endless hill constantly accumulates layers of snow, each generation of robots builds on advances in technology resulting in rapidly improving robotic capabilities. Through modern robotic interfaces, the surgical experience is streamlined as the surgeon is immersed into the digital world while remaining at a virtual operating table. The workstation has become not only an area for master control, but more importantly, a rich sensory environment for the quick and effective manipulation of information.

3.7 Acknowledgments

This work was supported by grants from the Canada Foundation for Innovation, Western Economic Diversification, Canada, and Alberta Advanced Education and Technology. Appreciation is extended to Claire Lacey, BA, MA, for her considerable help in preparing this manuscript.

3.8 References

Barker KJ, Davis K, Hoisie A, Kerbyson DJ, Lang M, Pakin S, and Sancho JC (2008), Entering the petaflop era: the architecture and performance of Roadrunner, *Proceedings of the 2008 ACM/IEEE conference on supercomputing*, IEEE Press, Piscataway, NJ, USA, pp. 1–11.

Baumgartner RW (1997), History of neurovascular ultrasonography, *Ther Umsch Rev Ther*, **54**, 24–30.

Chinzei K and Miller K (2001), Towards MRI guided surgical manipulator, *Med Sci Monit*, **7**, 153–163.

Dandy WE (1919), Roentgenography of the brain after the injection of air into the spinal canal, *Ann Surg*, **70**, 397–403.

Dirnhofer R, Jackowski C, Vock P, Potter K, and Thali M J (2006), VIRTOPSY: minimally invasive, imaging-guided virtual autopsy, *Radiographics*, **26**, 1305–1333.

Fankhauser H, Glauser D, Flury P, Piguet Y, Epitaux M, Favre J and Meuli RA (1994), Robot for CT-guided stereotactic neurosurgery, *Stereotact Funct Neurosurg*, **63**, 93–98.

Greer AD, Newhook P and Sutherland GR (2008), Human–machine interface for robotic surgery and stereotaxy, *IEEE/ASME Trans MRI Compatible Mechatron Syst*, **13**, 355–361.

Kwoh YS, Hou J, Jonckheere EA and Hayati S (1988), 'A robot with improved absolute positioning accuracy for CT guided stereotactic brain surgery', *IEEE Trans Biomed Eng*, **35**, 153–160.

Lang MJ and Sutherland GR (2010), Informatic surgery: the union of surgeon and machine', *World Neurosurg*, **74**, 118–120.

Le Roux PD, Das H, Esquenazi S and Kelly PJ (2001), Robot-assisted microsurgery: a feasibility study in the rat, *Neurosurgery*, **48**, 584–589.

Lee B and Newberg A (2005), Neuroimaging in traumatic brain imaging', *NeuroRX*, **2**, 372–383.

Li QH, Zamorano L, Pandya A, Perez R, Gong J and Diaz F (2002), The application accuracy of the NeuroMate robot – a quantitative comparison with frameless and frame-based surgical localization systems', *Comp Aid Surg*, **7**, 90–98.

Loomis JM (1979), An investigation of tactile hyperacuity, *Sensory Processes*, **3**, 289–302.

Masamune K, Kobayashi E, Masutani Y, Suzuki M, Dohi T, Iseki H and Takakura K (1995), Development of an MRI-compatible needle insertion manipulator for stereotatic neurosurgery, *J Image Guid Surg*, **1**, 242– 248.

Nathoo N, Cavuşoğlu MC, Vogelbaum MA and Barnett GH (2005), In touch with robotics: neurosurgery for the future, *Neurosurgery*, **56**, 421–433.

Pandya S, Motkoski JW, Serrano-Almeida C, Greer AD, Latour I and Sutherland GR (2009), Advancing neurosurgery with image-guided robotics, *J Neurosurg*, **111**, 1141–1149.

Prasad SM, Prasad SM, Maniar HS, Chu C, Schuessler RB and Damiano RJ (2004), Surgical robotics: impact of motion scaling on task performance, *J Am Coll Surg*, **199**, 863–868.

Shikhare D and Prakash PR (2004), *Introduction to parallel processing*, New Delhi, Prentice-Hall.

Stone R (2001), Haptic feedback: a brief history from telepresence to virtual reality, *Proceedings of the First International Workshop on Haptic Human–Computer Interaction*, **2058**, 1–16.

Stone R and Xin H (2010), Supercomputer leaves competition – and users – in the dust, *Science*, **330**, 746–747.

Sutherland GR, Kaibara T, Louw D, Hoult DI, Tomanek B and Saunders J (1999), A mobile high-field magnetic resonance system for neurosurgery, *J Neurosurg*, **91**, 804–813.

Sutherland GR, Newhook P, Feil G, Fielding T, Greer AD and Latour I (2008), An image-guided MR compatible surgical robot, *Neurosurgery*, **62**, 286–293.

Takakura K (2002), NeuRobot: telecontrolled micromanipulator system for minimally invasive microneurosurgery – preliminary results, *Neurosurgery*, **51**, 985–988.

Taylor R, Jensen P, Whitcomb L, Barnes A, Kumar R, Stoianovici D, Gupta P, Wang ZX, deJuan E and Kavoussi L (1999), A Steady-Hand robotic system for microsurgical augmentation, *Int J Robot Res*, **18**, 1201–1210.

Turk M (2004), Computer vision in the interface, *Commun ACM*, **47**, 60–67.

Vallbo AB and Johansson RS (1984), Properties of cutaneous mechanoreceptors in the human hand related to touch sensation, *Human Neurobiol*, **3**, 3–14.

Wachs JP, Kolsch M, Stern H and Edan Y (2011), Vision-based hand-gesture applications, *Commun. ACM*, **54**, 60–71.

Walker R (2003), Design of a dextrous hand for advanced CLAWAR applications, *Proceedings of the 6th International Conference on Climbing and Walking Robots (CLAWAR)*, Catania, Italy, *September* 17–19.

Zomaya AY (1996), Parallel processing for real-time simulation: a case study, *IEEE Parallel Distrib Technol*, **4**, 49–62.

4 Robotic systems for cardiovascular interventions

M. A. ZENATI and M. MAHVASH, Harvard Medical School, USA

Abstract: The evolving role of cardiac surgeons and cardiologists in performing cardiovascular interventions is examined and available commercial robots and proposed novel snake-like robots and robotic catheters for cardiovascular interventions are described.

Key words: minimally invasive surgery, catheter, medical robots, snake robots, continuum robots.

4.1 Introduction

The use of robotic systems for cardiovascular intervention is growing. There are several major heart conditions that require complex interventions and, unlike in the past, a growing number of interventions today can be performed by both cardiologist and cardiac surgeons (e.g. coronary revascularization, atrial ablation, pacing lead placement, and repair of intracardiac structural heart defect). A brief review of heart conditions and the roles of cardiologist and cardiac surgeons in each one of these conditions can help identify the robotic features required for cardiac interventions and determine if the use of the new robots can provide efficiency compared with the traditional minimally invasive cardiac approaches (endoscopic or catheter-based). We first review heart conditions and the various interventional approaches for palliative treatment. We then discuss available commercial robots and other robotic concepts recently proposed for cardiovascular interventions. Finally, a discussion of likely future trends in image-guided robotic surgery is presented.

4.2 Heart conditions and the evolving role of cardiac surgeons and cardiologists

The most common heart conditions that require intervention are: 1 blockage of the coronary circulation, 2 defect or failure of heart valves, 3 heart failure or heart disorder that reduces the ability of the heart to pump a sufficient amount of blood throughout the body, and 4 atrial fibrillation or abnormal heart rhythm.

The traditional paradigm in cardiovascular medicine until the early 1990s was that non-surgeons (cardiologists and electrophysiologists) were primarily providing *diagnostic* services (e.g. coronary angiograms, mapping, and echocardiography), whereas surgeons were the ones primarily performing *interventions* (e.g. coronary artery bypass graft (CABG) surgery, aortic and mitral valve repair/replacement, correction of congenital cardiac anomalies, and Maze procedure for atrial fibrillation).

Training background was also vastly different: cardiologists were required to complete training first in general medicine and then cardiology, whereas cardiac surgeons first had to complete general surgery training and then cardiothoracic surgery. Each specialist was receiving little or no exposure to the knowledge base of the other 'camp'. These traditional boundaries between cardiovascular surgical and medical specialties are being redefined and new training programs are being developed. Today, non-surgeons are performing an increasing number of complex structural heart interventions that previously were exclusively limited to surgeons, such as percutaneous coronary intervention (PCI), transcatheter aortic valve interventions (TAVI), percutaneous mitral valve repairs, closure of atrial septal defects, and atrial fibrillation ablation. Conversely, cardiac surgeons are now increasingly trained in interventional cardiology and catheter-based techniques and, since 2007, medical students in the USA can choose a training pathway in order to become board-certified cardiac surgeons that bypasses almost entirely general surgery and places increasing emphasis on interventional cardiology skills. There is also a growing worldwide trend of forming collaborative teams of surgeons and non-surgeons (the so called 'heart-team') working elbow-to-elbow in dedicated hybrid rooms.

The area where 'interventional' cardiology first successfully competed with surgery was coronary revascularization for ischemic heart disease. Thanks to the pioneering work of Dr Andreas Gruentzig, first in Zurich, Switzerland and then at Emory University in Atlanta, Georgia, in the late 1980s, coronary balloon angioplasty developed from an experimental technique into a mature therapeutic alternative to CABG. Using a series of catheters introduced into the bloodstream percutaneously, the blocked coronary artery can be dilated using an inflatable balloon (a technique called percutenous transluminal coronary angioplasty or PTCA); since 1995, following balloon dilatation, a metal stent is increasingly deployed to prop the vessel open (stents can be 'bare metal' or 'drug eluting' in order to decrease the risk of restenosis). Collectively, these techniques are called percutaneous coronary interventions (PCI). In 1996 for the first time, the worldwide number of PCIs was greater than CABG and, currently, PCI outnumbers CABG by 5:1. Cardiac surgeons have responded to this challenge by developing minimally invasive techniques for CABG, including hybrid coronary revascularization (HCR, combining minimally invasive CABG with PCI) and robotic totally endoscopic coronary artery bypass (TECAB) using the DaVinci robot (Intuitive Surgical).

With the success of PCI, in the early 2000s, a number of pioneer cardiologists identified structural heart conditions that were ripe for a transcatheter approach. Two common congential heart defects, atrial septal defect (ASD) and patent foramen ovale (PFO), are now routinely repaired percutaneously using implantable devices (e.g. Amplatzer, AGA Medical) thus avoiding open heart surgery. Another cardiac structure that is potentially amenable to the catheter approach is the aortic valve. Aortic valve replacement was the only available therapy for degenerative severe aortic stenosis until transcatheter aortic valve implantation (TAVI) was developed by non-surgeons (one of the pioneers was Alain Cribier, a French cardiologist), capitalizing on the previous experience with balloon aortic valvuloplasty (BAV) pioneered by Alain Cribier in France in 1985. Similarly, mitral valve therapies were the exclusive domain of cardiac surgery until percutaneous mitral valve repair became available with the Evalve system developed for the cardiologists by Edwards Lifesciences. Similar to the coronary revascularization challenge, cardiac surgeons developed minimally invasive approaches for aortic valve replacement (mini-sternotomy or mini-thoracotomy) and mitral valve repair/replacement (DaVinci robotic); in addition, cardiac surgeons began embracing percutaneous aortic valve approaches including the transapical aortic valve implantation.

Another area of cardiovascular medicine where a friendly competition developed is the non-pharmacologic (without drugs) treatment of atrial fibrillation, a growing epidemic now affecting up to 5 million Americans. Until the mid-1990s, the only effective therapy was the open-heart Cox Maze procedure developed by James Cox (Cox 2010). With the recognition that one type of atrial fibrillation (paroxysmal) (Haïssaguerre *et al.*, 1998) can be cured with a simpler catheter ablation technique, the open-heart Maze surgery was largely abandoned in favor of simpler catheter ablation. Minimally invasive versions of the Maze procedure have been developed on the beating heart without requiring open-heart surgery.

Whereas CABG surgery is performed 'outside' of the heart (coronary arteries lie subepicardially), valve repair/replacement and correction of congenital heart defects require true 'open-heart' surgery with the use of the heart–lung machine and cardioplegic cardiac arrest. The availability of transcatheter therapies as alternatives to open-heart surgery has provided therapeutic options for patients otherwise deemed 'inoperable' because of excessive operative risk (elderly patients or reoperations, for example). With the graying of the population, this trend is likely to increase in the future.

The increased 'competition' between cardiovascular specialists is good news for patients, because each advance in one field pushes more development in the competing one; given the fast pace of technological development, more effective and safer options for ever sicker patients are likely to be available in the near future.

The ever-increasing sophistication of cardiovascular interventions is also accelerating the development of other related fields: cardiovascular imaging in particular has evolved dramatically in the last few years. Cardiovascular interventional teams increasingly rely on computed tomography angiogram (CTA) for preprocedure planning and new generation machines such as the DynaCT (Siemens Inc) are available in the hybrid procedure suite.

4.3 Surgical robot requirements and availability for cardiovascular interventions

Medical robots assist either cardiac surgeons or cardiologists to perform cardiovascular procedures more efficiently than traditional endoscopic or catheter-based procedures. Medical robots allow surgeons to more dexterously manipulate surgical instruments or catheters inside the patient's body during minimally invasive surgeries. During robotic procedures, surgeons control the surgical instruments with joysticks or telemanipulators as easily as moving virtual objects in computer games.

A surgical robotic system is often a telerobotic system that consists of one or several patient-side robots (or slave robots) and one or several joysticks or master manipulators. The master manipulators capture the surgeon's hand motions and send them to the patient-side robots to be applied to small-scale surgical instruments that operate inside the patient's body. An optimal surgical system is often considered a telepresence surgical system 'telepresence' means 'feeling of actually being present' (Minskey, 1980). A telepresence surgical system is a telerobotic system which allows surgeons to feel as if their hands were present inside patient's body, performing surgery with small-scale surgical tools mounted on the tip of the patient-side robots. Hand motions of surgeons with a telepresence surgical system are intended to mimic the hand motions of the open procedures. A telepresence surgical system needs to provide sufficient tip dexterity for intended tasks and to provide transparent haptic feedback.

Enhanced tip dexterity has been achieved for several surgical robots such as da Vinci surgical system from Intuitive Surgical Inc. The da Vinci instruments follow the orientation and linear motions of the hands of the surgeon. Unfortunately, adding a transparent haptic feedback to da Vinci and surgical robotic systems of the same type is rather difficult and costly. This is because of the lack of accurate small-force sensors that can be mounted at the tip of the robot (Mahvash and Okamura, 2007), and because of high robot forces from the inertia and joint friction. These forces are so large than that a stable teleoperator controller with even a force sensor cannot sufficiently cancel them (Mahvash *et al.*, 2008). Also the flexibility of the robot shaft (Mahvash *et al.*, 2008) is high for most surgical environment.

Available commercial robots used for cardiovascular interventions can be divided into two groups of multilink arms and robotic catheters. Multilink arms reach the heart through multiple ports created on the chest wall of the patient. The da Vinci surgical system from Intuitive Surgical Inc. belongs to this group. The major benefits of using the da Vinci System for the surgeons are improved dexterity and enhanced three-dimensional (3D) vision. The da Vinci system has two master arms and three to four patient-side arms. Each patient-side arm has a tip with six degrees of freedom and a gripper motion (DiMaio *et al.*, 2010) (www.intuitivesurgical.com/products/davinci_surgical_system/). Although the DaVinci system was initially developed for cardiac surgery, the vast majority of procedures are performed in urology (prostatatectomy) and gynecology.

Robotic catheters access the beating heart through peripheral blood vessels, most commonly the femoral vein. Hansen Medical Inc. (www.hansenmedical.com) (Camarillo *et al.*, 2008) and Stereotaxis Inc. (www.stereotaxis.com/niobe) both develop robotic systems designed for accurate positioning, manipulation and stable control of catheters. Stereotaxis catheters have a magnetic tip, and are guided by a magnetic field surrounding the patient, whereas Hansen Medical catheters are controlled by several pull-wires that are attached to external motors to deflect the catheter tip. Hansen robotic catheters and Stereotaxis catheters have primarily been developed for treatment of atrial fibrillation and other electrophysiology applications. They allow performance of ablation inside blood vessels and heart easier and quicker than traditional catheters.

A major limitation of the da Vinci system is that it requires several (up to seven) access ports and direct access to the surgical targets from the ports of entry is required, resulting in a high potential for arm collision. One of the major limitations of current robotic catheters is the lack of strength and stiffness at their tips. For tissue manipulation tasks, such as tissue penetration and suturing, the tip of the robotic catheter should be stiff enough to apply sufficient force to manipulate tissue. These constraints of robotic catheters limit their applications. Hansen Medical Inc. and Stereotaxis systems are currently used clinically to perform atrial ablations that do not require significant contact force. All of these commercial robots are also expensive and the cost of surgical operation is more than traditional minimally invasive procedures or open surgeries.

4.4 Proposed novel robots for cardiovascular interventions

Snake-like robots and worm-like organ-mounted robots have been recently introduced for cardiovascular interventions. These robots have been proposed in order to expand the portfolio of heart conditions that can be treated, and to reduce the invasiveness of current multiport endoscopic procedures. Proposed snake-like robots can be divided into two types: surgical serpentine robots (Fig. 4.1 and 4.2) and continuum robots (Fig. 4.3).

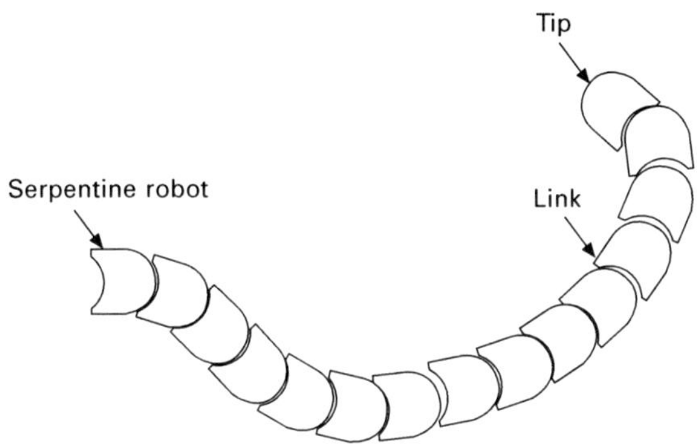

4.1 A serpentine robot consists of a series of rigid links.

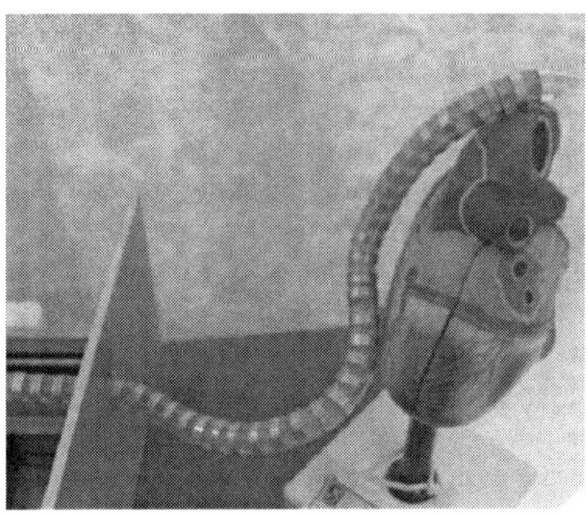

4.2 Highly Articulated Robotic Probe (Degani *et al.*, 2006).

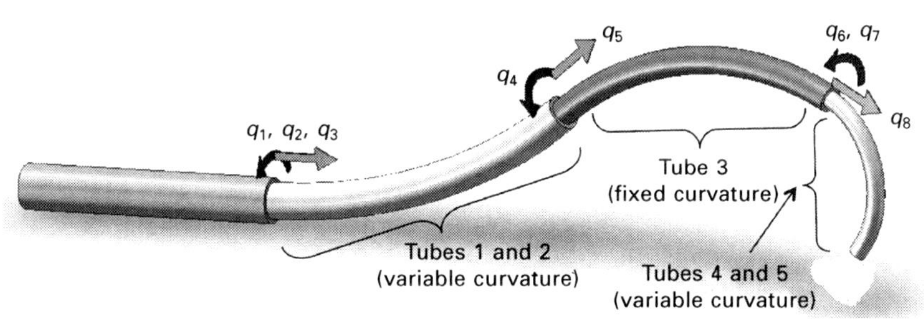

4.3 Concentric tube robot (Dupont *et al.*, 2010).

4.4.1 Surgical serpentine robots

These serpentine robots consist of a series of rigid links. The snake-like shape of the robot is formed by positioning the links of the robot in such a way that they create the desired snake-like shape (Fig. 4.1). Actuating the links of surgical serpentine robots is challenging. Two main approaches have been used: using conventional motors and transmission cables (Degani *et al.*, 2006) and shape memory alloy actuations (Ho and Desai, 2009). Medical robots based on shape memory alloy actuators generally suffer from slow response time, low contact force, and excessive heat.

Two proposed serpentine robots for cardiovascular interventions are: the highly articulated robotic probe (Degani *et al.*, 2006) or articulated robotic MedProbe (ARM) from Cardiorobotics Inc., Rynham, MA) (Ota *et al.*, 2009); and the multi-turn, tension-stiffening catheter. Both of these robots use conventional actuation and a cable tension-stiffening mechanism to locate the links of the robot in the planned positions and form a desired snake-like curve. Generally, four transmission cables are used to locate all links of the robots in the desired positions regardless of the number of robot links. The snake-like body of the ARM robot comprises two mechanisms, each mechanism comprising several rigid links connected with cables. The cables pass through all the links of the body and are tied to the last link at the tip of each mechanism. When the cables of a mechanism are pulled from the distal end, the mechanism becomes stiff. When one mechanism is stiff, the other one, which is limp, can slide along the stiff mechanism and extend over the length of the stiff mechanism preferably for one link length. By repeating this procedure, the combination of both mechanisms can eventually generate the planned snake-like body. Because serpentine robots are made of rigid links, they have high stiffness. However, one limitation is that they have relatively low tip dexterity. The ARM robot (Degani *et al.*, 2006) has 30 links and an outside diameter of 11 mm (Fig. 4.3). The ARM can take up any desired curve with minimum radius of curvature of 35 mm. The probe is made of concentric tubular links connected with cables. The multi-turn, tension-stiffening catheter has a smaller size than the ARM and it was proposed for intracardiac surgery (Chen *et al.*, 2007). The links of each mechanism are adjacent to each other.

4.4.2 Surgical continuum robots

Surgical continuum robots are made of flexible beams or tubes and they are curved by an actuation mechanism to form a snake-like shape. Medical continuum robots include: wired backbone robots, such as Hanson System and multibackbone robot (Simian *et al.*, 2004), concentric tube robots (Dupont *et al.*, 2010, Sears and Dupont, 2006 and Webster *et al.*, 2009) and shape memory actuated catheters (Veeramani *et al.*, 2008).

Both concentric tube robots and shape memory actuated catheters (Veeramani *et al.*, 2008) have been proposed for cardiovascular interventions. A concentric tube robot is constructed by telescopically extending concentrically combined precurved superelastic tubes. The robot's shape and tip location are controlled by rotating and translating of the tubes at their proximal ends (Dupont *et al.*, 2010). This robot has been proposed for intracardiac surgery. Because it is stiffer than conventional and robotic catheters, it provides more tip stiffness and it is expected to be able to perform intracardiac procedures that require higher tip contact force. However, by design, concentric tube robots are flexible and therefore have limited strength.

The shape-memory alloy continuum robot Veeramani *et al.*, 2008) is constructed from a backbone flexible beam and serially connected bending segments actuated by internal SMA tendons (Fig. 4.4). As the tendons contract because of the heat, they produce bending moments and, consequently, the catheter bends. This robotic catheter is proposed for the treatment of atrial fibrillation.

4.4.3 Hybrid snake robot

Recently, a hybrid snake robot for cardiovascular surgery was proposed (Mahvash and Zenati, 2011). This robot benefits from mechanisms of a concentric tube robot and a highly articulated robotic probe (Fig. 4.5). The

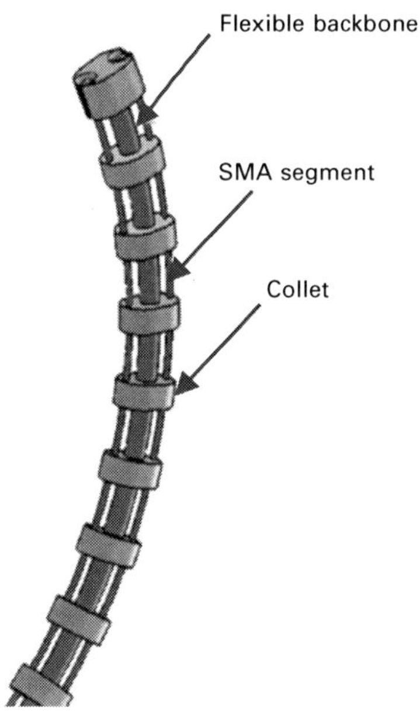

4.4 The shape-memory alloy continuum robot (Veeramani *et al.*, 2008).

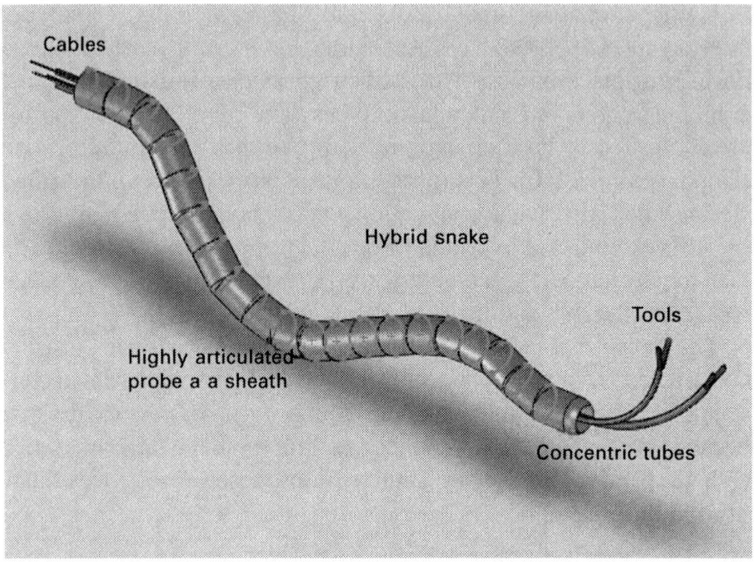

4.5 A hybrid snake robot consists of a highly articulated robotic probe and two sets of concentric tubes.

hybrid snake robot is expected to provide simultaneously high tip stiffness and dexterity that cannot be obtained by the single use of any of two robots. The hybrid snake robot was proposed for single port cardiac surgery when complex tissue manipulation such as blunt dissection of virtual spaces of the heart is required.

4.4.4 Worm-like organ-mounted robots

The HeartLander robot (Patronik *et al.*, 2009) is an organ-mounted inchworm-like robot that can move (or 'crawl') over the surface of the beating heart and delivers minimally invasive therapies (Fig. 4.6). The HeartLander adheres to the surface of the heart using suction, and navigates via inchworm-like locomotion, using flexible push wires. Because it adheres to the heart surface, it is not disturbed by the beating motion of the heart. The robot consists of two segments that adhere to the heart by suction (Fig. 4.6). The locomotion of the robot is generated by alternating the suction to the sections, while changing the distance between them. Suction is controlled by air pressure and the distance between the bodies is controlled by pushing and pulling the wires that connect the segments. The HeartLander has been proposed for ablation for ventricular arrhythmia (tachycardia), lead placement for biventricular pacing, and delivery of myocardial regenerative treatments. The HeartLander allows stable tissue penetration of the heart because it is not disturbed by heart motion. However, the HeartLander is not designed

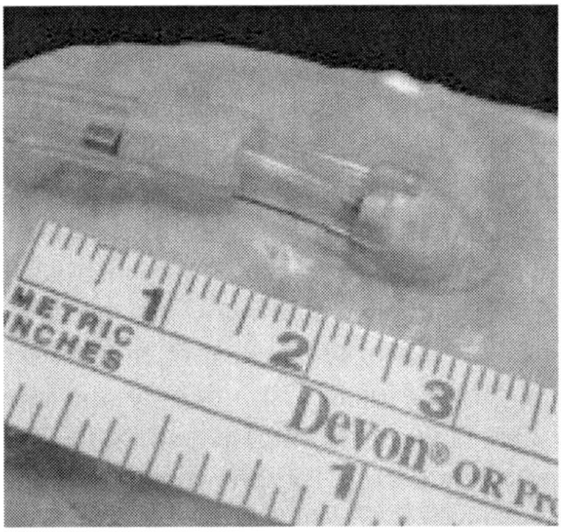

4.6 HeartLander, miniature heart-mounted robot (Patronik *et al.*, 2009).

to perform complex manipulation tasks over the heart surface and is not suitable for atrial interventions.

4.4.5 Millimeter-scale active catheters

Millimeter-scale active catheters have been suggested for intracardiac interventions. These active catheters have a very small size (less than 3 mm OD). Various actuation mechanisms have been used to control shape and the tip of these catheters including: external magnetic fields, and smart materials such as shape memory alloy and ionic polymer–metal composite (Fu *et al.*, 2009).

4.5 Future trends

Catheter-based procedures are truly minimally invasive and are preferred instead of minimally invasive surgeries if the same patient outcomes are expected. In the future, it is expected that the robotic catheters and small-scale smart tools deployable by these catheters will allow more cardiac conditions to be effectively treated (Dupont *et al.*, 2010; Suematsu and del Nido, 2004). It might be difficult to have a robotic catheter with sufficient dexterity and stiffness for all intracardiac tasks performed with conventional tools. However, it is possible to use new smart end effectors such as microelectromechanical (MEMS) tools to perform complex intracardiac tasks with robotic catheters that do not necessarily provide enhanced tip dexterity and high tip stiffness (Butler *et al.*, 2011; Gosline *et al.*, 2012).

There are many heart conditions that cannot be treated by using catheters. Open surgery or minimally invasive surgery is then required. Minimally invasive robotic cardiac surgery is expected to become less invasive and to be extended to more procedures. Dexterous stiff snake robots that can reach the pericardial sac through a single subxiphoid port are less invasive and may provide adequate tip dexterity and stiffness (Mahvash and Dupont, 2011) required for performing more complex tissue manipulation tasks.

We also believe that image-guidance will have an important role in the future of robotic cardiovascular surgery. Traditionally, imaging has been used for diagnostic proposes. The next advance will allow the use the imaging tools for therapeutic purposes. For example, the use of real-time magnetic resonance imaging (MRI) to provide clear definition of the anatomy as well as function, perfusion and device tracking; physiologic imaging for revascularization and computer modeling for preoperative planning and intraoperative assessment (McVeigh *et al.*, 2006).

4.6 Sources of further information and advice

For general information about cardiac conditions and the role of surgeons and cardiologists in interventional therapies refer to Berlinger (2006) and Gharagozloo *et al.* (2009). For more information about snake-like robots for surgery, refer to the proceedings of the ICRA Workshop (2009) http://www.bu.edu/biorobotics/icra10workshop/icra10workshop/Description.html. For more information about concentric robots refer to Dupont *et al.* (2010), for surgical serpentine robots to Degani *et al.* (2006), for organ-mounted robots to Patronik *et al.* (2009), for Hanson multibackbone continuum robots to Camarillo *et al.* (2008) and Simian *et al.* (2004), for SMA robots to Veeramani *et al.* (2008), and for active catheter mechanisms to Fu *et al.* (2009).

4.7 References

Berlinger NT. Robotic surgery: squeezing into tight places. *New Engl J Med*, 2006; **354**: 2099–2101.

Butler E, Folk C, Cohen A, Vasilyev N, Chen R, del Nido P and Dupont P. 'Metal MEMS tools for beating-heart tissue approximation'. Conf Proc IEEE International Conference on Robotics and Automation 2011, 411–416.

Camarillo D, Milne C, Carlson C and Salisbury KJ, 'Mechanics modeling of tendon-driven continuum manipulators', *IEEE Trans Robot*, 2008; **24**(6): 1262–1273.

Chen Y, Chang JH, Greenlee AS, Cheung KC, Slocum AH and Gupta R, 'Multi-turn, tension-stiffening catheter navigation system', IEEE 2008 International Conference on Robotics & Automation, Anchorage, AK, pp. 5570–5575 May, 2007.

Cox JL, 'The longstanding, persistent confusion surrounding surgery for atrial fibrillation', *J Thorac Cardiovasc Surg*, 2010; **139**: 1374–1386.

Degani A, Choset H, Wolf A, and Zenati M, Highly articulated robotic probe for minimally invasive surgery, Proc 2006 IEEE International Conference on Robotics and Automation, Orlando, USA, May 2006.

DiMaio S, Hanuschik M, and Kreaden U, 'The da Vinci surgical system', in *Surgical robotics: systems applications and visions*, J Rosen, B Hannaford, RM Satava, Springer, 2010.

Dupont P, Lock J, Itkowitz B, and Butler E, 'Design and control of concentric tube robots', *IEEE Trans Robotics*, 2010; 26(2): 209–225.

Fu Y, Liu H, Huang W, Wang S, and Liang Z, 'Steerable catheters in minimally invasive vascular surgery', *Int J Med Robot Comp Assist Surg*, 2009; **5**(4), 381–391.

Gharagozloo F, and Najam F, *Robotic surgery* McGraw-Hill Medical, 2009.

Gosline AH, Vasilyev NV, Butler E, Folk C, Cohen A, Chen R, Lang N, del Nido PJ, Dupont PE, 'Percutaneous intracardiac beating-heart surgery using metal MEMS tissue approximation tools', *Int J Robot Res*, 2012; doi: 10.1177/0278364912443718.

Haïssaguerre M, Jaïs P, Shah DC, Takahashi A, Hocini M, Quiniou G, Garrigue S, Le Mouroux A, Le Métayer P and Clémenty J, 'Spontaneous initiation of atrial fibrillation by ectopic beats originating in the pulmonary veins', *New Engl J Med*, 1988; **339**(10): 659–666.

Ho M, and Desai JP, 'Characterization of SMA actuator for application in robotic neurosurgery', in International Conference of the IEEE Engineering in Medicine and Biology, pp. 6856-6859, September, 2009.

Mahvash M, and Okamura A, 'Friction compensation for enhancing transparency of a teleoperator with compliant transmission', *IEEE Trans Robot Autom*, 2007; 23(6): 1240–1246.

Mahvash M, Gwilliam J, Agarwal R, Vagvolgyi B, Su L, Yuh D, and Okamura A, 'Force feedback surgical teleoperator: controller design and palpation experiments', Symposium on haptic interfaces for virtual environments and teleoperator systems, 2008.

Mahvash M, and Dupont PE, Stiffness control of surgical continuum manipulators, *IEEE Trans Robot*, 2011; **27**(2): 334–345.

Mahvash M, and Zenati M, 'Toward a hybrid snake robot for single-port surgery', 33rd Annual International Conference of the IEEE Engineering in Medicine and Biology Society, Boston, 2011, pp. 5372–5375.

Minsky M, Telepresence. *Omni*, 1980; **2**: 44–52.

McVeigh E, Guttman M, Lederman R, Li M, Kocaturk O, Hunt T, Kozlov S, and Horvath K, 'Real-time interactive MRI-guided cardiac surgery: aortic valve replacement using a direct apical approach', *Magn Reson Med*, 2006; **56**(5): 958–964.

Sears P, and Dupont P, 'A steerable needle technology using curved concentric tubes', in IEEE/RSJ Int Conference on Intelligent Robots and Systems, Beijing, 2006, pp. 2850–2856.

Simian N, Taylor R and Flint P, 'A dexterous system for laryngeal surgery', in *Proc IEEE Intl Conf on Robotics and Automation*, New Orleans, April 2004, pp. 351–357.

Suematsu Y, and del Nido PJ, 'Robotic pediatric cardiac surgery: present and future perspectives', *Am J Surg*, 2004; **188**: 98–103.

Ota T, Degani A, Schwartzman D, Zubiate B, McGarvey J, Choset H and Zenati MA, 'A highly articulated robotic surgical system for minimally invasive surgery. *Ann Thorac Surg*, 2009; **87**: 1253–1256.

Patronik NA, Ota T, Zenati MA and Riviere CN, 'A miniature mobile robot for precise and stable access to the beating heart', *IEEE Trans Robot*, 2009; **25**(5) 1109–1124.

Webster R, Romano J, and Cowan N, 'Mechanics of precurved-tube continuum robots', *IEEE Trans Robot*, 2009; **25**(1): 67–78.

Veeramani AS, Buckner GD, Owen SB, Cook RC and Bolotin G, 'Modeling the dynamic behavior of a shape memory alloy actuated catheter', *Smart Mater Struct*, 2008; **17**(1): 5037.

5
Robotics in orthopaedic surgery

A. HODGSON, UBC Mechanical Engineering, Canada

Abstract: Robots that have been designed for orthopaedic applications and developed to the point of commercial release are described and the evidence for benefits or undesirable consequences is considered. Five orthopaedic robots are currently known to be available commercially: ROBODOC, ACROBOT/Sculptor, Mako RIO, Mazor SpineAssist and Praxim iBlock. Although several of these robots have demonstrated improved accuracy relative to conventional procedures, and some preliminary evidence of some functional benefits is starting to emerge, there have also been reports of lengthened surgical times and increased use of preoperative computed tomography scanning, along with the increased cost of the robotic system itself. In addition, only one of the robots has been explicitly compared with an alternative to conventional surgery (such as computer-assisted navigation), so even where improvements relative to the conventional surgery can be demonstrated, it is difficult to conclude that the robot itself is necessary to achieve these gains. Evidence supporting the use of orthopaedic robots is still modest, although use of some of the robots may be justified on the basis that they enable less invasive types of surgery, which are difficult or impossible to do otherwise; this is the fundamental argument in terms of using the ACROBOT/Sculptor or the Mako RIO to perform unicompartmental knee replacements or the Mazor to do less invasive spinal surgeries.

Key words: orthopaedics, medical robotics, surgical robotics, computer-assisted surgery, minimally invasive surgery.

5.1 Introduction

Orthopaedic surgeons treat a broad range of musculoskeletal disorders including joint diseases (e.g., osteoarthritis), congenital abnormalities (e.g., scoliosis), tumours, and injuries. Although most orthopaedic problems are not life-threatening, they can be seriously debilitating and so can have an immense impact on public health, though the degree of impact is often underappreciated. The United Nations declared 2000–2010 the Bone and Joint Decade in order to raise public awareness of these conditions.

Disclaimer: The author was involved in designing the iBlock robot discussed in this chapter and is listed as a co-inventor with a Praxim employee on a patent application they have jointly filed. However, he currently has no direct financial interest in Praxim, nor in any of the other companies discussed in the paper.

Musculoskeletal disorders affect hundreds of millions of people around the world and represent the leading cause of disability in developed countries (Woolf and Pfleger 2003). In the USA, musculoskeletal problems resulted in more physician visits than any other class of disease at an estimated cost of over $200B, according to the Arthritis Foundation (see http://www.arthritis.org/bone-joint-decade.php). These impacts are expected to increase significantly as baby-boomers age.

Given the significant and rising impact of musculoskeletal disorders, many researchers have explored various technological approaches to improve treatment. In particular, the healthcare system faces challenges related both to quality and quantity of care. Although orthopaedics is generally considered a mature surgical discipline, meaning that effective and reliable treatments exist for many degenerative conditions and acute injuries, the sheer number of people affected and their desire to live a full and active life in their senior years provides considerable incentive both to drive the failure rate of treatment down even further and improve the functional outcomes for the patients as much as possible. Furthermore, over the coming decade, the number of patients is expected to increase significantly, e.g., the number of arthroplasty patients in the USA is expected to double in ten years (Fehring *et al.*, 2010) while the number of practicing orthopaedic surgeons is predicted to decline by close to 20%, resulting in treatment capacity less than 50% of anticipated demand (Fehring *et al.*, 2010) by as early as 2016.

These demand factors have encouraged researchers to consider potential applications of navigation and robotic technologies to orthopaedic problems such as hip and knee arthroplasties, spine surgeries and fracture repair procedures, amongst others. Navigation technologies are sometimes referred to as global positioning systems (GPS) for the body; the idea is that by using optical or electromagnetic tracking systems to monitor the spatial positions of tools and anatomical structures, surgeons can more accurately execute their desired surgical plans and thus improve functional outcomes for patients and longevity of the implants. Ideally, these systems would also speed up surgical procedures so as to improve time efficiency and enable a surgeon to perform a greater number of procedures.

In a recent review, Hodgson (2008) discussed evidence for improvements produced by navigation technologies alone. In this chapter, we consider whether incorporating robots into surgical procedures can improve the accuracy and repeatability of implementing a desired orthopaedic intervention and decrease the invasiveness of surgery and, if so, if the use of robots can produce detectable improvements in the outcomes of surgery. We particularly focus on those robots which have developed to the point where they have been released commercially, as these are the main ones for which cadaveric or clinical results are available.

5.2 Existing orthopaedic robotic systems

Pott *et al.* (2005) surveyed the entire field of surgical robotics and presented a comprehensive list of all known surgical robotic systems at the time, whether used for research or in production. Overall, they identified almost 160 different robotic systems across the fields of imaging, abdominal and thoracic surgery, ear, nose and throat (ENT), oral and maxillofacial surgery (OMS), neurosurgery, orthopaedic surgery, radiosurgery, trauma surgery, and urology, and 31 systems specifically in the field of orthopaedic surgery. Of these, only four were at the time commercially available: the ACROBOT (now called Sculptor, UK), Galileo (Switzerland), Medacta (Switzerland) and ROBODOC (USA) systems. Since the time of Pott's survey, a number of additional systems have been developed in research settings, but only three additional systems have been introduced commercially: the Mazor SpineAssist (Israel), Mako RIO (USA) and Praxim iBlock (France). Note that the iBlock system was originally known as Praxiteles. Following Praxim's acquisition by OMNIlife Science (USA) in 2010, the iBlock has recently been renamed Apex Robotic Technology (ART); in this chapter, we have retained the name most commonly used in the published literature (i.e., iBlock). Two previously available systems appear to be no longer available (Galileo and Medacta; the Galileo system was originally produced by Plus Orthopaedics and acquired by Smith and Nephew in 2007), so there are currently only five robotic systems on the market in the field of orthopaedic surgery.

In this chapter, we first characterize some of the more well-known orthopaedic robotic systems according to their design features and then move on to an assessment of studies that evaluated the benefits and costs of these systems. The primary design features that differentiate orthopaedic robots relate to their mechanical architecture, controller design, and anatomical interface. Before describing these features in detail, a summary is given in Table 5.1 of the characteristics of the five commercially available systems identified above.

5.2.1 Mechanical architecture

The mechanical architecture of a robot refers to the configuration of the links which comprise the moving parts of the robot. The two primary architectures

Table 5.1 Primary design features of commercially available orthopaedic robots

System	Architecture	Control type	Anatomical interface
ROBODOC	Serial	Autonomous	Bedside, bone clamps
ACROBOT/Sculptor	Serial	Active constraint	Bedside, bone clamps
Mako	Serial	Active constraint	Bedside, realtime tracking
Mazor	Parallel	Passive Toolholder	Bone-mounted
iBlock	Serial	Passive Toolholder	Bone-mounted

are called *serial*, in which the links form a chain extending from the robot's base to its end-effector, much the way our own arms do, and *parallel*, in which linear actuators directly connect the base to the end-effector; this configuration is typically used in aircraft simulator platforms. In a serial robot, each joint normally adds one degree of freedom relative to the fixed base, so for full control of the position of the end-effector, six joints are needed (to allow for arbitrary translation and rotation of the end-effector, within limits). In a parallel robot, each linear actuator adds one controllable constraint between the base and the end-effector, so six actuators need to be added to completely constrain the motion of the end-effector relative to the base.

Hybrid architectures are also possible in which both serial and parallel components are combined. In some cases, is useful to mount a small parallel actuator at the end of the larger serial arm; this configuration is called a macro–micro architecture and is used to allow the positioning of a high accuracy end effector at relatively arbitrary positions in a large workspace.

5.2.2 Controller design

The word *robot* implies some capacity for the device to move under its own power. In the popular press, robots are most frequently portrayed either as autonomous creatures with human-like movement and manipulation capabilities or as industrial automatons which perform various assembly processes on manufacturing lines. In both these situations, the robot may be regarded as autonomous; that is to say, capable of moving and executing its desired task without intervention or supervision by a human. In the case of an industrial robot, there is frequently a process of either pre-programming or training the robot to do a particular task, after which it is activated to execute the task on its own. The ROBODOC system, discussed later, is an example of an autonomous robot used in a surgical task.

In the surgical domain, cutting tasks are frequently more complex and the anatomical structures less uniform than those normally encountered in an industrial setting. Because of this, and because the consequences of making a mistake are typically so much greater in the surgical setting, few surgeons are prepared to trust a robot to perform a surgical procedure autonomously. Instead, they prefer to retain a substantial measure of control during actual cutting or milling processes. Three main classes of robot controllers have been designed to allow this kind of sharing of responsibilities during the surgical procedure.

Passive toolholders

At the most basic level, a robot is used to move a cutting jig into position, at which point the robot motors are deactivated and the device becomes essentially a fixed stand for the jig. In knee surgery, for example, the jig consists of a cutting block which has slots cut in it, through which the surgeon inserts the blade of an oscillating saw to make the actual bone cuts. Such systems are frequently referred to as passive because the robot's motors are not engaged during the cutting task. The iBlock and Mazor robots are examples of this type of robot.

Teleoperators

Teleoperators are robotic devices that are typically controlled from a different location by a surgeon operating a remote input device; normally, the surgeon-side controller and the patient-side end-effector are linked by an electronics communications channel. The patient-side device replicates the motions of the surgeon's hand and arm at the operating console, frequently scaled down. Similarly, forces generated at the patient side can, in some designs, be played back by motors on the input side so that the surgeon is able to appreciate and monitor the tissue interaction forces; these designs are known as force-reflecting teleoperators. The most well known surgical teleoperator is the da Vinci system made by Intuitive Surgical Systems. Its primary applications are in the domain of minimally invasive (laparoscopic) procedures in the abdomen. There is currently no commercially available teleoperator in the field of orthopaedic surgery, though there are examples of research systems being developed for applications in long bone fracture reduction (Westphal *et al.*, 2009).

Active constraint robots

A third class of robot which shares control between the surgeon and the robot is frequently referred to as an *active constraint* (or sometimes a *semiactive* or *collaborative*) device. In such robots (exemplified by the commercially available ACROBOT/Sculptor system from the UK and the Mako system from the USA), the robot is responsible for presenting boundaries to the motions of the end-effector, while the surgeon is free to move the cutting tool anywhere within these boundaries. In the ACROBOT and Mako systems, the position of the end effector is continuously monitored and motors are engaged when the end effector approaches a boundary to apply a force opposing further movement across the boundary. The most compelling orthopaedic application proposed to date has been the milling of the cavity for a unicompartmental knee replacement, especially for bone-conserving implants in which the bed for the implant is not prepared with straight cuts, but rather curved ones, and in which it is desirable to significantly limit the invasiveness of the surgical approach.

5.2.3 Anatomical interface

A third characteristic that differentiates orthopaedic robots relates to how they attach to the patient. The two major design approaches are either to mount the robot to a movable cart which is positioned at the bedside and (usually) clamped to the patient using screws or bone clamps, or to mount it directly to the bone itself, if the robot is designed to be sufficiently small (e.g., the iBlock and Mazor systems). In some designs (e.g., the Mako RIO robot; Pearle *et al.*, 2010), the physical clamping to the bone is replaced by realtime optical or electromagnetic tracking of the bone relative to the robot and a realtime controller, which continuously drives the end-effector into the appropriate relative position; this approach can reduce the invasiveness of the surgery and reduce the setup time, but requires greater device complexity.

5.3 Evaluation of impact of orthopaedic surgical robots

Although hundreds of studies have been carried out on the design and testing of surgical robots for orthopaedic applications, relatively few have explicitly evaluated their benefits and costs. In this section, we assess what is currently known about the few systems which have been deployed clinically, and focus on the five commercially available systems introduced earlier. For each of these systems, we describe benefits such as new procedures enabled, reduction in surgical invasiveness, increased accuracy and repeatability, improvements in functional outcomes for patients, decreases in radiation exposure for the surgical team and/or the patient, decreases in the learning curve for procedures, and ergonomic benefits for the surgeon. We also describe costs associated with the use of such systems, including purchase, commissioning and operating costs, reimbursement restrictions, complications, increases in setup and procedure time, and the need for specially-trained personnel.

To begin this review, we conducted a PubMed literature review in August 2011 using the search terms 'orthopaedic robot', which yielded 113 hits. We extended the search slightly by perusing some of the related links and ended up with 123 papers, which we then classified as shown in Fig. 5.1. Of the 123 papers, 58 either primarily focused on robotic technologies rather than clinical assessment or discussed non-clinical or non-orthopaedic applications. Of the remaining 65 papers, 54 discussed specific systems and applications and 11 represented general reviews.

Of the 54 papers which discussed specific clinical applications, four main applications emerged: knee, hip, trauma and spine (Fig. 5.2). Two papers discussed applications to anterior cruciate ligament (ACL) repair.

The time course of these papers is also interesting to consider. Figure 5.3 illustrates the publication dates of the papers related to technology and

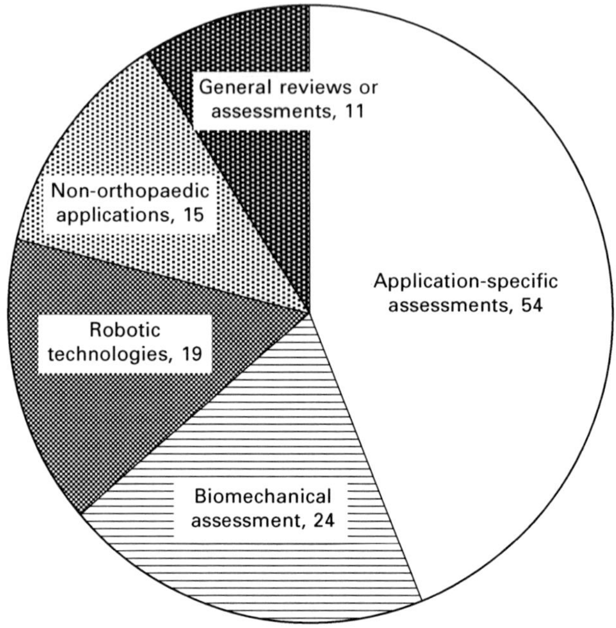

5.1 Categories of papers found in literature review (numbers of papers given).

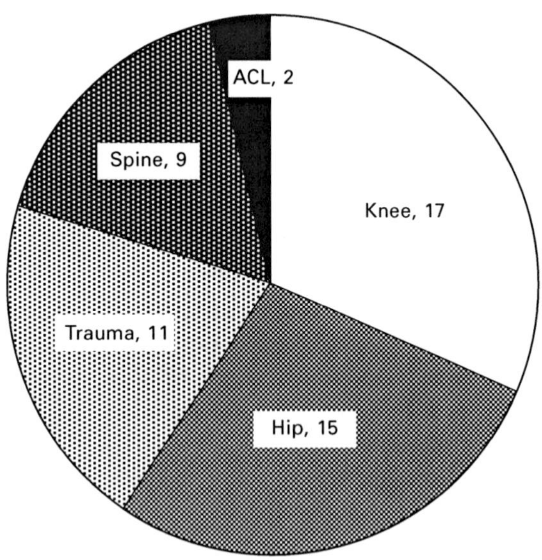

5.2 Specific clinical application areas of papers found in literature review (numbers of papers given).

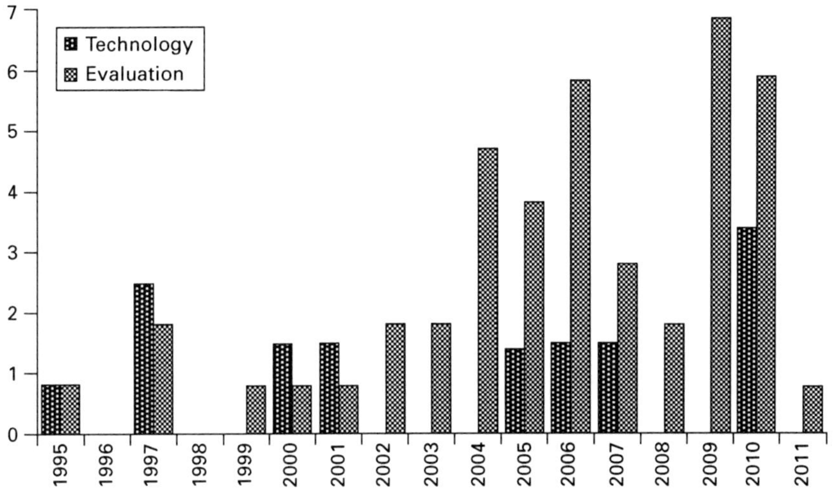

5.3 Time distribution of publications in orthopaedic robotics that focus on technology and evaluation.

evaluations. Although the technology papers are not exhaustive (much of the literature is to be found in engineering journals rather than the more medically-focused journals indexed in PubMed), there are two main spikes in the evaluation literature: the one in the mid-2000s primarily represents literature related to ROBODOC and ACROBOT, whereas the more recent rise is related primarily to the Mako, Mazor and iBlock systems, together with reports of clinical trials of research robots being used in trauma applications (fracture reduction and distal locking of intramedullary nails).

These trends are further visible in Fig. 5.4, which shows that interest in robot systems for hip surgery was greatest in the middle part of the last decade, whereas recent interest is more broadly spread. Given this overview, we can now give specific consideration to the five commercially available robots.

5.3.1 Summary of findings

Overall, we found that relatively little has been reported about the impact of these technologies. When comparative studies have been done, they have tended to compare the use of the robot to conventional surgical procedures, rather than to potentially less costly competitive technologies such as navigation systems alone or, more recently, patient-specific templates (PSTs) which use rapid prototyping technologies to create custom cutting jigs from preoperative computed tomography scans of the patient. Table 5.2 shows which differences from conventional surgical approaches have been

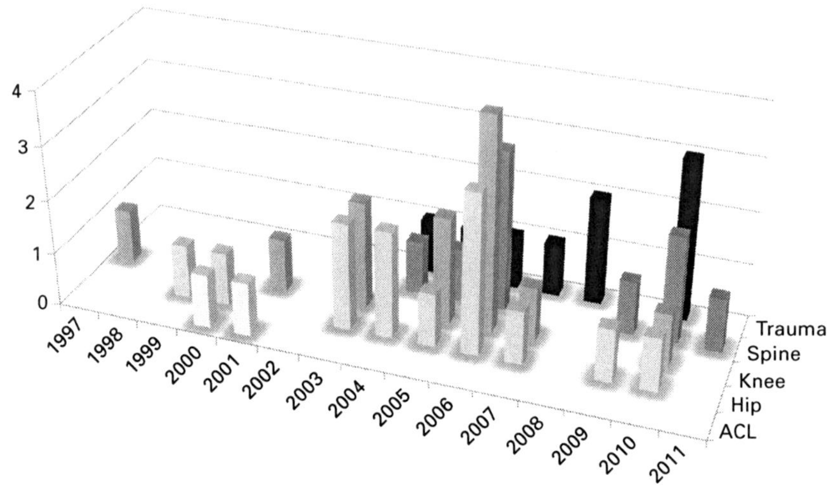

5.4 Time distribution of publications in orthopaedic robotics by clinical areas of application.

Table 5.2 Comparison of five commercially available robots for orthopaedic surgery

System	New procedures	Accuracy	Function	Radiation	Time	Complications
ROBODOC		++	+		–	+(?)
ACROBOT	++	++	++	–	– –	
Mako	++	+		–	–	
Mazor	+	++		++		+
iBlock		++			++	

Note: '+' and '–' symbols indicate the direction and strength of the evidence in favour of particular benefits or costs of each type of robot. '+' indicates a benefit and '–' indicates a cost, double symbols ('++' or '––' indicate stronger evidence, and a blank space indicates no significant evidence either way.

demonstrated. We now discuss these results in more detail in the context of specific systems.

5.3.2 Curexo ROBODOC

ROBODOC is one of the earliest orthopaedic surgical robots and probably the first to have been commercialized (Fig. 5.5). It was originally designed to mill the femoral cavity for total hip replacement surgery and was first used in 1992 by Dr William Bargar in Sacramento, California. The robot was developed in a collaboration between researchers at University of California, Davis, and IBM, it was subsequently commercialized by Integrated Surgical Systems

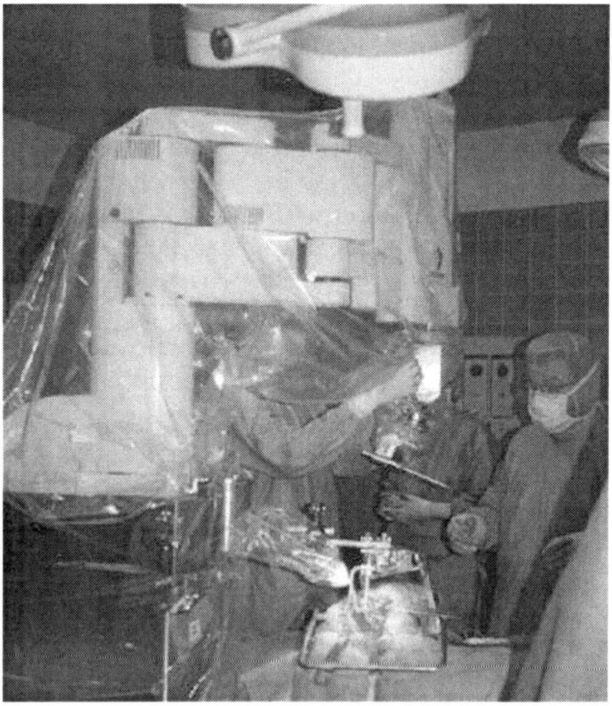

5.5 ROBODOC system (image courtesy of Professor Peter Kazanzides, Johns Hopkins University).

and is now available through Curexo Technology Corporation. ROBODOC was originally based on a conventional industrial robot, augmented with specialized control systems to provide the level of redundancy and safety required for a medical application. It has subsequently undergone a number of design iterations and is now essentially a purpose-built robot.

Given its relatively long history, there are a number of evaluation studies which have appeared, along with some meta-analyses. A relatively comprehensive review was compiled by Schräder (2005); in this report, he identified 60 publications and reports, including two randomized control trials and three health technology assessments. Schräder concluded that, at the time, there was no proof of clinical benefit, but some evidence of an increased incidence of complications. For example, Honl *et al.* (2003) reported a higher dislocation rate (20% versus 4%) and revision rate (13% versus 0%) for robotic compared with conventional surgery, with gluteus medius tendon rupture occurring in all revision cases.

Since Schräder's study, there have been several further reports. Nishihara *et al.* (2006) compared 77 robotically performed cases with 72 conventional controls. They found that numerous technical measures such as gap size between implant and bone were significantly improved using the robot, although Nogler *et al.* (2004) found that improvements in controlling gap size did not necessarily translate to measurable improvements in primary stability. Nishihara *et al.* also found slightly improved hip function scores after two years (17.4 versus 17.1 on the Merle D'Aubigne metric), though no improvement earlier, 20% longer operating time (122 min versus 102 min), 25% less blood loss, an increase in the proportion of patients who could walk within 13 days (53% versus 36%), no significant difference in thigh pain levels, a decreased intraoperative fracture rate (0% versus 6%) and better preoperative estimation of the required implant size (100% versus 91%).

Schulz *et al.* (2007) reported on 97 cases performed with the ROBODOC system. Although there was no control group, they claimed results similar to the conventional technique, but note a relatively high rate of technical complications (>9%) attributable to the use of the robot.

The most significant recent study by Nakamura *et al.* (2010), describes a randomized control trial in which 146 hip surgeries were done in two hospitals; 75 procedures were done by the robot and 71 using a conventional procedure. They found that the Japanese Orthopaedic Association (JOA) scores were slightly elevated at 2 and 3 years (of the order of 1–2 points on a 100 point scale, where the conventional procedure produced a before–after operation difference of close to 50 points), but no significant difference was found after 5 years. The robotic technique also reduced limb length variance (though the average discrepancy was equivalent) and produced less stress shielding in the bone. The operating time was modestly longer with the robot (120 min versus 108 min), but it eliminated intraoperative fractures (0% versus 7%). These results were largely consistent with previous studies (Bargar *et al.*, 1998; Honl *et al.*, 2003).

Other studies have identified other possible concerns and benefits. Zipper and Püschmann (2005) noted a nerve injury rate of 10% in a series of 30 procedures, which was described as being higher than the traditional experience of about 3% in conventional procedures. Nogler *et al.* (2001a) noted the presence of knee pain caused by the fiducial marker in the medial femoral condyle and, in a separate study, they discussed the contamination risk to the surgical team owing to the use of a high-speed cutter (Nogler *et al.*, 2001b). On the positive side, Hagio *et al.* (2003) found in a study of 75 cases of hip surgery, 50 of which were done by robot, that pulmonary embolism events were reduced when using the robot.

In summary, ROBODOC appears to offer improved technical outcomes (primarily in terms of implant fit to cavity), modestly enhanced functional outcomes (as measured by hip scores and time to walking) and decreased intraoperative fracture risk, but these benefits come at the cost of slightly increased operative time, along with variable experience with a range of potential complications.

5.3.3 Stanmore ACROBOT/Sculptor

The ACROBOT system was originally designed to prepare bone surfaces for total knee replacement procedures (Fig. 5.6). It was the first orthopaedic robot to use the concept of active constraint, in which the robot's cutting tool (a milling cutter) is mounted to the end of the robot and manipulated by the surgeon. The system tracks the relative position of the milling cutter and the patient's bone and activates motors attached to the robot's links if the surgeon attempts to move the cutter beyond the permitted regions. These permitted cutting regions are defined in advance of the procedure based on preoperative computed tomography (CT) images and a three-dimensional (3D) surgery planning system.

Although the original research laboratory implementations of this system were extremely bulky, the design was gradually refined as the development was taken over by the ACROBOT corporation and the focus shifted towards unicompartmental implants and less invasive surgical approaches; the latest version of the system, now named Sculptor, was recently purchased by Stanmore Implants (UK). Although this device is commercially available, relatively few systems are in use. This is also evident from the fact that the published peer-reviewed studies available on the ACROBOT/Sculptor are exclusively from the developers. This consists of roughly a dozen studies, most of which focus on technical or procedural issues. Two studies (Rodriguez *et al.*, 2005 and Cobb *et al.*, 2006) present the results of a randomized control trial that compared 15 conventional unicompartmental knee arthroplasties (UKAs) with 13 robotically performed procedures.

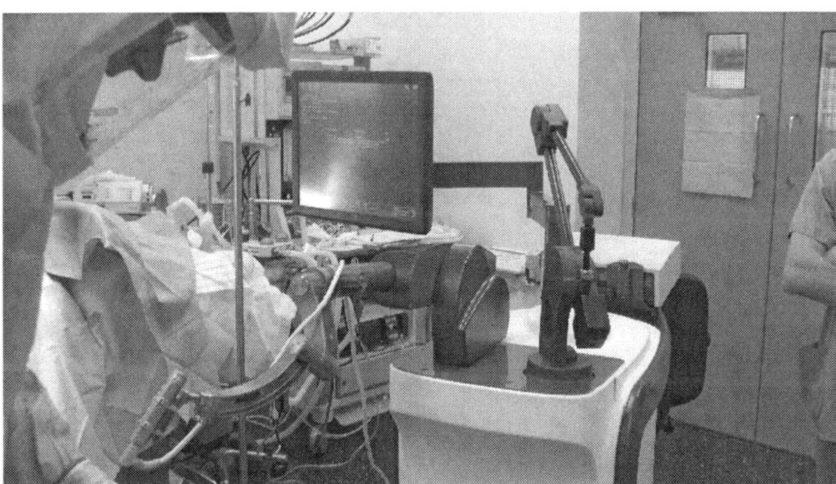

5.6 ACROBOT/Sculptor robot (image courtesy of Professor Brian Davies, Imperial College, London).

The robot demonstrated significantly improved alignment accuracy (all 13 cases were within 2° in varus/valgus orientation, versus 6 out of 15 of the conventional cases). More significantly, the robot produced a highly significant improvement in functional outcome as measured by the change in the American Knee Society (AKS) Score: the median/mean changes were +62/+65 points for the robot versus +19/+33 for the conventional procedure; this represents arguably the strongest evidence from any of the robotic systems for a substantial benefit in outcome by using a robot. Figure 5.7 illustrates the relationship between the orientation error and the change in AKS score for the two types of procedures; note how the robotically performed procedures cluster towards the upper left, indicating comparatively lower alignment errors and larger improvements in function.

However, the robot took approximately 18% longer than the conventional procedure (104 min versus 88 min for skin-to-skin time), but there were no significant differences in complication rates or adverse event rates between the two types of procedures.

5.3.4 Mako RIO

The Mako Robotic Arm Interactive (RIO) orthopedic system (Fig. 5.8) is similar to the ACROBOT/Sculptor in that it is an active-constraint-type robot designed primarily for preparing the bone surface for UKA. As with the ACROBOT, the surgical plan is derived from a preoperative CT scan. The Mako system is relatively newer than the Sculptor (the ACROBOT Company was founded in 1999, whereas Mako was founded in 2004), and

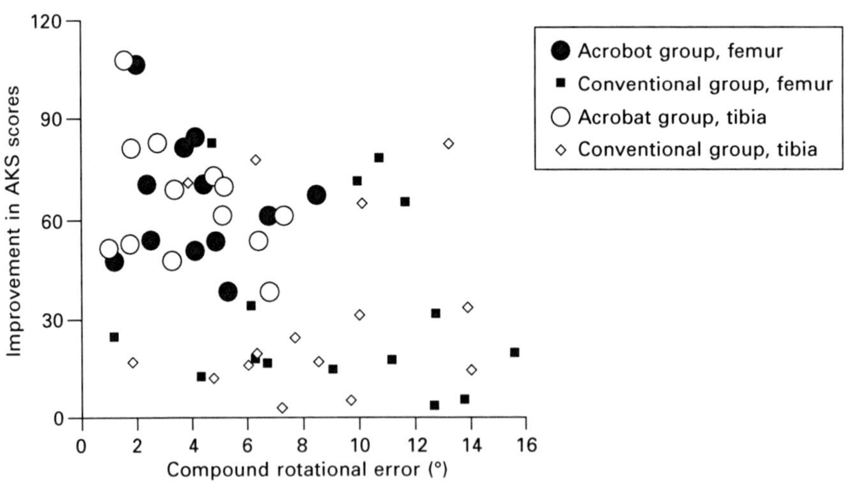

5.7 Comparison of alignment error and functional improvement for robotic and conventional UKA surgeries.

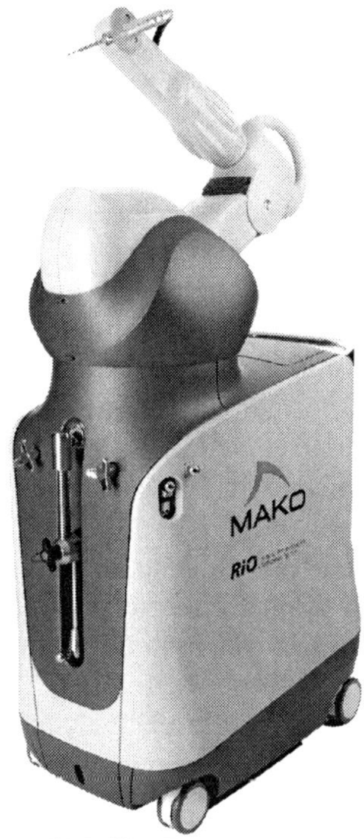

5.8 Mako RIO robot (image courtesy of Mako Surgical Corp.).

relatively few studies evaluating the performance of the Mako system have been published yet, though numerous clinical trials are currently underway. We identified approximately 15 studies explicitly describing either the design philosophy behind the Mako system (e.g., Banks, 2009; O'Loughlin *et al.*, 2009) or clinical experiences with it. Many of these were descriptive and lacked any control group, but several presented some early case series, e.g., Pearle *et al.* (2010) describes the first clinical series of 10 UKA patients).

Some of the early findings from Pearle's study include relatively lengthy setup time (41 min with trained technician), over 40 min required for registration and burring, total surgical time of about 140 min at the beginning, dropping later to about 120 min, and accurate component placement (tibiofemoral varus/valgus errors typically under 1°). In discussing these results, the authors speculate that not needing to directly clamp to the bone may be beneficial, though no direct evidence of benefit has yet been produced. The authors also suggest that the robotic technique may enable better preservation of bone stock and may enable minimally invasive surgery with similar outcomes to more open procedures. However, they also acknowledge that costs are high and draping is more complicated.

Despite these higher costs at present, Swank *et al.* (2009) made a detailed economic argument for adopting the Mako system by modelling the impacts of using robotics throughout all stages of care from admission to discharge and predicts that cost recovery for the system will occur within 2 years after introduction of the robot.

We identified three studies that compared results of UKA procedures using the Mako robot to those of conventional manual procedures. Coon (2009) demonstrated in a study involving 36 robotic procedures and 45 manual ones that the learning curve with the robot was relatively short and that the robot could produce markedly more consistent and accurate component placement (reductions in error and variability by factors of 2.5–3.2 times). Lonner *et al.* (2010) likewise showed significant improvements in component placement accuracy and repeatability in 31 robotic UKA procedures versus 27 conventional ones and found similar results in a related study (Lonner, 2009).

In summary, the Mako system is a well funded, commercially available device that has demonstrated markedly improved control over implant alignment in UKA procedures, but there is as yet little direct evidence of improvement in functional outcomes such as those we saw in the one study presented for the Sculptor system. However, given the relatively high number of Mako systems currently in service, we expect to see many more clinical studies being published in the coming years.

5.3.5 Mazor SpineAssist

The Mazor SpineAssist is a small bone-mounted robot (50 mm diameter by 80 mm long, 250 g, Fig. 5.9) intended primarily for use in inserting pedicle

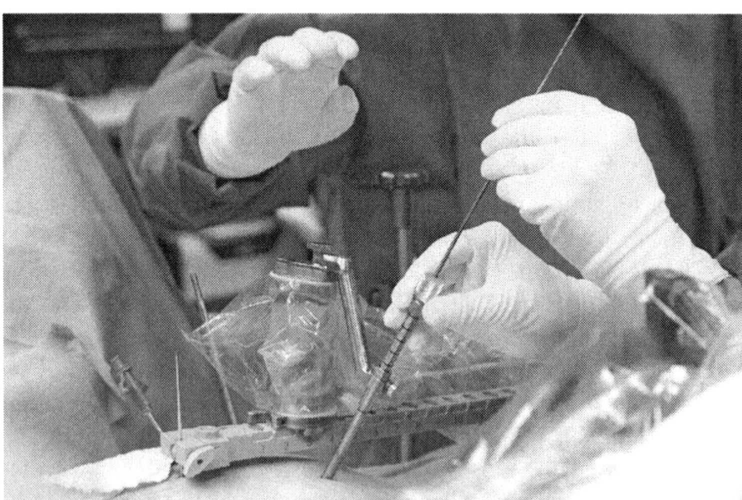

5.9 Mazor SpineAssist robot (image courtesy of Mazor Robotics).

screws during spinal surgeries. The device consists of a base which is clamped to the spinous processes, six linear actuators configured in parallel, and an end-effector to which is attached a drill guide. The workflow consists of the following steps:

1. obtain a preoperative CT scan of the patient and plan the insertion trajectories;
2. intraoperatively, mount a frame and image-acquisition targets to the patient's spine (this can be done using percutaneous techniques);
3. obtain two fluoroscopic shots of the system from different angles (ideally, substantially orthogonally to one another) and use this information to register the mounting frame to the spine model extracted from the CT images;
4. attach the robot to the mounting frame and drive the drill guide to the desired position; and
5. drill through the guiding tube; repeat for additional holes.

The Mazor system is relatively new. The earliest studies describing the system were published in about 2004, and only a handful of clinical studies have yet been reported (e.g., Pechlivanis *et al.*, 2009; Shoham *et al.*, 2007; Sukovich *et al.*, 2006). A study by Barzilay *et al.*, (2008) reviewed the evidence available at the time and noted that '[A]ll data is based on cohort studies, and none compared the SpineAssist to other techniques, i.e. free hand, fluoroscopy guided, fluoro-navigation, other navigation systems, therefore, no superiority can be claimed and cost effectiveness cannot be calculated'.

The most important study since then was presented by Devito *et al.* (2010) (an overview of studies reporting clinical experiences with the Mazor SpineAssist is presented in Table 5.3), which was a major retrospective review covering 840 cases in 14 hospitals (~4000 screws total); 49% of the screws were placed percutaneously. 84% of the screws were placed fully under robotic control (90% in the last third of the study); 9% of the cases had registration problems, and 3% had other technology-related problems.

Of all screws inserted in the study, 98% were judged to have been placed acceptably. There were initial nerve deficits in four cases of 593 monitored

Table 5.3 Overview of studies presenting results for pedicle screw implantations using the Mazor SpineAssist robot

Study	Number of Patients/screws	Amount placed by robot (%)	Amount placed within 2 mm (%)
Sukovich *et al.* (2006)	14/49	93	96 (< 1 mm)
Shoham *et al.* (2007)	65/316	80	93
Pechlivanis *et al.* (2009)	31/133	~94	91.0–98.5
Devito *et al.* (2010)	840/4000	84–90	98

cases, but all were resolved following revision and there was no permanent damage. Devito *et al.* (2010) state that this experience is better than the injury rates of 0.5–5% reported in other studies using the standard technique, although, because they did not have a control group in their own study, they did not claim that this decrease in injury rate was proven. The time needed per screw for insertion decreased with the number of screws (vertebral levels) per case from about 12 min per screw with four screws inserted to about 4 min per screw with 12 or more per case; over the series, the time needed per screw improved somewhat for cases with seven or fewer screws inserted, but there was virtually no change in insertion time with experience for cases with eight or more screws inserted.

Because the overall success rate was high and half their cases were done percutaneously, they did suggest that this system was suitable for, and would likely be seen as most valuable in, less invasive or minimally invasive surgical (LIS/MIS) cases.

An additional benefit of using the Mazor robot is decreased use of radiation. Lieberman *et al.* (2007) presented a study in which 16 surgeons inserted a total of 217 screw in 11 cadavers. They found that cases performed using the robot used only ~2% of the radiation required with the standard fluoroscopically guided technique. Although this result has not yet been confirmed in clinical studies, it is probably true because the Mazor technique requires only two X-ray images for registration and two more at the end of the procedure for verification.

In summary, the Mazor SpineAssist robot has so far been shown to produce highly satisfactory outcomes in *in vivo* settings and, in a cadaver study, to significantly reduce radiation use. As Barzilay *et al.* (2008) noted, there are as yet no direct comparative studies with any other technique, either the conventional fluoroscopically guided procedure or any of the navigated procedures, so it is premature to make claims of superiority. However, we do note that several navigated approaches have all been shown to produce lower pedicle perforation rates than the conventional procedure (Tian *et al.*, 2011), so we expect that the robot will also be able to demonstrate improved performance relative to the conventional procedure. By virtue of making it easier to perform percutaneous screw placements, we believe that there are preliminary indications that the SpineAssist device may be able to enable new, less invasive procedures and decrease the complications associated with open procedures, although there is not yet direct evidence to back up these suggestions.

5.3.6 Praxim/OMNIlife Science iBlock

The iBlock (formerly Praxiteles) robot is the most recent commercial offering in the orthopaedic robotic field, with the first commercial systems having been made available only in the past year or two by Praxim/OMNIlife Science (Fig. 5.10). It is conceptually similar to the Mazor SpineAssist in that it is a small, bone-mounted robot designed as a cutting-guide positioner. It is intended primarily for use in total and unicompartmental knee procedures in which cuts are normally made with an oscillating saw, although it can also be configured to guide a milling tool (Plaskos *et al.*, 2005). The device is mounted directly into one of the condyles of the knee (normally the medial condyle) and manual adjustments are made under navigation guidance to align the axis of the robot to be perpendicular to the desired sagittal plane of the knee implant.

Following this, two drive motors control the rotational position and angular alignment of a slit-type cutting guide. For a standard total knee implant, the iBlock drives the guide through a series of five cuts corresponding to the anterior, distal, posterior and two chamfer cuts. In contrast to the SpineAssist, the iBlock has only two powered degrees of freedom. The device uses a serial architecture with two rotational joints, both driven through high-reduction gearing.

Studies on iBlock/Praxiteles are still relatively limited, with only two significant studies describing the system, one from a technical point of view (Plaskos *et al.*, 2005) and a recent study (Koulalis *et al.*, 2010a) comparing the accuracy and efficiency of the system to a standard navigated approach in a cadaveric setting. Koulalis *et al.* (2010a) showed that the iBlock took substantially less time than the navigated approach (5.5 min versus 13.8 min, $p<0.001$), largely owing to significant reductions in the time needed to attach, navigate and detach the conventional cutting block, as well as by eliminating the need for the 4-in-1 cutting block. In addition, the iBlock was

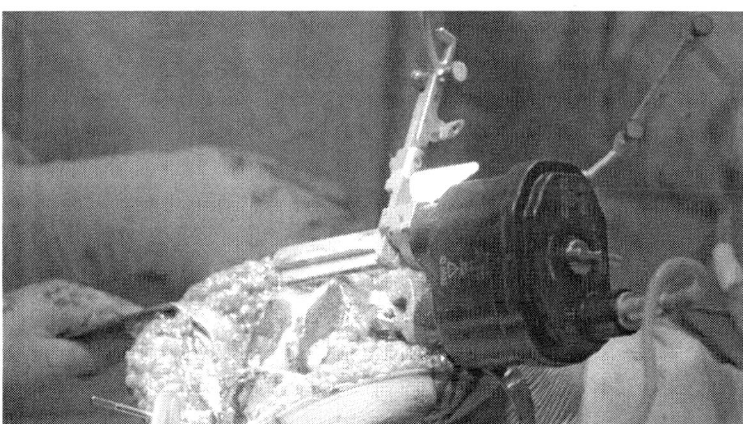

5.10 Praxim iBlock robot (image courtesy of Jan A. Koenig, MD, Mercy Medical Center, New York, and Christopher Plaskos, PhD, OMNIlife science).

more reproducible, producing deviations relative to the planned cuts which were only 35–50% of those produced by the navigated system. Koulalis *et al.* (2010a) concluded that the iBlock was both more efficient and accurate than navigation, though this has not yet been shown in a clinical trial. However, a study presented at the 2011 Computer-Assisted Orthopaedic Society (CAOS) conference showed results consistent with those of the cadaver study (Koenig *et al.*, 2011) and also suggested that the iBlock would prove less expensive than conventional navigation because of a reduction in the number of components in the surgical kit, which could translate into lower sterilization and other handling costs, though the evidence to support these predictions is not yet available.

An interesting challenge the iBlock system faces stems from another project by the same group. Koulalis *et al.* (2010b) recently presented a similar cadaver study evaluating the performance of an adjustable cutting guide compared with a conventional navigated guide (an adjustable cutting guide is a passive cutting guide with adjustment screws built in; they are adjusted under navigation guidance following fixation of the base to the bone). They found significantly improved performance of the adjustable guide relative to conventional blocks, and the level of improvement was as good or better than that of the iBlock; likewise, the adjustment time was substantially reduced using the adjustable guide – from over 6 min to about 2 min. They have not yet directly compared the iBlock with adjustable cutting guides.

In summary, the iBlock system has proven in cadaver studies to be both more accurate and time-efficient than conventional navigation, but clinical trials are only now starting to be reported in the peer-reviewed literature, and it has not been compared with alternative technologies such as adjustable cutting guides or patient-specific templates.

5.4 Conclusion

In this chapter, we review the state-of-the-art in orthopaedic robotics in terms of what is known about their potential advantages (benefits) and costs. Concentrating on the five commercially available systems (summarized in Tables 5.1 and 5.2), we found, by and large, that claims of improved accuracy have been substantiated, certainly against the conventional manual procedures, but also, in the case of the Praxim system, against standard computer-assisted navigation. Three of the systems can reasonably lay claim to changing the nature of surgical procedures and facilitating less invasive procedures: both the ACROBOT/Sculptor and the Mako systems enable advanced unicompartmental knee surgery and the Mazor appears to greatly facilitate percutaneous pedicle screw insertion.

Of the five, only the ACROBOT has shown evidence of significantly improved functional outcomes (2–3-fold improvements in the American

Knee Society scores), and the ROBODOC has demonstrated slight short- and medium-term increases in the Japanese Orthopaedic Association scores (1–2 points on a 100 point scale).

Three of the robots (ROBODOC, ACROBOT and Mako) achieve their increased accuracy by starting from a preoperative CT scan. Because such scans are not normally required for joint replacement procedures, these represent an additional cost and radiation hazard which must be included in any overall assessment of the value of these systems. The Mazor SpineAssist robot has been shown in a cadaver study that closely approximates the clinical situation to substantially eliminate the need for intraoperative fluoroscopy, whereas the Praxim iBlock is fully compatible with an image-free approach.

The ROBODOC, ACROBOT and Mako all appear to lengthen surgery somewhat, with the first two extending it by approximately 12–16 min, on average. The difference is less clear with the Mako, however, because all reported studies have been cohort studies, so no direct comparison is possible. The Mazor system likewise has not been compared with a control group, so it is difficult to make a claim one way or another. The Praxim iBlock is the only system which has shown a significant decrease in operating time (albeit in a cadaver trial); nonetheless, the reduction from 14 min to 5.5 min, if confirmed in clinical trials, would be clinically meaningful.

In terms of complications, most systems have shown either no evidence of problems or modest evidence of improvements. The SpineAssist system has apparently produced a large case series with a zero permanent nerve injury rate (lower than rates of 0.5–5% commonly reported for the conventional procedure). Likewise, the ROBODOC has virtually eliminated intraoperative femoral fractures, although there is some suggestion that soft tissue injuries can be increased (though this suggestion has been heavily disputed).

Finally, there is no convincing evidence of decreased cost for any of the systems, although one economic model has been presented to argue that the Mako system is cost-effective overall. It will be interesting to see more evidence on this point in coming years.

Overall, the evidence to justify the use of orthopaedic robots remains modest. In particular, most studies to date have been cohort studies or have compared the use of the robot to conventional manual procedures. However, there are frequently alternative technologies available for achieving a similar surgical goal, and, because robotic technologies tend to be relatively expensive, it will be important to determine if robots have any incremental advantage over standard navigation systems, the emerging patient-specific templates (i.e., custom jigs), or smarter cutting guides (in the case of iBlock). Until such comparisons are available, we expect to only see robots used in niche applications that are not well served by existing techniques or new applications where the robotic technology enables a surgeon to perform a procedure that would otherwise be technically impossible.

5.5 References

Banks SA (2009) Haptic robotics enable a systems approach to design of a minimally invasive modular knee arthroplasty. *Am J Orthop* **38**(2S): 23–7.

Bargar WL, Bauer A and Börner M (1998) Primary and revision total hip replacement using the Robodoc system. *Clin Orthop Relat Res*, (354): 82–91.

Barzilay Y, Kaplan L and Libergall M (2008) Robotic assisted spine surgery: a breakthrough or a surgical toy? *Int J Med Robot*, **4**(3): 195–6

Cobb J, Henckel J, Gomes P, Harris S, Jakopec M, Rodriguezy Baena F, Barrett A and Davies B (2006) Hands-on robotic unicompartmental knee replacement: a prospective, randomised controlled study of the acrobot system. *J Bone Joint Surg, Br Vol*, **88**(2), 188–97, doi:10.1302/0301-620X.88B2.17220.

Coon TM (2009) Integrating robotic technology into the operating room. *Am J Orthop*, **38**(2S): 7–9.

Devito DP, Kaplan L, Dietl R, Pfeiffer M, Horne D, Silberstein B, Hardenbrook M, *et al.* (2010) Clinical acceptance and accuracy assessment of spinal implants guided with Spineassist Surgical robot: retrospective study. *Spine*, **35**(24): 2109–15, doi:10.1097/BRS.0b013e3181d323ab.

Fehring TK, Odum SM, Troyer JL, Iorio R, Kurtz SM and Lau EC (2010) Joint replacement access in 2016: a supply side crisis. *J Arthroplasty*, **25**(8): 1175–81.

Hagio K, Sugano N, Takashina M, Nishii T, Yoshikawa H and Ochi T (2003) Effectiveness of the ROBODOC system in preventing intraoperative pulmonary embolism. *Acta Orthop Scand*, **74**(3): 264–9.

Hodgson AJ (2008) Computer-assisted orthopaedic surgery. In *Image-guided interventions*. Peters T and Cleary K (eds), Springer Science + Business Media, LLC, pp. 333–86.

Honl M, Dierk O, Gauck C, Carrero V, Lampe F, Dries S, Quante M, Schwieger K, Hille E and Morlock MM (2003) Comparison of robotic-assisted and manual implantation of a primary total hip replacement. A prospective study. *J Bone Joint Surg Am*, **85**-A(8): 1470–8.

Koenig JA and Plaskos C (2011) Surgical accuracy and efficiency of computer-automated total knee arthroplasty – a report on the first 80 cases. 11th Annual Meeting of computer Assisted Orthopaedic Surgery-International, London, UK, June 15–18, 2011.

Koulalis D, O'Loughlin PF, Plaskos C, Kendoff D, Cross MB and Pearle AD (2010a) Sequential versus automated cutting guides in computer-assisted total knee arthroplasty. *Knee*, **18**(6): 436–42.

Koulalis D, O'Loughlin PF, Plaskos C, Kendoff D and Pearle AD (2010b) Adjustable cutting blocks for computer-navigated total knee arthroplasty: a cadaver study. *J Arthroplasty*, **25**(5): 807–11.

Lieberman I, Hardenbrook M, Wang J, Guyer RD and Khanna AJ (2007) Radiation exposure using miniature robotic guidance for spinal surgery. *Spine J* **7**(5) 152S–3S, DOI: 10.1016/j.spinee.2007.07.362.

Lonner JH, John TK and Conditt MA (2010) Robotic arm-assisted UKA improves tibial component alignment: a pilot study. *Clin Orthop Relat Res*, **468**(1): 141–6.

Lonner JH (2009) Robotic arm-assisted unicompartmental arthroplasty. *Sem Arthroplasty*, **20**(1): 15–22.

Nakamura N, Sugano N, Nishii T, Kakimoto A and Miki H (2010) A comparison between robotic-assisted and manual implantation of cementless total hip arthroplasty. *Clin Orthop Rel Res*, **468**(4): 1072–81, doi:10.1007/s11999-009-1158-2.

Nishihara S, Sugano N, Nishii T, Miki H, Nakamura N and Yoshikawa H (2006) Comparison between hand rasping and robotic milling for stem implantation in cementless total hip arthroplasty. *J Arthroplasty*, **21**(7): 957–66.

Nogler M, Maurer H, Wimmer C, Gegenhuber C, Bach C and Krismer M. (2001a) Knee pain caused by a fiducial marker in the medial femoral condyle: a clinical and anatomic study of 20 cases. *Acta Orthop Scand*, **72**(5): 477–80.

Nogler M, Polikeit A, Wimmer C, Brückner A, Ferguson SJ and Krismer M (2004) Primary stability of a ROBODOC implanted anatomical stem versus manual implantation. *Clin Biomech*, **19**(2): 123–9.

Nogler M, Wimmer C, Lass-Flörl C, Mayr E, Trobos S and Gegenhuber C. (2001b) Contamination risk of the surgical team through ROBODOC's high-speed cutter. *Clin Orthop Relat Res*, **387**: 225–31.

O'Loughlin PF, Pearle AD, Fyhrie DP and Long F (2009) Arthroscopic robotic arm-assisted unicompartmental knee arthroplasty. *J Am Acad Orthop Surg*, **17**: 266–9.

Pearle AD, O'Loughlin PF and Kendoff DO (2010) Robot-assisted unicompartmental knee arthroplasty. *J Arthroplasty*, **25**(2): 230–7, doi:10.1016/j.arth.2008.09.024.

Pechlivanis I, Kiriyanthan G, Engelhardt M, Scholz M, Lücke S, Harders A and Schmieder K (2009) Percutaneous placement of pedicle screws in the lumbar spine using a bone mounted miniature robotic system: first experiences and accuracy of screw placement. *Spine*, **34**(4): 392–8, doi:10.1097/BRS.0b013e318191ed32.

Plaskos C, Cinquin P, Lavallée S and Hodgson AJ (2005) Praxiteles: a miniature bone-mounted robot for minimal access total knee arthroplasty. *Int J Med Robot*, **1**(4): 67–79.

Pott PP, Scharf HP and Schwarz ML (2005) Today's state of the art in surgical robotics. *Comput Aided Surg*, **10**(2): 101–32.

Rodriguez F, Harris S, Jakopec M, Barrett A, Gomes P, Henckel J, Cobb J and Davies B (2005) Robotic clinical trials of uni-condylar arthroplasty. *Int J Med Robot Comp Assist Surg*, MRCAS, **1**(4): 20–8, doi:10.1002/rcs.52.

Schräder P (2005) [Technique evaluation for orthopedic use of Robodoc]. Zeitschrift für Orthopädie und ihre Grenzgebiete, **143**(3): 329–36, doi: 10.1055/s-2005-836458.

Schulz AP, Seide K, Queitsch C, von Haugwitz A, Meiners J, Kienast B, Tarabolsi M, Kammal M and Jürgens C (2007) Results of total hip replacement using the Robodoc surgical assistant system: clinical outcome and evaluation of complications for 97 procedures. *Int J Med Robot*, **3**(4): 301–6.

Shoham M, Lieberman IH, Benzel EC, Togawa D, Zehavi E, Zilberstein B, Roffman M, Bruskin A, Fridlander A, Joskowicz L, Brink-Danan S and Knoller N (2007) Robotic assisted spinal surgery: from concept to clinical practice. *Comput Aided Surg*, **12**(2): 105–15.

Sukovich W, Brink-Danan S and Hardenbrook M (2006) Miniature robotic guidance for pedicle screw placement in posterior spinal fusion: early clinical experience with the SpineAssist. *Int J Med Robot Comp Assist Surg* MRCAS, **2**(2): 114–22, doi:10.1002/rcs.86.

Swank ML, Alikire M, Conditt MA and Lonner JH (2009) Technology and cost effectiveness in knee arthroplasty: computer navigation and robotics. *Am J Orthop*, **38**(2S): 32–6.

Tian NF, Huang QS, Zhou P, Zhou Y, Wu RK, Lou Y and Xu HZ (2011) Pedicle screw insertion accuracy with different assisted methods: a systematic review and meta-analysis of comparative studies. *Eur Spine J*, **20**(6): 846–59.

Westphal R, Winkelbach S, Wahl F, Gösling T, Oszwald M, Hüfner T and Krettek C (2009) Robot-assisted long bone fracture reduction. *Int J Robot Res*, **28**(10), 1259–1278.

Woolf AD and Pfleger B (2003) Burden of major muscoskeletal conditions. *Bull World Health Organ*, **81**: 646–56.

Zipper SG and Püschmann H (2005) Nerve injuries after computer-assisted hip replacement: case series with 29 patients. *Z Orthop Ihre Grenzgeb*, **143**(4): 399–402 (In German).

6
Robotic-assisted knee replacement surgery

C. PLASKOS, OMNIlife Science, Inc., USA,
J. A. KOENIG, Winthrop University Hospital, USA and
C. E. PONDER, Oklahoma Sports and Orthopedics Institute, USA

Abstract: An overview is presented of robotic and computer-assisted surgical (CAS) technologies, which have remarkable potential to enhance the precision and the quality of total knee arthroplasty (TKA). A detailed description is given of an exemplary imageless CAS TKA system that is based on bone-morphometric planning software combined with miniature robotic cutting-guide technology. The application of this technology in the clinical setting is discussed as it pertains to surgical accuracy and efficiency, surgeon learning curve, clinical utility in complex cases and severe deformities, and minimally invasive surgical (MIS) techniques.

Key words: robotic-assisted surgery, robotics, computer-assisted surgery, computer navigation, total knee replacement, knee arthroplasty.

6.1 Introduction

Technologies for robotic and computer-assisted surgery (CAS) have remarkable potential to enhance the precision and the quality of orthopaedic surgery. This may improve functional outcomes and quality of life for patients undergoing knee arthroplasty (Ishida *et al.*, 2011; Longstaff *et al.*, 2009), and may prolong prosthesis longevity (Ritter *et al.*, 1994; Sharkey *et al.*, 2002). Robotic and CAS technologies can also allow less invasive surgical techniques, which have been shown to accelerate functional recovery and shorten hospital stays (Dutton *et al.*, 2008), and enable the use of new implant designs that preserve bone (Banks, 2009). Other theoretical benefits include reduced costs to healthcare and greater overall efficiency (Swank *et al.*, 2009).

The prevalence and impact of degenerative joint diseases such as osteoarthritis (OA) warrant the advancement and use of joint replacement technologies such as CAS. Approximately one in three people in the United States over the age of sixty suffer from OA of the knee (Iorio *et al.*, 2008; Lawrence *et al.*, 1998), which can mean discomfort, pain, loss of motion, and a reduced quality of life for tens of millions of Americans. In order to accommodate the growing population, the number of total knee arthroplasty (TKA) procedures has been increasing at a dramatic rate. In the USA, the number of TKAs performed over the last decade has grown by approximately

250%, from 252 241 in 1998 to 616 342 in 2009 (Bozic, 2012), and this figure is expected to surpass one million TKAs per year by 2016 (Iorio *et al.*, 2008). Importantly, today's arthroplasty patients are younger and demand more from their procedures. Although the elderly population is growing at a faster rate, the percentage of TKAs being performed in patients between the ages of 55-64 has increased, from about 20% in 1998 to 29% in 2009 (Bozic, 2012). Because younger patients are more active, live longer, and want to return to a productive lifestyle sooner, they place greater demands on their joint replacements and may wear them out sooner. Robotics and CAS may therefore be of even greater value in this patient group.

In order to become adopted on a widespread scale, CAS technology must demonstrate sufficient added value such that its benefits outweigh any added cost or burden imposed on the healthcare system (Beringer *et al.*, 2007). Historically, the prevalence of CAS in joint-replacement procedures has been very low in comparison to conventional surgery despite more than fifteen years of ongoing research, development and commercialization efforts. To some degree this is because of the difficulty the clinical and scientific community has had in demonstrating improved outcomes, with the majority of randomized controlled studies showing improvements in knee implant alignment accuracy with CAS (Mason 2007) but not in clinical outcomes as evaluated by knee function and patient scores. Moreover, prior generation robotic and CAS systems may have been cumbersome and expensive to use, adding significant time and cost to the case and often requiring a substantial capital investment from the hospital, Table 6.1 (Bellemans *et al.*, 2007; Slover *et al.*, 2008; Swank *et al.*, 2009). In particular, earlier CAS systems that positioned conventional fixed cutting blocks using freehand navigation and pinning methods were found to be frustrating and less accurate to use (Klima *et al.*, 2008; Koulalis *et al.*, 2010b). However, CAS technology is continuously advancing, becoming ever more efficient, useful, and cost effective. A recent survey conducted by the American Association of Hip and Knee Surgeons (AAHKS) indicated that 14% of respondents 'strongly believed in CAS technologies' and use it in almost every TKA case (Berry and Bozic, 2010), which is substantially higher than the 3–5% usage rate quoted in the past. We believe that the value and usage of robotic and CAS technologies will continue to increase as the technologies advance because of the potential benefits they offer:

- greater accuracy in implant alignment and overall positioning in all planes;
- real-time feedback on knee kinematics, ligament balance, and stability;
- increased confidence and safety in less invasive surgical techniques where visualization may be limited;

Table 6.1 Summary of publications providing approximate capital costs and per case costs associated with various passive CAS and robotic knee arthroplasty systems

Technology (system or manufacturer)	Capital costs[1]	Cost per case[1]	Reference
Passive CAS			
Passive CAS	\$150 000–\$300 000	Not disclosed	Swank *et al.*, 2009
Passive CAS	\$140 000 plus \$48 000/year[2]	Not disclosed	Slover *et al.*, 2008
Passive CAS	Not disclosed	\$600–\$2000	Beringer *et al.*, 2007
Passive CAS	Not disclosed	\$1500	Novak *et al.*, 2007
Passive CAS	Not disclosed	\$300–\$400	Dong and Buxton, 2006
Active robotic			
Active robotic (ROBODOC)	\$635 000 – \$1500 500	\$150[3]	Bargar *et al.*, 2007
Active robotic (CASPAR)	\$545 000	\$1360[3]	Bellemans *et al.*, 2007
Semiactive robotic			
Semiactive robotic (MAKO)	\$941 000	Not disclosed[3]	Lang *et al.*, 2011
Semiactive robotic (MAKO)	\$800 000	Not disclosed[3]	Lonner *et al.*, 2010 Swank *et al.*, 2009
Patient-specific instruments			
Patient-specific instruments	\$0	\$2500 (\$1500 for instruments plus \$1000 for CT imaging)	Slover 2012

[1]All amounts are in US dollars.
[2]Includes annual maintenance costs for computer hardware (\$20 000) and software (\$8000) and the service contract (\$20 000) over a five-year period.
[3]Does not include cost related to preoperative imaging.

- greater efficiency during surgery;
- fewer manual instruments required in the OR, reducing costs and logistics; and
- quantitative electronic reporting of the surgery.

In this review we first provide background information on conventional and minimally invasive TKA, followed by an overview of some of the developments in the field of computer and robotic-assisted TKA. A detailed discussion is then provided on the technological development and validation of an exemplary CAS system for TKA that is based on imageless morphometric planning software combined with miniature robotic cutting-guide technology (Praxim navigation with Apex robotic technology, or ART, from OMNIlife Science Inc., Massachusetts). The application of ART in the clinical setting is described as it pertains to surgical accuracy and efficiency, surgeon learning curve, clinical utility in complex cases with severe deformities, and minimally invasive surgical (MIS) techniques. Finally, we conclude with our view on future developments in this field.

6.1.1 Total knee replacement

TKA was pioneered in the late 1960s with the goals of relieving pain and restoring knee joint function to patients with end stage knee OA (Freeman *et al.*, 1973; Gunston, 1971; Ranawat *et al.*, 1976). This is accomplished by replacing the worn articular surfaces of the knee with artificial metal and plastic (polyethylene) bearing surfaces, Fig. 6.1. Implant design, surgical technique and instrumentation, and patient selection are a few of the many factors that play an important role in the outcome of TKA. Although knee implant designs and materials markedly progressed over the decades that

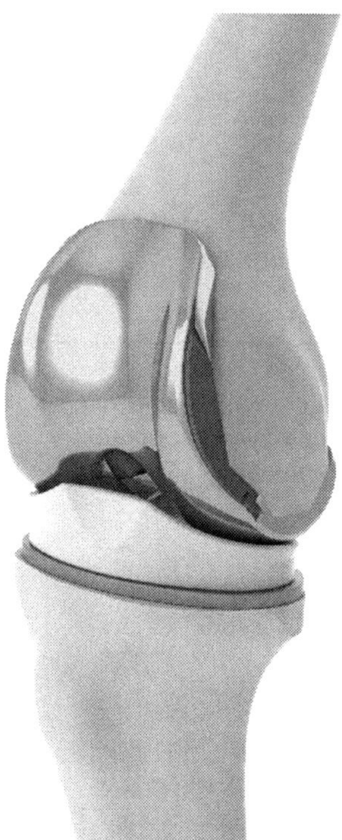

6.1 Total knee arthroplasty (TKA) is a procedure in which the three compartments of the knee are replaced with a metal and plastic (polyethylene) implant. At least five planar bone cuts are required on the femur and one on the tibia in order to insert the implant (© 2012 OMNIlife science, Inc.).

followed their introduction, the manual instruments that most surgeons use to perform TKA even today are akin to those used 25 years ago. Surgeons need to have an exceptional degree of surgical skill in order to perform knee replacement accurately and consistently with manual instrumentation. Technique-related factors that can affect the success of TKA include: implant sizing, positioning, and alignment in the coronal, sagittal, and rotational planes, soft-tissue balance, range of motion and patellar tracking. Although modern TKA is considered to be a very successful procedure overall with a survival rate in the 90th percentile beyond ten years (Rasquinha *et al.*, 2006), premature and preventable failures do still occur, even for experienced surgeons. In a review of 212 revision TKA procedures, Sharkey *et al.* (2002) reported that more than half of all revisions were performed within 2 years of the index operation, and as many as 50% of those premature failures were caused by factors related to surgical technique, such as implant malalignment, malpositioning, and instability.

Why robotics?

TKA is an attractive application of robotic assistance for a number of reasons. Firstly, knee malalignment of as little as 3° in the frontal plane has been correlated to increased polyethylene stresses and early clinical failures, so a high degree of implant placement accuracy is key for good clinical results (Liau *et al.*, 2002; Longstaff *et al.*, 2009; Ritter *et al.*, 1994, Sharkey *et al.*, 2002). Secondly, conventional TKA instrumentation systems that rely on sequential mechanical jigs to aid bone resurfacing are known to produce variable results with respect to implant alignment and fit of the femoral component (Bathis *et al.*, 2005; Huddleston *et al.*, 2005; Koulalis *et al.*, 2010a; Laskin, 1991; Lennox *et al.*, 1988; Plaskos *et al.*, 2002). Furthermore, manual instrumentation systems usually require that a number of guides be available in the operating room to cover the entire range of implant sizes (typically one template for each of the six to eight sizes), which can occupy valuable space around the operating table and increase sterilization costs.

6.1.2 Conventional and minimally invasive surgery (MIS) techniques

In conventional TKA, the surgeon strives to achieve accurate alignment by adequately exposing the knee joint and using an intramedullary or extramedulary alignment guide to orient cutting blocks across the exposed aspects of the bones. The standard approach has been described as a 15–25 cm anteromedial or midline skin incision extending proximally from just distal to the level of the tibial tubercle, followed by a medial parapatellar arthrotomy that extends superiorly through the quadriceps tendon, Fig. 6.2.

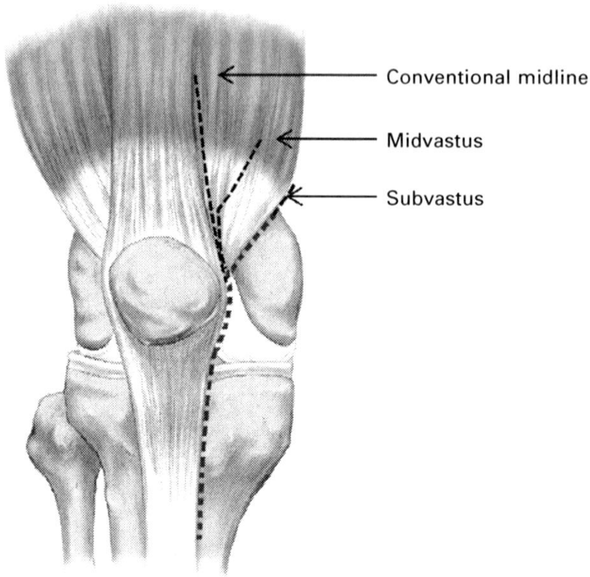

6.2 Surgical approaches and muscle exposure in conventional TKA midline, midvastus, and subvastus.

The extent of the incision allows for lateral eversion and dislocation of the patella, thus exposing most of the structures in the knee joint. Although dividing the quadriceps muscle in this manner has been shown to have no significant long-term effects on the outcome of TKA, various short-term repercussions have been reported in some studies. These include increased pain, blood loss and time to ambulation, prolonged postoperative hospital stay and rehabilitation, and decreased the range of motion and knee strength (Laskin, *et al.*, 2004; and Tria Coon 2003).

MIS TKA has been classified as a procedure in which the knee arthrotomy minimizes quadriceps damage and avoids patella eversion (Laskin, 2003). Certain techniques such as the subvastus (Hofmann *et al.*, 1991) or minisubvastus (Schroer *et al.*, 2008) preserve the quadriceps mechanism entirely, whereas others utilize a ~2 cm vastus medialis snip to facilitate patellar subluxation, Fig. 6.2 (Scuderi *et al.*, 2004). Femoral cuts are made from the anterior or medial side through a 6–14 cm 'mobile' incision that is moved to expose different aspects of the joint by flexing and rotating the knee. Approaching the bone cuts obliquely or medially circumvents the need to evert the patella, potentially reducing morbidity and trauma to the extensor mechanism, and improving postoperative knee function, recovery rate, and pain.

MIS TKA remains a controversial procedure with several studies showing no difference in patient outcomes beyond the 6 week to 3 month follow-up period (Smith *et al.*, 2012). Critics of MIS TKA argue that the decreased exposure restricts visibility and access to the knee, making it difficult to attain precise bone resections, implant placement, soft-tissue balance, and adequate application and removal of excess bone cement. In a randomized control study comparing radiographic leg alignment accuracy, Chin *et al.* (2007) reported that MIS side cutting techniques where the bone cuts are performed from medial to lateral, resulted in 56% of cases within ±3° of mechanical alignment versus 83% in the conventional and MIS midvastus techniques.

6.1.3 Robotics, navigation, and patient-specific instruments

Robotic and computer-assisted surgery systems have been classified as active, semiactive, or passive systems (Delp *et al.*, 1998, Stindel *et al.*, 2002; Bargar, 2007; Bellemans *et al.*, 2007). Active robotic systems were the earliest systems developed and the most complex to use. These employed preoperative computer tomography (CT) based planning systems and large robotic arms that performed bone cutting (milling) autonomously without direct surgeon interaction. Development of the first active robotic system for orthopaedics (ROBODOC) began in 1986 and was directed at total hip replacement surgery, with the first operation being performed in a human patient in 1992 (Bargar, 1998; Paul *et al.*, 1992). Despite the extreme accuracy that active robotic systems offered in TKA (Table 6.2), the excessive operating

Table 6.2 Summary of clinical studies on active robotic systems used in total knee arthroplasty

Reference	System used	Type of study	Number of patients	Accuracy	Mean operation time (range)	System failure (abort) rates
Siebert *et al.*, 2002	CASPAR	Prospective	70	0.8° (0–4.1°)	135 min (80–220) approx. 90 min after learning curve	1/70 reported
Bellemans *et al.*, 2007	CASPAR	Prospective	25	< ±1°	195 min (130–255 min)	12%
Chun *et al.*, 2011	ROBODOC	Retrospective consecutive case study	62 (TKA)	N/A	186 min	34% (21/62)

time and complexity associated with the use of these systems, as well as their extremely high operational costs (Table 6.1) have led some clinicians to abandon their use and direct their interests more towards smart semiactive systems (Bellemans *et al.*, 2007).

Semiactive robotic systems do not carry out surgical operations on their own, but interact synergistically with the surgeon to perform a task. Semiactive systems can vary in both form and function. Active constraint or haptic systems employ a robotic arm that allows the surgeon to operate a surgical tool or burr freely within a predetermined safe zone and provides resistance when the surgeon approaches the boundary. Two systems that have been developed for partial (uni- and bicompartmental) knee resurfacing applications are the Acrobot Sculptor (now Stanmore Sculptor, from Stanmore Implants Worldwide, Ltd.) initially developed at Imperial College, London (Davies *et al.*, 1997; Jakopec *et al.*, 2001; Cobb *et al.*, 2006) and the Robotic Arm Interactive Orthopaedic system, RIO®, (Mako Surgical Corp, Fort Lauderdale, FL) Fig. 6.3 (Lonner *et al.*, 2010; Pearle *et al.*, 2010). These systems use either mechanical or optical tracking devices to track the motion of the bone during the robot-assisted burring process, thereby overcoming some of the limitations of earlier robotic systems in which the bones had to be immobilized on the operation table (Siebert *et al.*, 2002; Cobb *et al.*, 2006). The integration of tracking with robotic systems also permits the use of ligamentous gap information for planning the position of the components, which can be important for achieving a well-balanced knee.

A different approach to guide bone-sculpting operations is to incorporate the robotic control directly into the surgeon hand-piece (Brisson *et al.*, 2004). The precision Freehand Sculptor (Bluebelt Technologies Inc., Pittsburgh, PA), Fig. 6.4, uses rotational speed control and a burr that retracts into a protective sleeve to prevent it from deviating outside of the 'safe zone'. This is an attractive solution because of its compact size and potentially lower cost in comparison to the larger and more sophisticated robotic-arm systems.

Semiactive systems can also limit the placement of surgical tools such as cutting or drilling guides, thereby allowing the surgeon to manually perform the resection using the positioned guide (Matsen *et al.*, 1993; Ritschl *et al.*, 2004; Plaskos *et al.*, 2005). The PI Galileo robot mounts on the anterior aspect of the femur using a clamp, and has a linear 2 degree of freedom architecture that displaces a saw-guide in the proximal–distal and anterior–posterior (AP) directions, Fig. 6.5. An advantage of miniature robotic cutting guides integrated with CAS systems is that they can improve the accuracy and efficiency of guide placement compared with conventional jigs while occupying a smaller space in the operating room than larger floor-standing robots. However, a significant design challenge for bone-mounted systems is to minimize the amount of soft-tissue exposure required to secure the device to the bone.

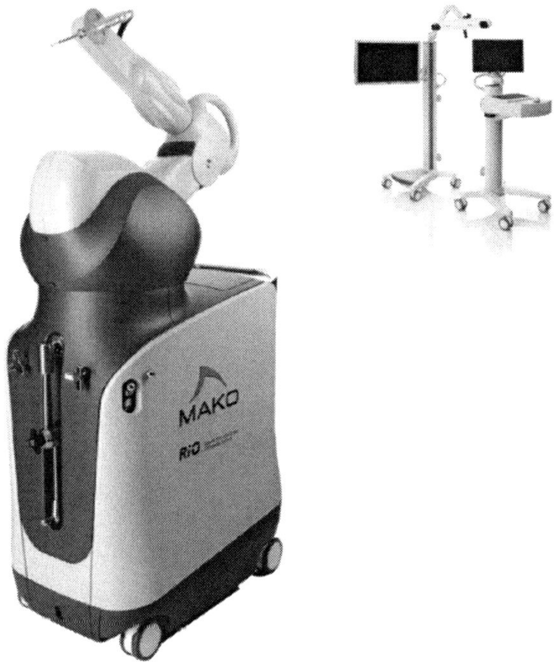

(a)

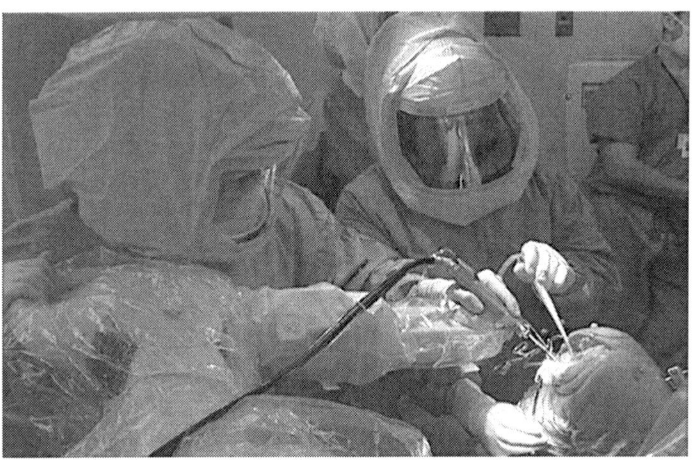

(b)

6.3 The Robotic Arm Interactive Orthopaedic system, (RIO®) is a semiactive robotic system for partial knee resurfacing (a). A tactile arm is used to constrain the position of the surgeon's burr within a pre-defined region or 'safe zone' (b). The system integrates robotics with optical tracking for patient CT-based registration and bone tracking during the burring procedure. Images provided by MAKO, © MAKO Surgical Corp.

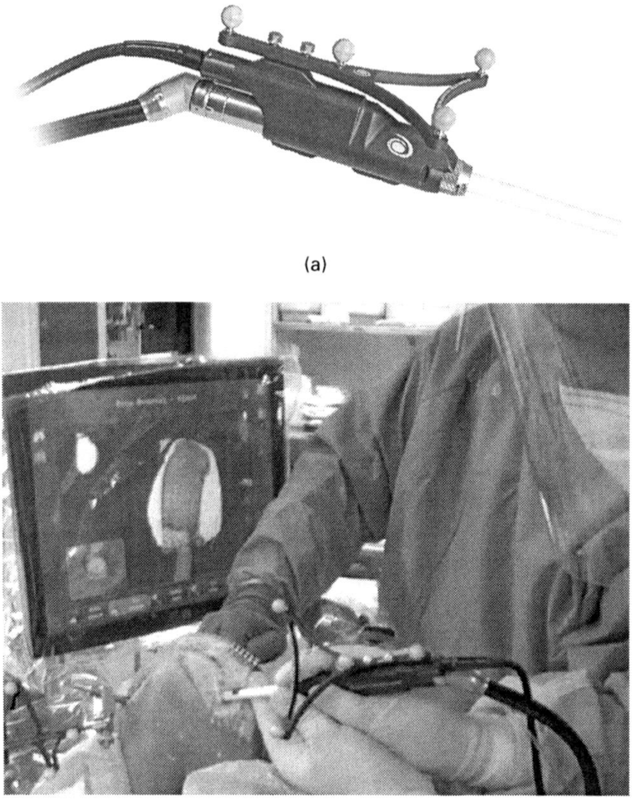

6.4 (a) The Precision Freehand Sculptor (PFS) is a handheld device that uses speed control and a retractable cutter to prevent the burr from overcutting bone. (b) The PFS is integrated into a surgical navigation system for a uni-compartmental knee arthroplasty. (Images provided by BlueBelt, © 2011 BlueBelt Technologies, Inc.)

CAS or computer-navigation systems that do not use robotic assistance are considered passive and are far more prevalent than robotic systems in TKA. CAS employs three-dimensional (3D) localization to measure the 6 degrees of freedom position of rigid objects in space. In TKA, CAS is used to register the anatomy of the patient, measure knee alignment and joint kinematics, plan the position and size of the prosthesis, position cutting guides, and check the final result obtained (Siston *et al.*, 2007; Stindel *et al.*, 2002; Stulberg *et al.*, 2002). Although the development of both imageless and image-based CAS systems began in the mid- to late 1990s, image-based systems did not gain adoption because they added substantial time and cost to the procedure and increased the radiation burden to the patient. To our knowledge, the first clinical use of CAS in TKA occurred in January

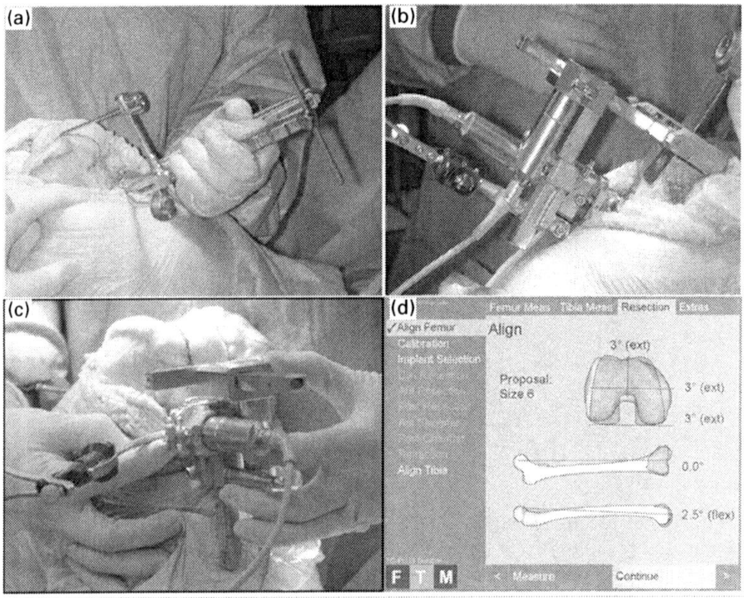

6.5 The Galileo miniature robot for TKA from Precision Instruments (now Smith and Nephew): (a) The robot is mounted onto the anterior cortex of the distal femur using a bone clamp; (b) the robot employs a linear two degree of freedom architecture that displaces a saw-guide from anterior to posterior and from proximal to distal; (c) view from anterior; (d) software planning interface.

1997 in Grenoble, France, using an imageless navigation system that was developed by researchers and clinicians from Praxim, the TIMC (techniques for biomedical engineering and complexity management) laboratory at the University of Joseph Fourier, and Aesculap (Leitner *et al.*, 1997). Several navigation systems have since been commercialized and used in hundreds of thousands of TKA procedures throughout the world.

Several different localization technologies for CAS have been proposed, including mechanical linkages (Yen and Davies 2010), optical, electromagnetic and ultrasound tracking, although nearly all orthopaedic CAS systems used today employ either passive or active optical tracking technology (Glossop 2009). Optical tracking has become the current standard in orthopaedics because of its large working volume, high (submillimetric) accuracy and robustness (Elfring *et al.*, 2010). However, inconveniences such the requirement for line-of-sight and high camera costs have motivated the development and commercialization of new technologies such as accelerometer based systems. The KneeAlign (Orthalign Inc, CA) is a handheld accelerometer-based surgical navigation device for making the proximal tibial and distal femoral resection in TKA, Fig. 6.6 (Nam *et al.*, 2011).

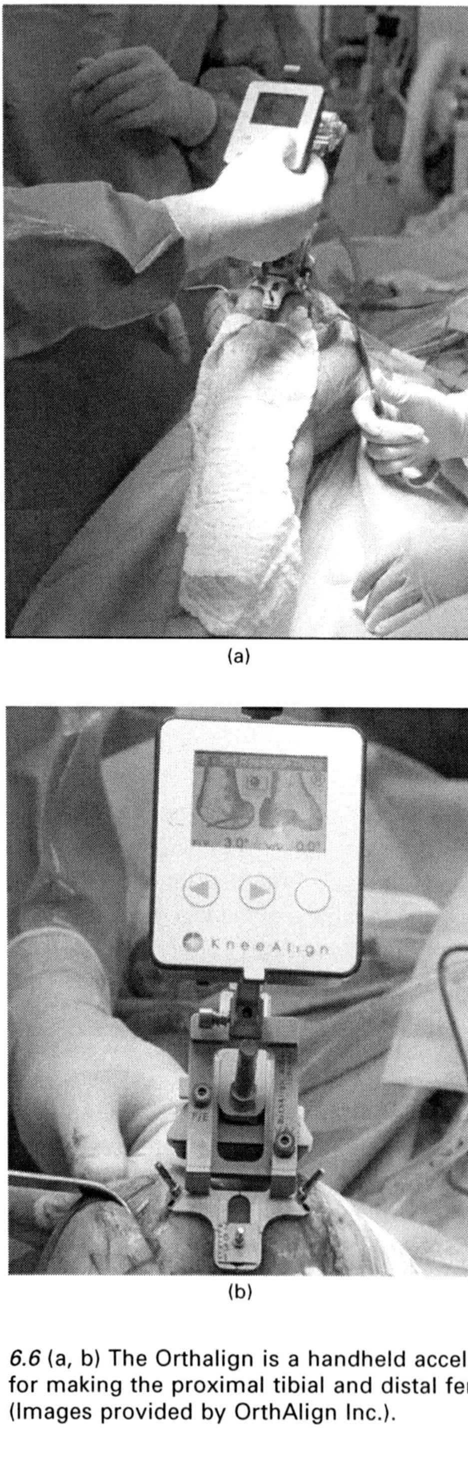

(a)

(b)

6.6 (a, b) The Orthalign is a handheld accelerometer-based system for making the proximal tibial and distal femoral resection in TKA (Images provided by OrthAlign Inc.).

Individual templates or patient-specific instrumentation use a preoperative CT or MRI scan to generate a model of the patient's knee joint from which a surgical plan is established and then reviewed by the surgeon before surgery (Radermacher *et al.*, 1998). Single-use patient specific drill guides or cutting blocks are then designed and manufactured so that they fit on the patient's bone or cartilage anatomy in a unique position, thereby aligning the cutting guide surface with the planned location of the bones cut (Fig. 6.7). Despite the dramatic uptake of patient specific TKA instruments in recent years, there

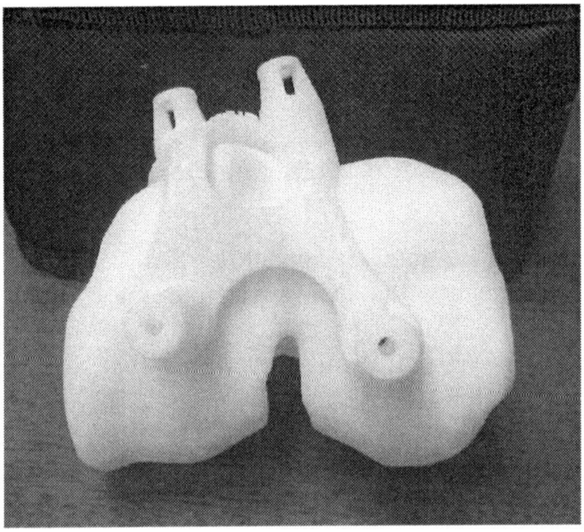

(a)

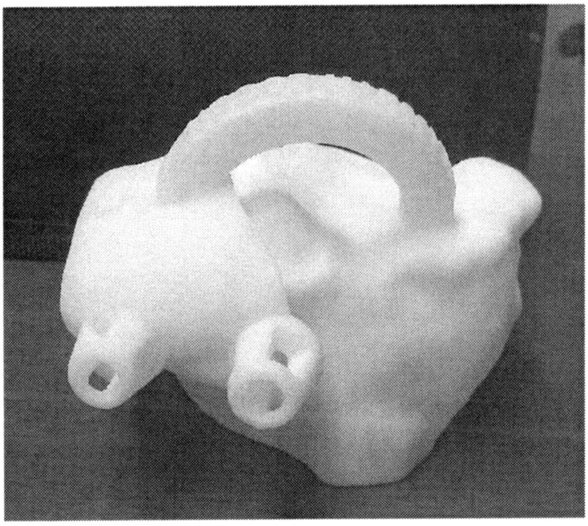

(b)

6.7 Patient specific instruments position cutting guides: (a) on the femur and (b) on the tibia according to a preoperative plan that is based on MRI or CT scans.

are few clinical studies that evaluate the accuracy of these techniques (Nunley *et al.*, 2012a, 2012b; Ng *et al.*, 2012; Gonzales 2010). While Ng (2012) demonstrated improved limb alignment using patient specific instrumentation over the conventional technique, others have reported outliers greater than ±3° in 32%–37% of cases (Gonzales 2010; Nunley *et al.*, 2012a, 2012b). This led those authors to conclude that patient-specific instrumentation provided similar accuracy to conventional instrumentation and that the routine use of this new technology may not be cost-effective in its current form.

6.2 Apex robotic technology (ART)

Apex robotic technology (ART), Fig. 6.8, is a computer-assisted TKA surgery system that encompasses the following design characteristics and capabilities:

- real-time kinematic measurement capabilities;
- imageless 3D morphometric modeling technology for virtual surgical planning;
- accurate and robust registration procedures that are quick and straightforward to perform;
- surgeon driven bone resections;
- miniature robotic cutting guide for efficient and accurate execution of bone resections;

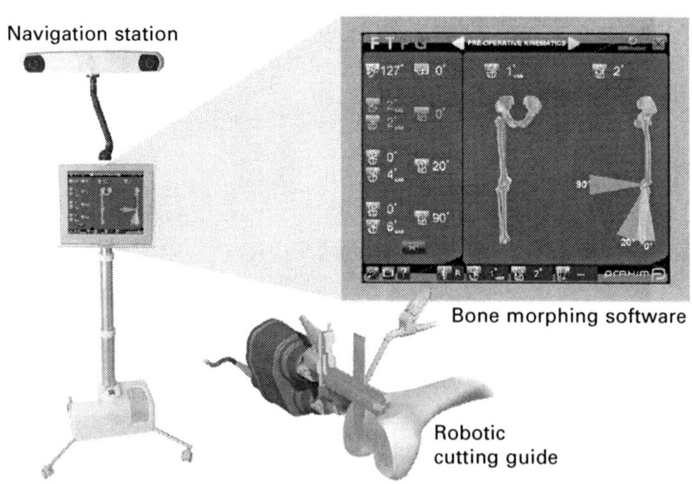

6.8 Apex robotic technology (ART) components include a navigation station with a 3D optical localizer, BoneMorphing software, and a robotic cutting guide (© 2011 OMNIlife Science, Inc.).

- compatibility with both measured resection and ligament balancing techniques;
- constant computer feedback and monitoring via quick and simple validations; and
- compatibility with both conventional and less invasive surgical techniques.

The following sections describe the system software and hardware.

6.2.1 Software

Software is a core component of all computer-assisted surgery systems. It performs several key functions such as: providing an interface between the surgeon and the machine, controlling how data are acquired, processed and presented into useful clinical information that the surgeon can use to plan and perform the surgery, and controlling the communication between the computer and peripheral devices such as the 3D localizer, foot pedal, touchscreens, remote controls, and robotic devices. CAS software must continuously relay important information to the surgeon through a clear and easy to read graphical user interface (GUI), while not overloading the user with information that is not essential to the current step of the procedure. It must also provide flexible surgical workflows, quick, accurate, and robust anatomical registration techniques, and safety checks throughout the surgery. In the following sections, we describe the ART approach for 3D registration, implant planning and gap balancing, and workflow.

Registration

Registration is the process of spatially aligning a model of the patient's anatomy to their physical position in 3D space. In TKA, the anatomical model of the knee must also include the mechanical axis of the leg, which is defined by the vectors joining the hip, knee and ankle centers.

Hip center

The center of the hip joint is determined using a kinematic approach. A key challenge in accurately identifying the kinematic hip center is to mathematically compensate for motions of the pelvis with respect to the OR table, Plate II (see colour section between pages 136 and 137). In addition, the patient may have a pathological hip anatomy that is not perfectly spherical in shape, or they may have limited range of motion. Therefore, the kinematic model needs to be more complex than a simple ball-and-socket joint model in order to function reliably. ART software uses an algorithm that has been designed to compensate for pelvic motion, non-spherical joint morphologies, and localizer measurement noise. Once the femoral reference array is attached, the surgeon moves the femur throughout a range of motion (ROM) of the hip and the computer indicates when sufficient data are acquired. The mathematical algorithm then searches for a point in the 3D space of the femur that exhibits the least amount of motion with respect to the operating table during the acquisition. In particular, the optimization routine minimizes a cost function that takes into account the length of the trajectory of the point being located. In a computer simulation study, this algorithm has been shown to be accurate and robust in a wide range of clinical scenarios that included various degrees of pelvic motion, localizer measurement noise, and ROM limits (Stindel *et al.*, 2005).

Ankle center

Both kinematic and digitization methods have been proposed and evaluated for determining the center of the ankle joint complex (Leitner *et al.*, 1997; Siston *et al.*, 2005). Although some studies have shown that kinematic methods are capable of determining the center of the ankle with sufficient accuracy for TKA, particularly if a biaxial model is used, the kinematic method is generally more cumbersome and time-consuming because a third reference is required and the foot needs to be mobile with respect to the tibia. Therefore, most contemporary CAS systems determine the ankle center by direct digitization of the medial and lateral malleoli.

Either the most extreme or the most distal point pairs can used, and the software calculates either the midpoint or an adjusted center-point between the digitized points as the distal mechanical axis point of the tibia. This method has been tested and validated using CT, MRI, and radiographic data (Siston *et al.*, 2005; Stindel *et al.*, 2002; Suero *et al.*, 2011a). In a radiographic study of 40 TKA patients, Suero *et al.* (2011a) found no clinically significant divergence from the anatomic center of the ankle in the mediolateral direction when using the Extremes Midpoint technique (mean divergence=0.2° lateral or varus; SD=0.5°) or the Distal Midpoint technique (mean divergence=0.2° lateral; SD=0.6°), Fig. 6.9. BMI also had no significant effect on the divergence from the true ankle center for either technique.

Knee center

A unique feature of ART is how the software distinguishes the preoperative and postoperative centers of the knee. In the preoperative or pathologic knee, the knee center is defined by direct digitization on the tibia and the femur. This center is used to calculate the preoperative knee kinematics, which is

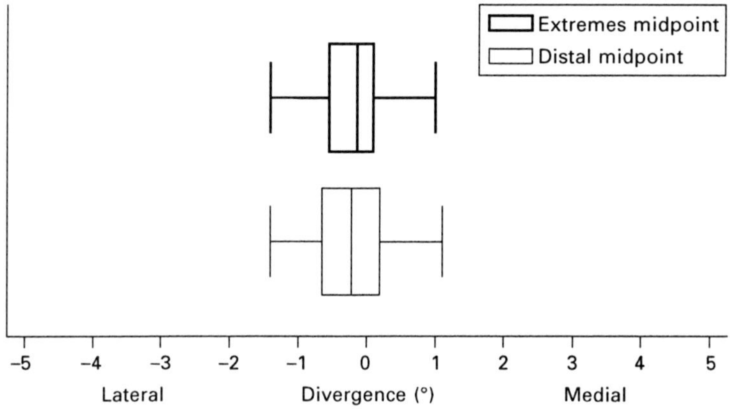

6.9 Ankle center digitization: either the most extreme or the most distal points of the medial and lateral malleoli can provide sufficient accuracy for registering the tibial mechanical axis (Suero *et al.*, 2011a); lateral–varus, medial–valgus.

useful for evaluating the initial stability and the degree of deformity in the coronal and sagittal planes. The software then allows planning of the position of the components in six degrees of freedom on 3D models of each bone (as described in the following subsections). The virtual center of the planned prosthesis then defines the postoperative mechanical axis. This provides increased accuracy in postoperative alignment, especially in severely deformed knees in which the discrepancy between the preoperative and postoperative knee centers can lead to errors in mechanical axis alignment as high as 2.4° varus (Takasaki *et al.*, 2010).

BoneMorphing®

At the core of ART software is a proprietary 3D morphometric imageless reconstruction technology called BoneMorphing®. The BoneMorphing process consists of the deformation of a generic 3D model of a bone to an intra-operatively acquired sparse-point dataset using elastic registration techniques (Szeliski and Lavallee, 1996). After the knee is exposed, a few hundred points are rapidly acquired on the bone surface using the point probe. The probe has a ball-end tip allowing it to glide smoothly over the bone surface in order to facilitate rapid scanning. The surgeon is prompted by the software to acquire points in key predefined areas where a high degree of accuracy is required for implant planning and visualization. As points are being collected they are continuously processed in real-time and evaluated according to predetermined mathematical criteria. Once the system has determined that a sufficient density and distribution of data has been collected in any particular zone, the system automatically indicates to the surgeon using visual and audible feedback that they can proceed to the next zone until all important areas are complete, Fig. 6.10a. From this dataset of points, a complete reconstructed 3D model that is specific to the

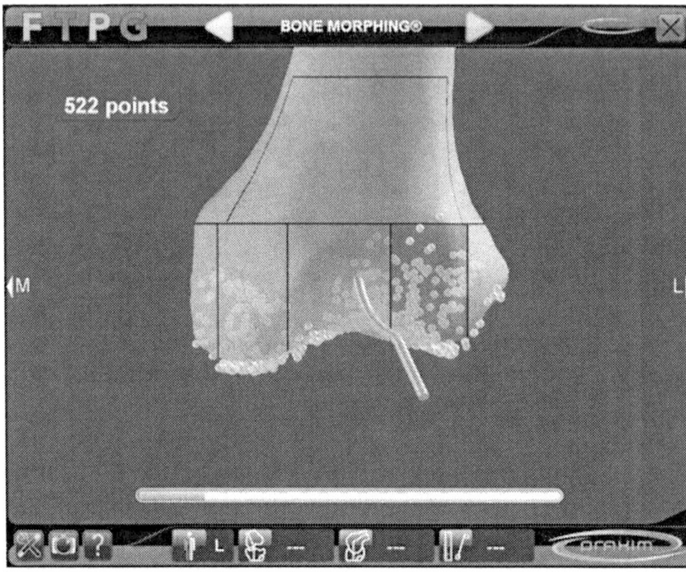

(a)

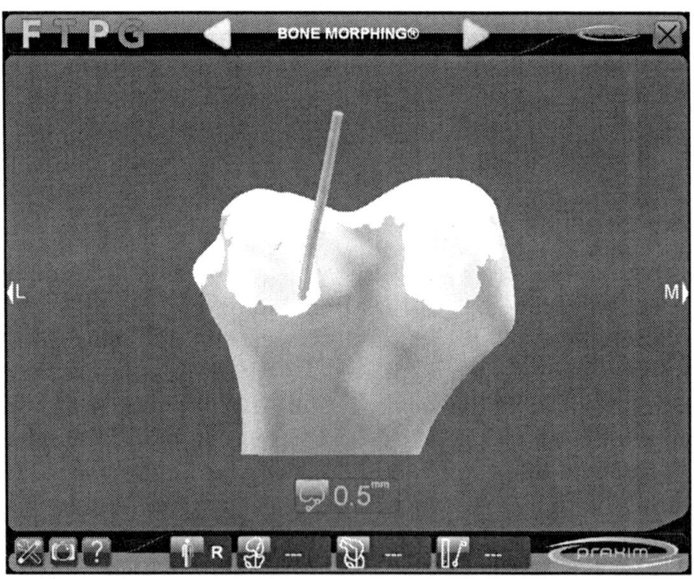

(b)

6.10 Imageless anatomical registration with BoneMorphing®: (a) the software automatically indicates to the surgeon once sufficient data has been acquired in any particular zone; (b) the accuracy of registration can be checked at any point during the procedure.

patients' unique anatomy is then computer generated in less than 3 s. The BoneMorphing acquisition process takes approximately 1 min on the femur and 1 min on the tibia, and approximately 3 min in total to complete the entire registration process including the mechanical leg axis. Once the process is complete the surgeon can verify the accuracy of the model at any location and at any time by placing the tip of the probe on the bone surface, Fig. 6.10b. BoneMorphing has proven stable and robust over tens of thousands of surgeries, and is accurate to within about 1 mm or less in any area that the surgeon can acquire points.

ART software automatically computes certain key bone landmarks and cut-height values directly from the 3D bone models, such as the most distal and most posterior points on the femoral condyles. Thus, the surgeon is not tasked with having to visually and subjectively estimate where the most posterior or distal points are on the bone surface. This makes the system less susceptible to user error than point-based systems, where the surgeon must manually identify landmark points (Perrin *et al.*, 2005). In a cadaver study comparing the accuracy and repeatability of BoneMorphing to freehand point-based digitization of boney landmarks, Perrin *et al.* (2005) demonstrated implant positioning to be significantly more accurate and robust using the BoneMorphing techniques. This was attributed to the high inter- and intrauser variability associated with landmark-based approaches, Plate III.

3D implant planning and visualization

One of the advantages of using complete 3D bone models in computer-assisted TKA is that they provide for virtual planning of component placement in all six degrees of freedom simultaneously. This allows the surgeon to visualize in real time how each parameter changes not only the depth of the resections but also the geometry of the resection contours on the bone surface, Fig. 6.11. This therefore allows the surgeon to optimize and customize the plan to the specific 3D anatomy of each individual patient, aiding them to optimize the fit of the implant while maintaining appropriate biomechanical positioning.

Optimization of femoral sizing and positioning

Femoral component sizing is traditionally determined by the AP dimension of the femur. Here, the surgeon aims to determine the best size of femoral component that will appropriately reconstruct the femoral posterior condyles and the tibial–femoral flexion gap, while not overstuffing the patella–femoral joint or notching the anterior cortex, Fig. 6.12. In manual TKA surgery, sizing is usually determined after the distal resection is made using an AP sizing instrument that is based off of an anterior or a posterior referencing principle. However, because the anatomy of each patient is different, and

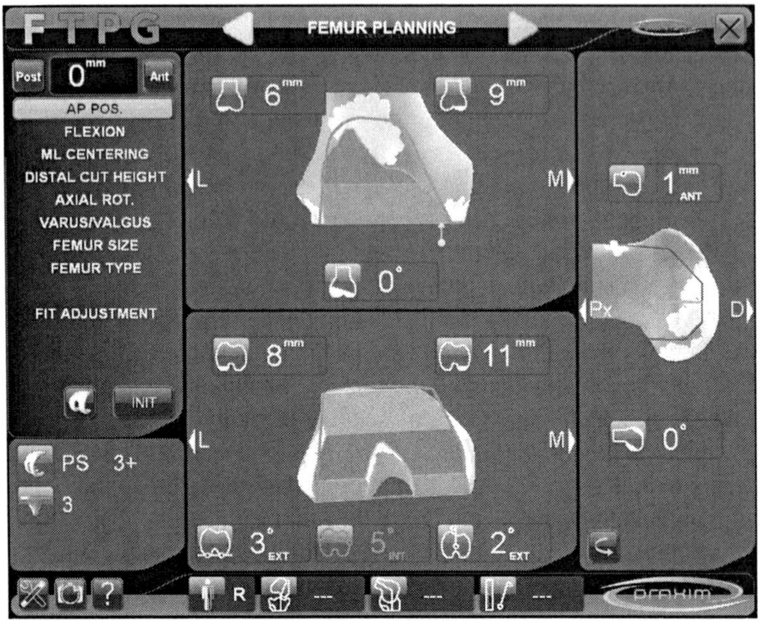

6.11 Virtual femoral surgery: image-free computer-assisted planning from 3D BoneMorphing anatomical reconstructions.

because implants are provided in discrete sizes, the true AP dimension of the femur usually falls somewhere between two implant sizes. Thus, the objective for the surgeon is to select the most appropriate size and position of the femoral component that best fits that specific patient. After the computer suggests an initial plan based on the surgeon's pre-established preferences, 3D planning software allows the surgeon to fine-tune component flexion and AP positioning to determine the best compromise between component sizing and positioning. This is not possible in manual surgery because typically the distal cut has already been performed and component flexion has been established before the implant sizing step. In addition, femoral component rotation, flexion, and AP positioning can be adjusted to achieve the optimal anterior cut profile while monitoring posterior condylar resection values, rotation relative to the posterior and epicondylar axes, Whiteside's line, and the flexion gap. 3D implant planning allows for the optimization of component sizing, AP positioning and flexion simultaneously such that appropriate resection depths and coverage can be obtained on both the posterior condyles and the anterior cortex.

Gap balancing

Soft tissue balance is crucial to the success of TKA. Traditionally, ligament balancing is a subjective procedure in which the surgeon relies on their feel

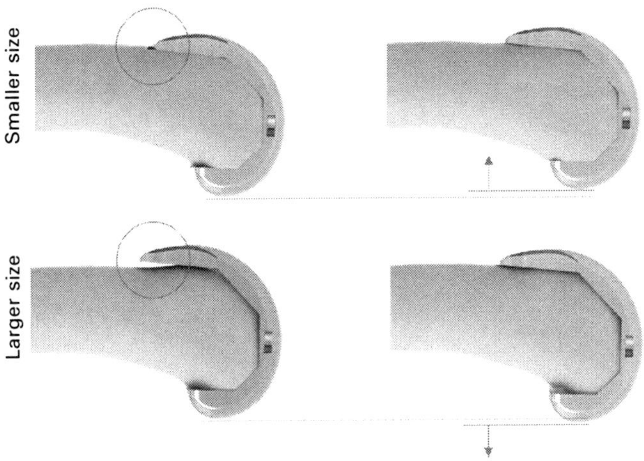

(a)

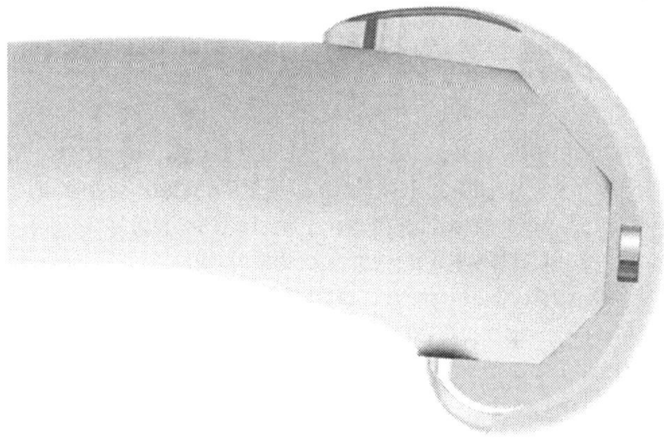

(b)

6.12 Posterior referencing aims to reconstruct the posterior condyles, which may tend to over-resect (notch) or under-resect the anterior cut if the bone is between two implant sizes. Similarly, anterior referencing may tend to compromise the posterior compartment, either under-stuffing or over-stuffing the flexion gap in order to have a flush anterior resection. Computer-assisted planning allows for the 3D optimization of component sizing, AP positioning and flexion simultaneously in a hybrid approach, such that appropriate resection depth and coverage is obtained on the posterior condyles and anterior cortex (© 2012 OMNIlife science).

in order to assess and attain soft tissue balance. CAS technologies provide surgeons with real-time feedback tools to quantify gap kinematics both pre- and postresection (Fig. 6.13), enabling them to use gap data to help plan

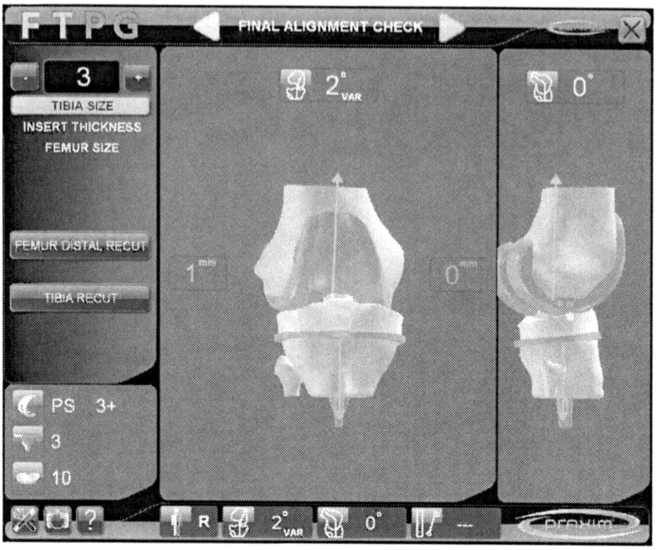

6.13 CAS ligament balancing software allows the surgeon to both plan femoral component positioning and rotation using gap data, and to evaluate the intra-implant gap throughout flexion once the components are in place.

optimal component position, and to assist gap balancing at any flexion angle once the prosthesis is in place. Ishida *et al.* (2011) demonstrated significantly better mid-term 5-year clinical results, including ROM and Knee Society Scores when using CAS with a ligament-balancing approach versus manual TKA. Most CAS systems, however, do not yet permit surgeons to standardize the amount of force applied during the ligament tensioning and evaluation phases. Dynamic intraoperative force and pressure sensing tools remain an important area for future development in CAS TKA (D'Lima *et al.*, 2007, Mayman *et al.*, 2009).

Customizable computer-assisted surgical protocols

Orthopaedic surgeons generally have different preferences as to how they would like to perform the procedure, and navigation software must cater its workflow to accommodate a wide variety of surgical techniques and user preferences. ART software is customizable to the preferred workflow of the surgeon and stores his or her workflow in their personal profile. In a multifactorial efficiency study of 90 TKA patients, Stiehl *et al.* (2009) reported that by streamlining the navigation protocol based on the surgeon's specific technique and workflow, a time saving of 15 min was observed in comparison to standard navigation and 4–5 min compared with conventional surgery (prenavigation), Table 6.3.

Table 6.3 Comparison of means for total time in the operating room, surgical procedure time, and tourniquet time

Navigation group	Total time (min)	Surgery time (min)	Tourniquet time (min)
Pre-non-navigated	131 +/–21	94 +/–17	64 +/–12
Medtronic	139 +/–21	101 +/–15	75 +/–12
Praxim custom	126 +/–15	86 +/–12	60 +/–9

Note: (data courtesy of Dr James Stiehl, MD, see Stiehl *et al.* (2009) for complete study details)

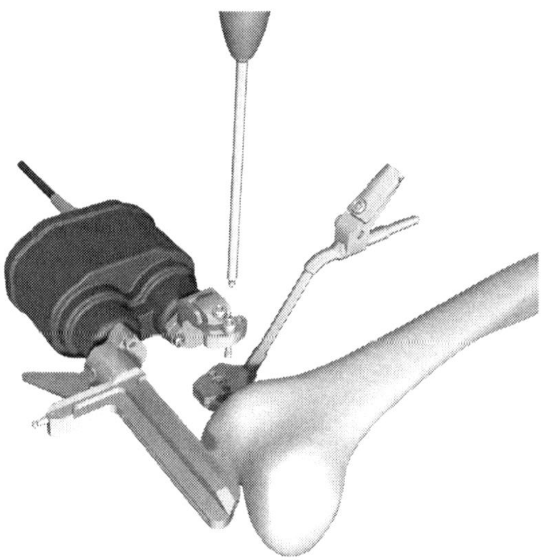

6.14 ART is a compact bone-mounted robotic-cutting guide that is fixed to the side of the knee using the same two pins that are used to secure the femoral reference array.

6.2.2 Intelligent instrumentation

A robotic cutting guide and adjustable cutting guides are now examined.

Robotic cutting guide

The ART robotic cutting guide is a compact bone-mounted two degree of freedom device that is fixed to the side of the knee with two 5.5 mm diameter cancellous bone screws, Fig. 6.14. Because of its miniature size, it is small enough to mount on the same two fixation pins that are used to secure the reference array to the femur so that no other femoral pins are required. Once mounted, the robot is manually aligned in the frontal and axial planes under navigated control. The robotic unit then automatically positions a single cutting guide in the sagittal plane for each of the five femoral cuts, automating guide positioning in the flexion, cut height, and anteroposterior directions. The cutting plane locations for each implant are programmed into the software, allowing the guide to be used for all implant sizes and shapes.

In a bilateral cadaver study, the robotic cutting guide demonstrated significantly improved precision in guide positioning, bone cutting, and final implant placement over conventional sequential blocks navigated freehand, Plate IV (Koulalis *et al.*, 2010a). Moreover, the duration for femoral preparation was significantly more efficient (5.5 min versus 13.8 min) using the robotic cutting guide because of the fewer steps required.

Motion control and safety features

Robotic devices that operate in the OR must be designed so that they safely interact with the surgeon, patient, and OR staff. Several safety features have been designed into ART, including a dual-mode positioning control scheme for low-torque and high-torque dynamic positioning. For low-torque dynamic positioning, the electrical current is limited during positioning in case of collision with bone or with soft tissues. The robotic cutting guide moves in a low-power mode and is continuously monitoring the current consumed during movement. If the system detects an increased torque greater than a predetermined threshold (for example, if it inadvertently collides with the femur when advancing from one cut to the next), the system automatically stops and reverts to a 'passive' mode where it can be repositioned away from the bone by hand. Audible and visual alerts are also provided to the OR team. A 'dead-man' switch has also been implemented such that the operator must hold down the foot pedal or onscreen button in order to initiate and maintain motion of the guide. If released before the guide reaches the target position, the guide automatically reverts to the passive mode.

For high-torque static positioning, once the robotic cutting guide is aligned with the desired cutting plane, it switches to a static positioning control mode. The system continuously monitors the guide position and if the surgeon applies excessive force on the guide during the bone-cutting process, the system detects any motion forced upon the guide and servo back to the aligned cut-plane position. They system will also alert the surgeon that they are applying too much force.

Adjustable cutting blocks

Adjustable cutting blocks allow the surgeon to manually fine-tune the position of the cutting guide plane after it is fixed to the bone (Klima *et al.*, 2008; Koulalis *et al.*, 2010b). The Praxim Nanoblock® incorporates three color-coded adjustment screws that allow the user to adjust the orientation

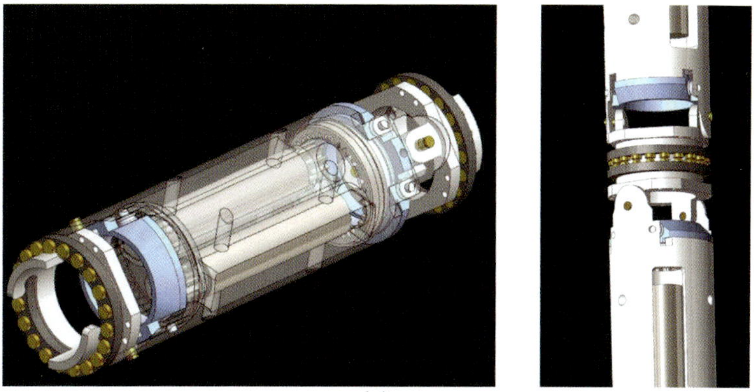

(a)

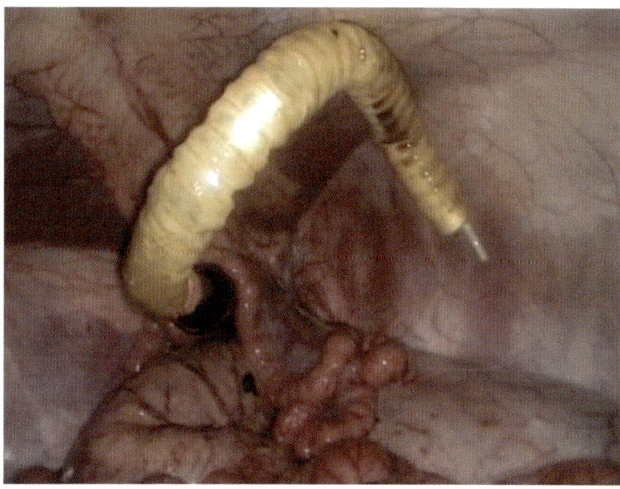

(b)

Plate I The i-Snake® robot for flexible access surgery: (a) modular joint design; (b) completely retroflexed robot configuration during an *in vivo* transvaginal tubal ligation procedure on a porcine model.

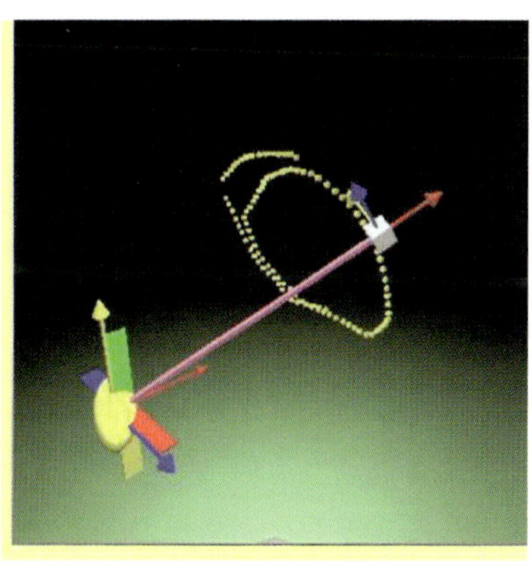

Plate II The hip center is a mobile point in space because of the motion of the pelvis. The Praxim hip center algorithm has been shown to be robust to measurement noise, pelvic motion, and restricted hip ROM, while providing subdegree accuracy in registration of the mechanical axis (see Stindel *et al.*, 2005 for complete study details (image provided by Dr Eric Stindel)).

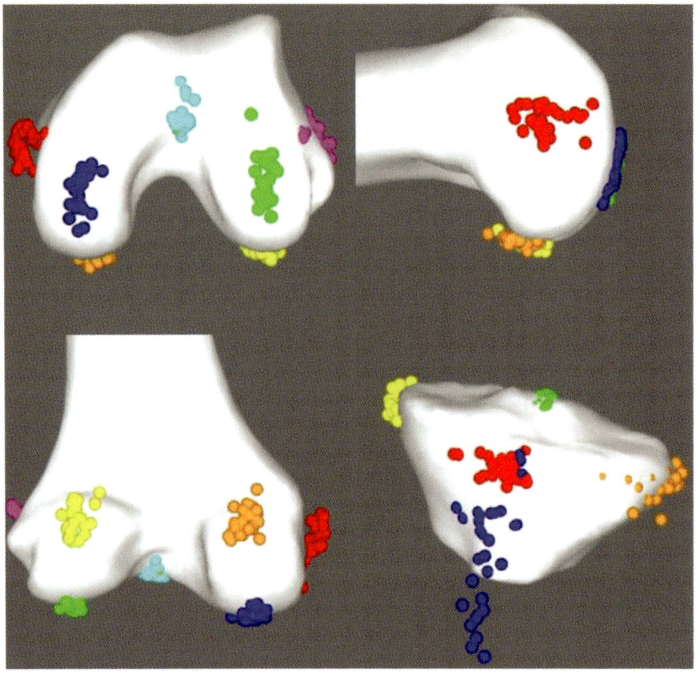

Plate III 3D visualization of the large variability for various landmarks acquired manually. In a cadaver study, implant positioning was significantly more reproducible with BoneMorphing® than with manual digitization of landmarks (reprinted from Perrin *et al.*, 2005).

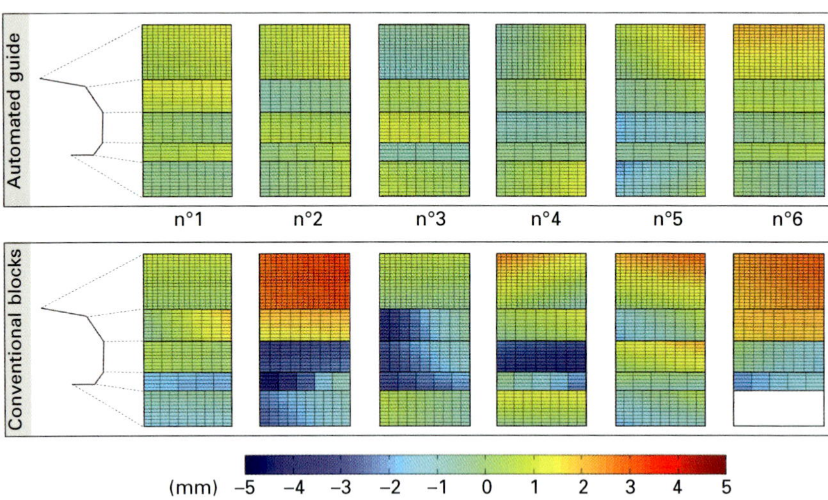

Plate IV Accuracy of bone resections prepared with the ART robotic cutting guide versus conventional blocks navigated free-hand. The mean deviation between the measured and the planned cutting planes was 0.6 mm for the robotic cutting guide and 1.4 mm for the conventional blocks ($p = 0.011$) (reprinted from Koulalis *et al.* (2010a), © 2010, with permission from Elsevier.

of the cutting guide slot relative to the fixation base after the guide has been pinned onto the bone, Fig. 6.15. The application software includes a specially designed interface that decouples the three prescribed screw

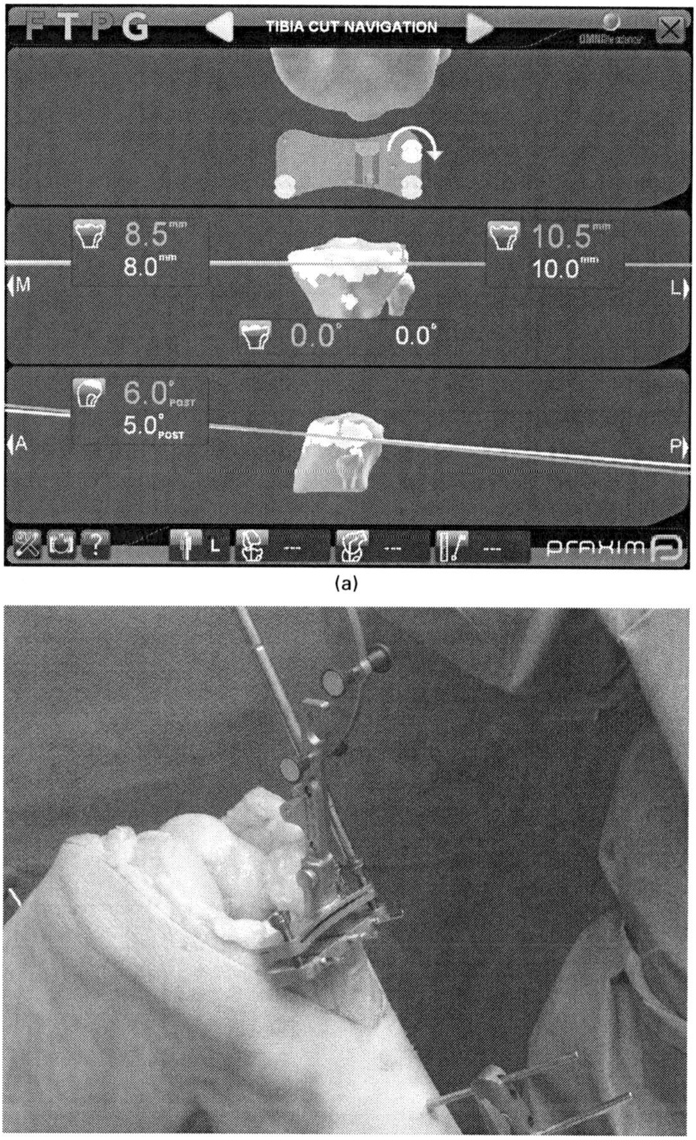

(a)

(b)

6.15 Following directions from the navigation system (a), the target alignment of the bone cut is precisely obtained by turning the screws on the Nanoblock (b). Once the target alignment has been set the surgeon may initiate the cut (reprinted from Suero *et al.* (2011b), © 2011, with permission from Springer Science.

adjustments from the target values in each anatomical plane; that is, the display indicates to the user, in real time, which screw needs to be turned, and to what degree, to reach the target position postosseous fixation. Once the surgeon has made all of the necessary adjustments to the screws, the color of the screws and the targeting lines turn green on the visual display unit, indicating that the guide is within 0.5°/mm of the planned target. In a clinical study of 94 patients who underwent navigated TKA, Suero *et al.*, (2011b) reported improved limb alignment accuracy (1.7° versus 2.7° SD) and a 14 min reduction in tourniquet time when using the Nanoblock versus conventional fixed blocks to perform the proximal tibial and distal femoral resections, Figure 6.16.

6.3 Clinical experience

The long term success of TKA relies on a combination of factors including: restoration of the proper mechanical alignment, correction of deformities and intraoperative balancing of the soft tissues and ligaments, in both the coronal and sagittal planes. When this is performed accurately we know TKA to be a highly successful operation, restoring knee function, ROM, and providing relief from the pain for the vast majority of patients.

The clinical literature provides proof that passive CAS technologies can significantly improve overall limb alignment in TKA, but at the expense of added time to complete the surgical procedure (Mason *et al.*, 2007; Bauwens

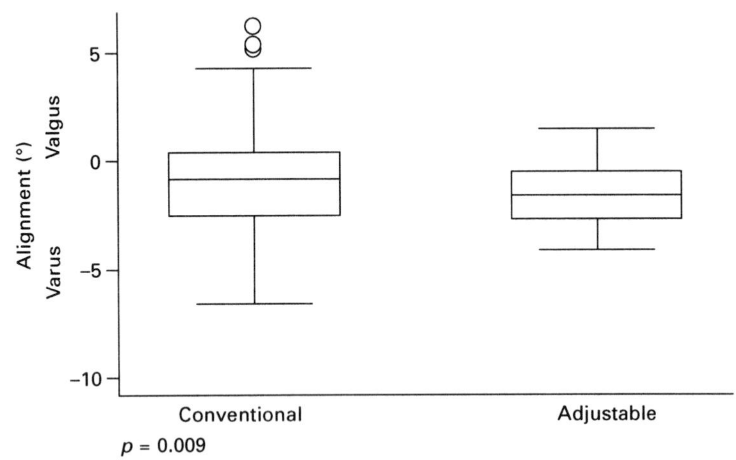

6.16 In a clinical study involving 94 patients, the use of adjustable blocks significantly reduced postoperative mechanical alignment variability and tourniquet time by 14 min compared with conventional blocks navigated freehand (reprinted from Suero *et al.* (2011b), © 2011, with permission from Springer Science.

et al., 2007). In a meta-analysis of alignment outcomes comparing CAS to manual TKA, Mason *et al.* (2007) identified 29 studies involving 3437 patients and found that mechanical axis malalignment greater than 3° occurred in 9.0% of CAS versus 31.8% of conventional TKA patients. The meta-analysis of Bauwens *et al.* (2007) also demonstrated that navigated surgery had a lower risk of malalignment at critical thresholds of >3° and >2°, but reported a mean increase of 23% in the duration of navigated surgery.

Conversely, there are few clinical studies on robotic-assisted TKA in the peer-reviewed English language literature (Bellemans *et al.*, 2007; Chun *et al.*, 2011), probably because there are few systems commercially available for clinical use in the USA. In 2005, one of the present authors (JAK) decided to adopt CAS in their practice only after CAS with integrated robotics became available (Ritschl *et al.*, 2004). Since then, over 1000 cases have been performed with this robotic TKA technique with no reported cases of early revision owing to aseptic loosening, malalignment or instability. Third generation CAS-TKA systems such as ART are now available and feature imageless 3D BoneMorphing reconstruction combined with miniature robotic cutting guides (Fig. 6.17) that are compatible with less invasive surgical approaches. In this section we describe the initial clinical experiences of the authors (JAK and CEP) during the first 500 cases of use.

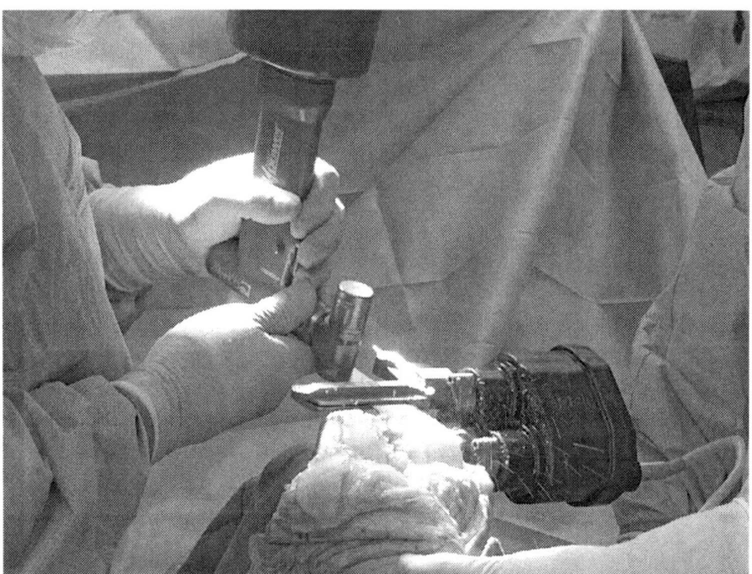

6.17 The Praxim robotic cutting guide aligns a single saw-guide to all five femoral resections for any planned femoral component placement and size. © OMNIlife science.

6.3.1 Clinical accuracy and the learning curve

Our first objective was to determine the clinical accuracy and efficiency of TKA performed with ART (Koenig and Plaskos 2011). Specifically, we asked how reproducible the resections are and how long they take to perform. We also wished to determine if there were any significant effects of the learning curve on the accuracy and efficiency of the procedure.

Clinical study methods

Patients

This was a retrospective single-center Institutionnal Review Board (IRB) approved study of 108 consecutive patients undergoing unilateral CAS TKA during the period of June 2010 to March 2011, beginning with the introduction of the system at Mercy Medical Center (NY, USA). To investigate the effect of the learning curve, patients were classified into four consecutive groups according to their chronological order starting with the first patient operated on with the system: Group I (cases 1–25), Group II (cases 26–50), Group III (cases 51–75), and Group IV (cases 76–108).

Training

Before performing the first surgery, the surgeon and OR staff were trained on two cadaver specimens in a laboratory setting, and five different OR technicians scrubbed-in on the first 10 cases to further educate the staff. All surgeries in this series were performed by a single experienced arthroplasty surgeon (JAK), who had extensive experience with other CAS TKA systems, but was using ART and the Apex total knee implant system for the first time.

Accuracy measurements

Pre- and postoperative overall mechanical alignment of the leg and individual component alignment of the tibia and femur were evaluated on standing long-leg radiographs by two independent observers, Fig. 6.18. Postoperative radiographs were taken at least 6 weeks post-op. Evaluable postoperative standing long-leg radiographs were available for 77 patients.

Time measurements

Tourniquet time was defined as the time from tourniquet inflation (before the skin incision) to deflation (after cementing of the implants and final kinematic validation). Robot-use time was defined as the time required to mount and adjust the orientation of the robot on the femur and to complete

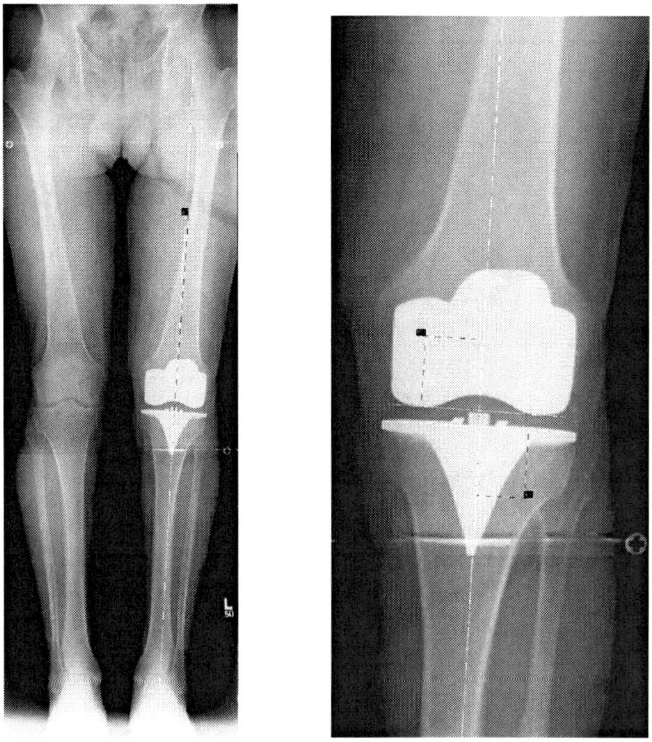

(a) (b)

6.18 Postoperative (a) overall alignment and (b) individual femoral and tibial component alignment in the coronal plane were measured relative to the mechanical axis on standing long-leg radiographs (© OMNIlife Science, Inc.).

all five femoral resections until they were ready to be validated with the system cut-check paddle.

Accuracy and learning curve results

Accuracy of overall leg alignment and individual component alignment

Mean preoperative long-leg radiographic alignment ranged from 21.5° varus to 14.5° valgus. Intraoperative femoral component alignment, tibial component alignment and final leg alignment were within 3° of neutral in 100%, 99%, and 97% of cases, respectively (Table 6.4). Postoperative mean radiographic alignment across all groups was 1.1° varus ± 1.7° SD (range: 4.5° valgus – 4.5° varus), with 91% (70/77) of knees within ±3° of neutral alignment. 99% (76/77) and 93.5% (72/77) of femoral components were within ±3° and ±2° of neutral alignment, respectively. 99% (76/77) and 92% (71/77) of tibial components were within ±3° and ±2° of neutral alignment, respectively.

Table 6.4 Intraoperative and computer data and radiographic data

Radiographic alignment	Intraoperative computer data (% of cases within 3° [Range])	Radiographic alignment data (% of cases within 3° [Range])
Femoral component alignment	100% (103/103) [2.0° valgus to 2.0° varus]	98.7% (76/77) [2.0° valgus to 3.5° varus]
Tibial component alignment	99% (102/103) [3.5° valgus to 1.5° varus]	98.7% (76/77) [4.0° valgus to 2.5° varus]
Final limb alignment	97.2% (104/107) [2.0° valgus to 3.5° varus]	90.9% (70/77) [4.5° valgus to 4.5° varus]

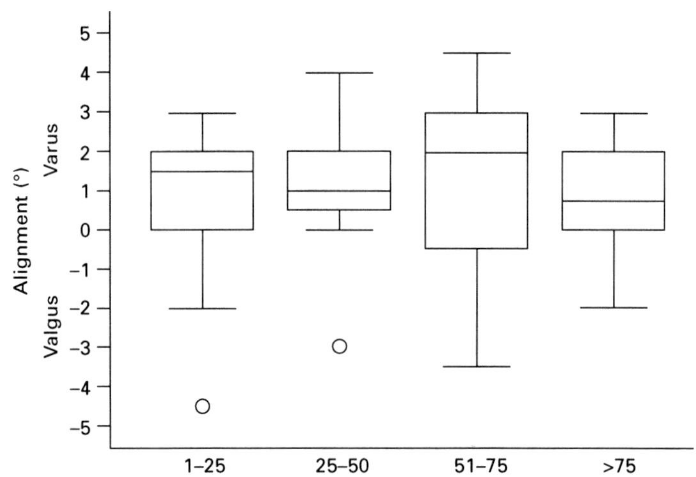

6.19 Postoperative overall limb alignment to the mechanical axis in the coronal plane for the individual groups of successive cases (© OMNIlife Science, Inc.).

There were no significant differences in mean accuracy, variability, or number of outliers between the first group of 25 patients and the remaining three groups for overall leg alignment or individual component alignments, Fig. 6.19 ($p > 0.05$).

Efficiency and the effect of the learning curve

Tourniquet time and robot-use time were both significantly longer in the first group of 25 patients than in the other three groups. Mean tourniquet time was 56 min for the first group and approximately 49 min for the subsequent groups ($p < 0.0001$), Fig. 6.20. Tourniquet time tended to be slightly longer in obese patients by 2.4 min ($p = 0.108$). On average, it took a total of 7 min to use the robot for the first 25 patients, which subsequently decreased to approximately 5 min ($p < 0.0001$).

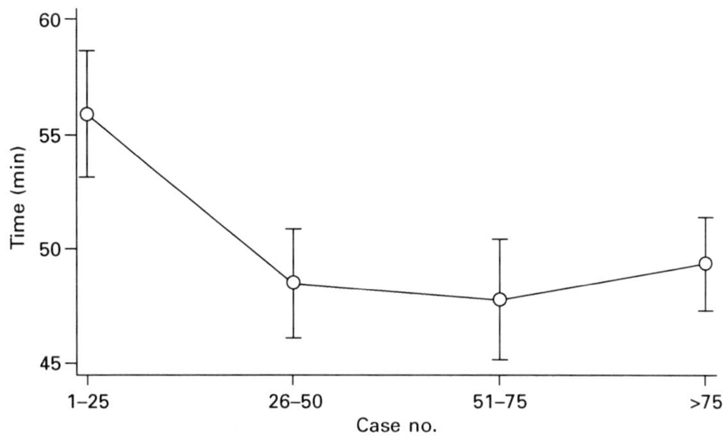

6.20 Effect of the learning curve on surgical efficiency: mean adjusted tourniquet time by case group. Error bars represent 95% confidence internal (© OMNIlife Science, Inc.).

Effect of patient factors on efficiency

Tourniquet time was 5.3 min shorter for females than for males ($p < 0.001$), and tended to be slightly longer in obese patients by 2.4 min ($p = 0.108$).

Complications and failures

There were no complications associated with the use of the system, including no fractures, notching, infection or wound healing issues. No lateral releases were performed for patellar maltracking, nor were there any postoperative patellar dislocations. In two cases the navigation system failed to establish a connection with the robotic cutting guide at the beginning of the procedure owing to a cable failure. On the first occurrence, the robotic procedure was aborted and the procedure was completed with manual instruments. This procedure was excluded from the present study. On the second occurrence, the resections were performed with the robot in a so called passive 'safety mode', where the guide can be manually navigated into position and fixed to the femur with two 3.2 mm diameter pins. This case was included in the study.

6.3.2 Clinical utility in severely deformed knees

In order to investigate the effects of preoperative coronal and sagittal deformities on postoperative alignment and surgery time, a second series of patients was analyzed after the learning curve phase (i.e. after the initial

25 cases). A total of 128 patients were included in this second study, the mean age was 71 (range 53–93), avarage BMI 31.1 (20–44.3), 48 males and 80 females. Patients were stratified into three groups according to their preoperative coronal plane deformity: neutral or mild deformity of <10° (baseline group); severe varus deformity ≥10°; and severe valgus deformity ≥10°. Patients were also stratified according to the degree of flexion contracture: neutral or mild flexion from –5° hyperextension to 10° flexion (baseline group); hyperextension ≤–5°, and severe flexion ≥10°. The degree of deformity in the coronal and sagittal planes and the final postoperative alignment and extension angle achieved was measured intraoperatively using Praxim navigation with ART in all patients.

Effect of preoperative deformity on alignment

Mean postoperative alignment in the control group was 1.4° varus. Severe valgus knees were left closer to neutral (mean 0.4° varus, $p = 0.004$) whereas severe varus knees tended to be in slightly more varus than in the control group (mean 1.77° varus, $p = 0.111$). Postoperative alignment ranged from 2° valgus to 3.5° varus across all groups, Fig. 6.21, and final extension ranged from 4° flexion to –4° hyperextension. Preoperative flexion, obesity, and gender had no significant effect on alignment accuracy or final extension.

Effect of preoperative deformity on tourniquet time

Mean adjusted tourniquet time for the control group was 48.8 min (95%, confidence interval 45.3–52.4). Severe varus knees took 4.8 min longer than average ($p = 0.006$), whereas severe valgus knees took 2.9 min longer, Fig. 6.22, although the difference was not significant for valgus knees ($p = 0.260$). Flexion contractures ≥10° did not increase tourniquet time significantly in this group (mean increase was 3.8 min, $p = 0.152$). However, patients having a flexion contracture of 15° or more (five patients) took 10 min longer than average ($p = 0.033$).

6.3.3 Discussion

The use of computer-assisted surgery with virtual planning and robotics (CAS/VPR) in TKA has made it easier for the surgeon to perform highly accurate and efficient TKAs in cases with the smallest to largest deformities. It does so by acting as a constant intraoperative global positioning system (GPS) that gives continuous feedback and validation to the surgeon so that they can formulate an individualized intraoperative TKA plan and base their many intraoperative decisions on real-time dynamic data. Moreover, the consequences of very small 1–2 mm or 1–2° bone resection or soft-tissue

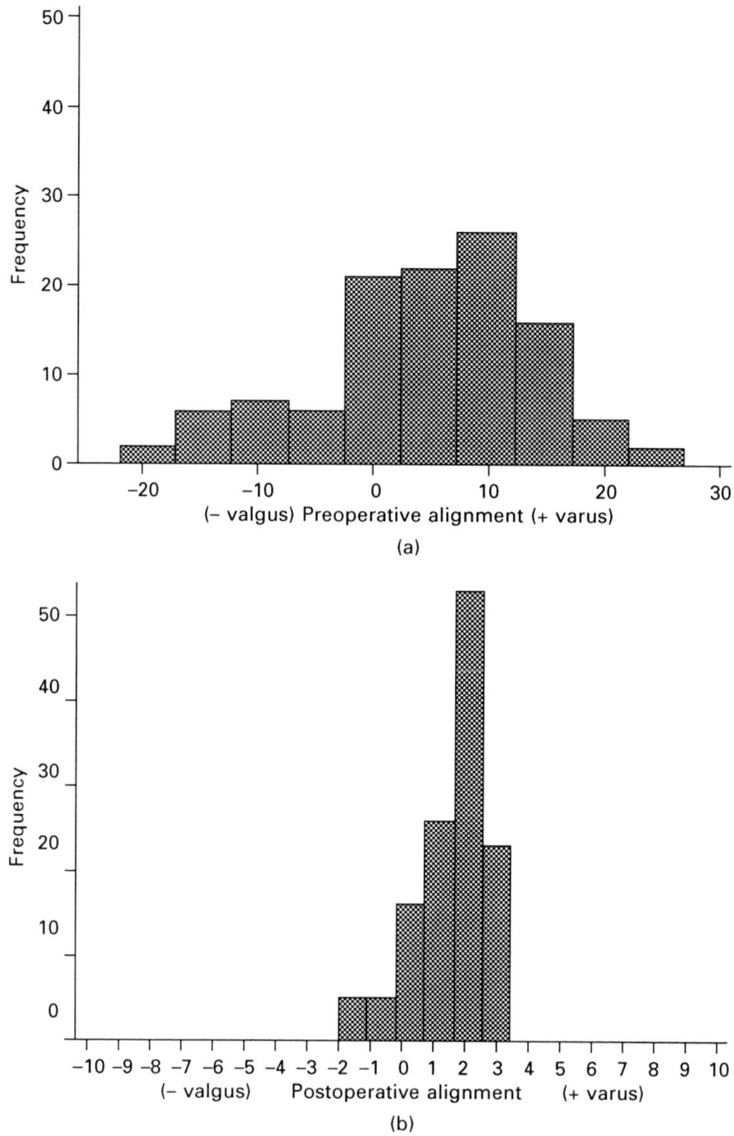

6.21 Distribution of: (a) preoperative and (b) postoperative alignment in 128 robotic-assisted TKAs.

release are instantly quantified, related and validated to the surgical team in an easily understood simple graphic fashion.

It was found that knees with a preoperative valgus alignment of 10° or more were significantly closer to neutral postoperatively than pre-op 'varus' knees and even pre-op 'neutral' knees. It is probable this bias toward varus

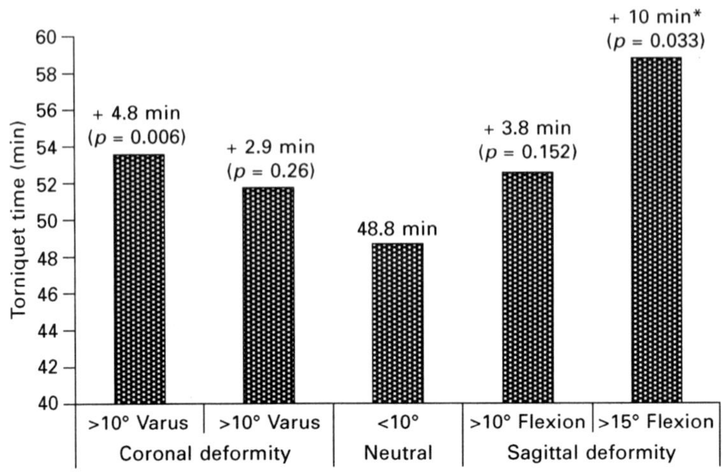

6.22 Effect of coronal and sagittal plane deformities on the efficiency of robot-assisted TKA surgery.

is not because of the bone cuts but to the initial preoperative deformity (Fig. 6.22a) and the resulting state of the soft tissues. There was an inclination to aim for a final intraoperative alignment that was within a 2° window from neutral, and to underrelease as opposed to overrelease the ligaments to avoid inadvertently creating instability; as a result this may have contributed to the post-op varus bias.

CAS/VPR not only helps to assure accuracy but can also save time and stress in difficult cases. Our results show that in one surgeon's hands, managing severe coronal plane deformities with CAS/VPR TKA takes only an additional 3–5 min on average. This is achieved by assessing the pre-resection kinematics, formulating a virtual plan, and executing and validating in real time that plan's execution. Important corrections, large or small, are achieved easily and quickly, such as re-cutting the distal femur or proximal tibia, adding slope or releasing soft tissues with real time CAS feedback and not just 'blind' visual confirmation or 'feel'. The final alignment page (Fig. 6.13) graphically quantifies the final intra-op coronal and sagittal alignment and soft tissue–ligament balance (i.e. the implant gap) of the TKA, assuring the surgeon that he or she achieved what they originally planned: good correction of the pre-op deformity, restoration of the proper mechanical alignment, and having a well-balanced knee with an improved arc of motion.

Many studies (including Mason *et al.*, 2007; Ritschl *et al.*, 2004; Stulberg *et al.*, 2002) have documented improvements in achieving mechanical alignment within 3° of neutral, with reported success rates in the ranges of 89–99%. CAS/VPR not only offers this degree of accuracy but also delivers this to a now quantifiable higher level of efficiency. Klima and Josten (2008) reported longer femoral guide-positioning times in performing CAS TKR than we observed in our study: 11 min for freehand navigation and 6 min for positioning adjustable blocks. With a robotic cutting guide, we have demonstrated that femoral preparation time can be reduced to 5 min on average, which includes the time to position the guide and to perform the resections. Our study has also shown that, after 20–25 cases, we were able to perform consistently efficient and accurate CAS/VPR TKAs in about 49 min of tourniquet time, even when teaching other surgeons how to use the system. Moreover, the small increases in tourniquet time we observed for severely deformed knees and for obese patients were not due to longer computer or robot-use times, but to more intensive surgical exposures, soft tissue releases, and removal of osteophytes, which are inherent to those more complex cases. It is likely that time was actually saved via more accurate planning of increased bone resections and ligament releases, and not having to 'recut' and 'rebalance' later. Importantly, the improved level of accuracy achieved as compared with conventional techniques was there from the first case to the last in the series, unlike studies published on patient-specific instruments that report an accuracy level that is similar to conventional TKA (Gonzales *et al.*, 2010; Nunley *et al.*, 2012b). The combination of a programmable streamlined workflow, intuitive GUIs, virtual planning with constant intra-op feedback, and robotic precision with fine surgical control has certainly led to this extreme level of accuracy, precision and efficiency.

Conventional TKA and patient-specific instruments cannot provide this highly accurate and valuable intraoperative feedback to the surgeon. It is important not only to consider surgical time when comparing patient-specific instruments against other surgical techniques as there is additional time associated with the surgeon logging onto a computer and doing his/her surgical plan statically outside of the OR, as well as the additional time required for the office to arrange and obtain authorizations for the scans as well as the patient's time and effort getting these scans. Using static technologies such as patient-specific instruments appears to remove one of the biggest benefits that technology affords us; without CAS/VPR one loses the dynamic feedback and intraoperative validation associated with the steps of planning, bone resecting, soft-tissue balancing and final implant placement. It is our belief that CAS/VPR TKA maximizes the technological benefits helping to make surgeons, better by providing constant feedback on bone resections and soft-tissue balancing procedures.

6.3.4 Surgical technique utilizing ART with a 'quad-sparing' subvastus approach

The subvastus approach to TKA has been proven to be a less invasive approach in terms of elimination of quadriceps tendon incision, limiting eversion of the patella, and less blood loss (Hofman *et al.*, 1991; Sastre *et al.*, 2009). When performed in conjunction with robotic-assisted surgery, the procedure can be performed in the least invasive and most precise way.

The skin incision is made along the medial border of the patella, extending from 2 cm superior to the superior pole of the patella to the distal aspect of the tibial tubercle, Fig. 6.23. With the knee fully extended, the vastus medialis obliquus (VMO) is exposed. The plane between the VMO and overlying skin and superficial fascia is developed. The knee is then flexed to 90°. The vertical limb of the arthrotomy starts at the inferior aspect of the VMO insertion on the patella and is carried distally the entire length of the skin incision. Care is taken to stay just medial to the patellar tendon. One of the key steps of this approach involves how the horizontal limb of the arthrotomy is performed. The goal is to incise the retinaculum 2 mm distal to the VMO muscle belly back to the medial intramuscular septum without cutting the capsule. The capsular incision is made vertically with sharp Mayo scissors up into the suprapatellar pouch. Using blunt finger dissection, the entire VMO is mobilized from the underlying tissue. The goal is to be able to fully sublux the patella into the lateral gutter without everting it. Once the quad is mobilized, we then proceed with the surgery the same way as a standard medial parapatellar approach. The only exception is that the patella is everted only when preparing it for the patellar prosthesis. Because the robotic cutting guide mounts to the medial aspect of the distal femur, the subvastus approach allows an easier application of the robotic cutting guide mount to the distal femur, Fig. 6.24.

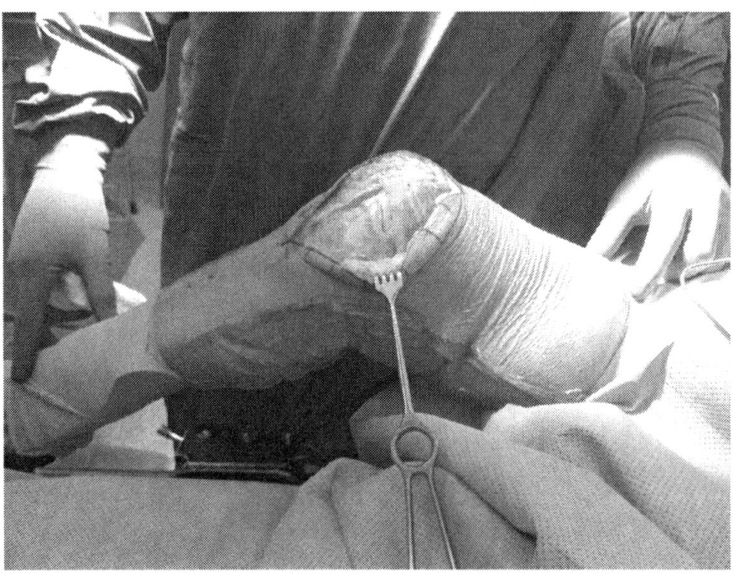

6.23 The subvastus surgical approach for TKA.

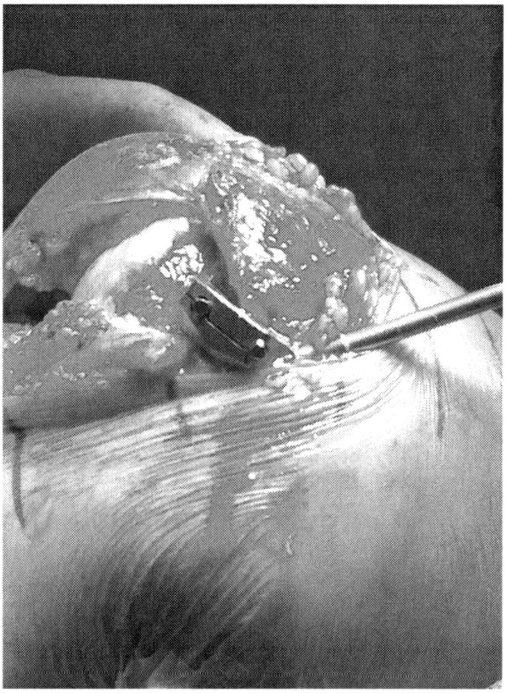

6.24 The subvastus approach allows for medial fixation of the robotic cutting guide base and femoral reference array without incision of the quadriceps or eversion of the patella.

Surgeons are advised to take caution in using this approach in certain patients. In particular, muscular males, severe valgus deformity, patients with prior open knee procedures, and any patient whose VMO attaches at or below the midsection of the patella should be avoided. Care should be taken to drop the tourniquet before closure and cauterize any vessels deep to the VMO as bleeding here can lead to severe bruising.

Closure is straightforward and closing the horizontal limb with #1 or #2 absorbable suture (Vicryl) is advised. Care should be taken to reapproximate the corner of the incision nicely. A running #2 Quill suture is used to close the remainder of the incision, oversewing the horizontal limb for additional support.

6.3.5 Adjusting the fit of the femoral component

One of the most unique features offered by the system is the ability to fine tune femoral fit (i.e. the tightness of the fit between the internal femoral implant surface and the resected femoral bone surface) according to surgeon preference. Surgeons have different preferences as to how tight they would like the femoral component to fit on the bone, and these preferences might vary from one surgeon to another, and they might depend on other factors such as the patient's bone quality. It is common practice in hip arthroplasty to classify bone type and quality to help guide the best choice for femoral stem (i.e. Dorr classification, Dorr *et al.*, 1993). In the knee, in order to achieve a specific fit in conventional surgery, some surgeons may use 'special' manual cutting guides in which the cuts have been adjusted during the design process to achieve a different or higher degree of press fit. However, this can be an expensive process as it requires special instruments to be designed and manufactured.

ART allows the surgeon to adjust the fit of the femoral components intraoperatively in increments of 0.25 mm (Fig. 6.25) according to their preferred parameters using flexible software. Bench testing conducted by OMNI and Praxim on the positioning accuracy of the robotic cutting guide has demonstrated an accuracy of –0.07 mm ± 0.14 (mean ± SD) in the AP dimension (i.e. from the anterior to the posterior resection). Intraoperatively, the tightness of the fit can be observed and assessed by the level at which the femoral component engages the bone (Fig. 6.26), and the amount of impaction force required to fully seat the component. Some orthopaedic surgeons seek a tight fit with the femoral trial in all bone types. The software allows for adjustment of the cuts and a reduction in the variability of the femoral trial fit. This is most noticeable in softer, less dense bone. Although this is understandable and also happens when using manual instruments, there were no other means to address this until now.

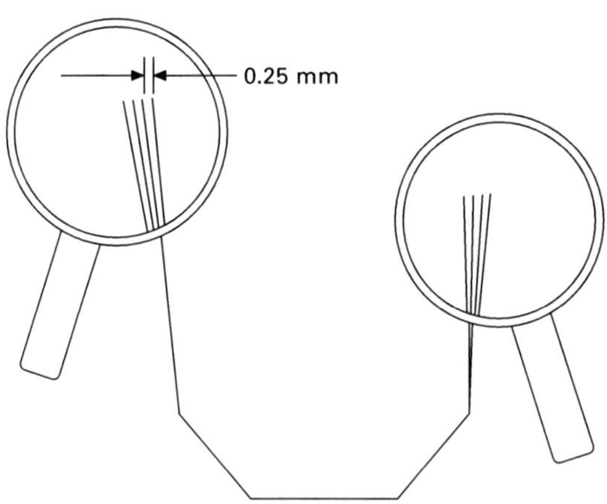

6.25 Using flexible software and a robotic cutting guide, the surgeon can intraoperatively adjust the tightness of the fit between the femoral component and the bone according to their own personal preference. The anterior and posterior resections can be adjusted in increments of 0.25 mm.

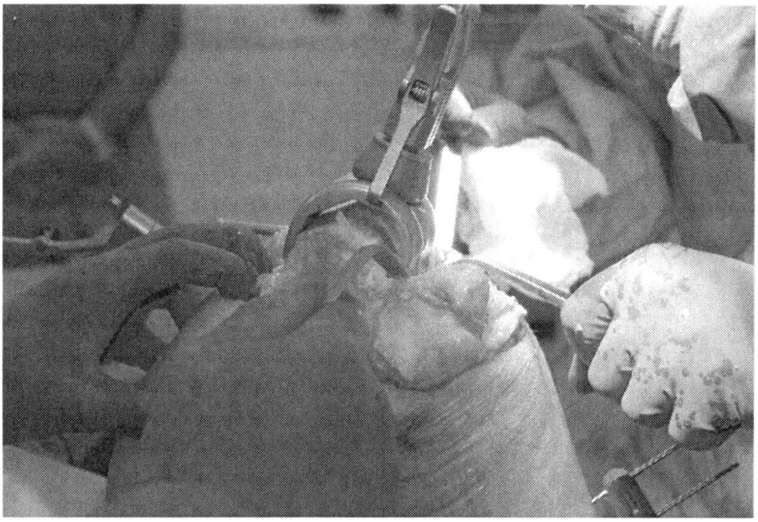

6.26 The tightness of the fit is assessed intraoperatively by the level at which the femoral trial component engages the bone and the amount of force required to fully seat the component.

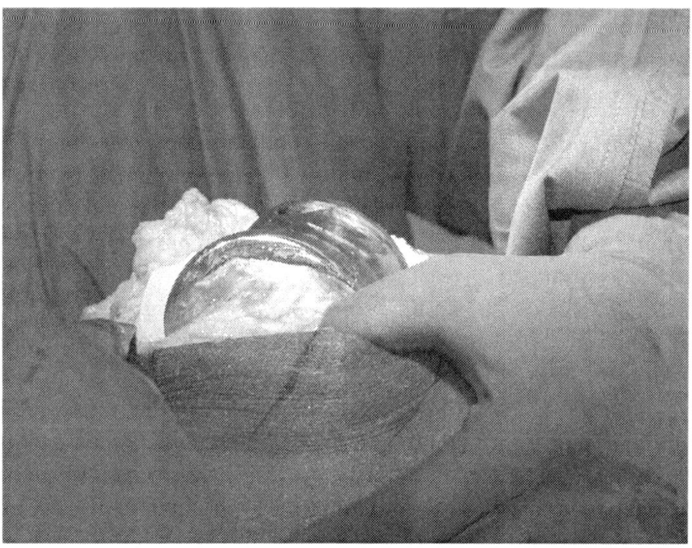

6.27 Intraoperative photograph illustrating the femoral component fit obtained when using a robotic cutting guide with adjustable fit software.

One of the coauthors (CEP) indicated: 'Since I have started adjusting my cuts using the software, every case has had a very satisfying femoral fit' (Fig. 6.27). By having the ability to adjust the AP cut height in increments of 0.25 mm, thereby cutting away less bone and adding a total of 0.5 to 1.5 mm in the AP direction, the surgeon is able to make intraoperative adjustments to ensure a better fitting femoral component. CEP routinely qualifies the bone quality after making the distal femoral cut: 'If the bone is soft, I will usually fit adjust to 1.5 mm'.

6.4 Conclusions and future trends

Robotics and CAS offer a quantitative and personalized approach to joint replacement surgery. Conceptually, the steps of surgical planning, execution, and control constitute a loop that is designed to improve the overall quality of knee arthroplasty for the benefit of patients, surgeons and healthcare as a whole. In order to gain widespread adoption, however, these technologies must add significant value to the intervention and they must prove cost-effective.

Steps are being made to accomplish these goals through:

1. patient-specific 3D planning that does not require costly preoperative scans or additional time spent outside of the OR;
2. compact robotic technology that is accurate and efficient to use and compatible with less invasive surgical approaches; and
3. real-time intraoperative feedback for evaluating knee kinematics and soft-tissue balance, and for validating and documenting the procedure.

Another objective is to increase cost-effectiveness by reducing fabrication costs such that CAS is of similar cost to conventional instrumentation. This allows CAS systems to be consigned in the same manner as conventional instruments are, i.e. without requiring any capital expenditures from the hospital and only a small per procedure fee for the disposables required to operate the system.

The field of robotic and computer-assisted knee arthroplasty will continue to bring innovative tools and new capabilities to surgeons. More convenient localization technologies that do not require line of sight are already being used in a limited capacity (Nam *et al.*, 2011) and, in the future, they may be capable of measuring kinematics in all six degrees of freedom. Automated distractors and digital force sensors are being incorporated into novel CAS instrumentation that the surgeon can use to intraoperatively quantify soft-tissue tension and the center of pressure in the knee (D'Lima *et al.*, 2007; Mayman *et al.*, 2009). This information can aid in achieving more precise soft-tissue balance, thereby improving joint stability, function, and patient satisfaction. Novel approaches to address the patella–femoral joint and to improve the accuracy of patellar resection are being explored (Anglin *et al.*, 2008; Fu *et al.*, 2012). New applications for robotics in knee arthropasty will also be developed, including robotic platforms for TKA revision procedures. It is likely that robotically assisted bone resections will markedly reduce the complexity of current manual revision surgery, enabling a greater number of surgeons to perform these technically challenging procedures.

In conclusion, the Praxim system with ART has been extensively tested and validated in simulation, cadaver, and clinical studies, and presents a unique and promising approach to TKA surgery. However, further clinical research is required to distinguish the value that this and other new robotic and CAS tools bring. In particular, high-quality randomized control trials and multicenter studies utilizing more sensitive and reliable outcome assessment methods (Scuderi *et al.*, 2012) will be needed to demonstrate the full potential and benefit that robotic and CAS technology bring.

6.5 Acknowledgments

We acknowledge the surgeons, scientific collaborators, and the employees at Praxim and OMNIlife science who have contributed to the system and data presented in this chapter. In particular, we gratefully acknowledge Dr Andrew Pearle, Dr Eric Stindel, and Dr James Stiehl for contributing scientific data, and Dr Eduardo Suero for his assistance with the statistical analysis and the radiographic measurements presented in Section 6.3.1. We also thank Robert Zoletti, Ed Cheal and Marty Nichols for their edits to the chapter text and Peter Cipolletti for generating the TKA renderings. Special thanks to our wives (Kathryn, Michelle, and Sara) for their neverending support and understanding during our robotic research and writing of this book chapter. JAK also acknowledges James Morimando PAC for his valued assistance and expertise in the operating room.

6.6 References

Anglin C, Ho KC, Briard JL, de Lambilly C, Plaskos C, Nodwell E and Stindel E. In vivo patellar kinematics during total knee arthroplasty. *Comput Aided Surg*, 2008 Nov; **13**(6): 377–91.

Banks SA. Haptic robotics enable a systems approach to design of a minimally invasive modular knee arthroplasty *Am J Orthop*, 2009; **38**(2 suppl): 23–7.

Bargar WL. Robots in orthopaedic surgery. Past, present, and future. *Clin Orthop Relat Res*, 2007; **463**: 31–6.

Bäthis H, Perlick L, Tingart M, Perlick C, Lüring C and Grifka J. Intraoperative cutting errors in total knee arthroplasty. *Arch Orthop Trauma Surg*, 2005 Feb; **125**(1): 16–20. Epub 2004 Nov 9.

Beringer DC, Patel JJ and Bozic KJ. An overview of economic issues in computer-assisted total joint arthroplasty. *Clin Orthop Relat Res*, 2007 Oct; **463**: 26–30.

Bauwens K, Matthes G, Wich M, Gebhard F, Hanson B, Ekkernkamp A and Stengel D. Navigated total knee replacement: a meta-analysis. *J Bone Joint Surg Am*, 2007; **89**: 261.

Bellemans J, Vandenneucker H and Vanlauwe J. Robot-assisted total knee arthroplasty. *Clin Orthop Relat Res*, 2007 Nov; **464**: 111–6.

Berry DJ and Bozic KJ. Current practice patterns in primary hip and knee arthroplasty among members of the American Association of Hip and Knee Surgeons. *J Arthroplasty*, 2010 Sep; **25**(6 Suppl): 2–4. Epub 2010 Jul 1.

Bozic KJ. TKR in the younger patient: happening but is it reasonable? 2012 Specialty Day Meeting of The Knee Society. San Francisco, California, Feb 11, 2012.

Brisson G, Kanade T, DiGioia AM and Jaramaz B. Precision freehand sculpting of bone. Proceedings of the 7th International Conference on Medical Image Computing and Computer-Assisted Intervention. 2004, pp. 105–112.

Chin PL, Foo LS, Yang KY, Yeo SJ and Lo NN. Randomized controlled trial comparing the radiologic outcomes of conventional and minimally invasive techniques for total knee arthroplasty. *J Arthroplasty*, 2007 Sep; **22**(6): 800–6. Epub 2007 Apr 20.

Chun YS, Kim KI, Cho YJ, Kim YH, Yoo MC and Rhyu KH. Causes and patterns of aborting a robot-assisted arthroplasty. *J Arthroplasty*, 2011 Jun; **26**(4): 621–5. Epub 2010 Aug 7.

Cobb J, Henckel J, Gomes P, Harris S, Jakopec M, Rodriguez F, Barrett A and Davies B (2006) Hands-on robotic unicompartmental knee replacement: a prospective, randomised controlled study of the acrobot system. *J Bone Joint Surg Br*, **88**: 188–97.

D'Lima DD, Patil S and Steklov N, Colwell CW Jr. An ABJS best paper: dynamic intraoperative ligament balancing for total knee arthroplasty. *Clin Orthop Relat Res*, 2007 Oct; **463**: 208–12.

Davies BL, Harris SJ, Lin WJ, Hibberd RD, Middleten R and Cobb JC Active compliance in robotic surgery: the use of force control as a dynamic constrant. *Proc Inst Mech Eng*, 1997; **211H**: 285292.

Delp SL, Stulberg SD, Davies B, Picard F and Leitner F, Computer assisted knee replacement. *Clin Orthop Relat Res*, 1998; **354**: 49–56.

Dorr LD, Faugere MC, Mackel AM, Gruen TA, Bognar B and Malluche HH. Structural and cellular assessment of bone quality of proximal femur. *Bone*, 1993 May–Jun; **14**(3): 231–42.

Dong H and Buxton M. Early assessment of the likely cost-effectiveness of a new technology: a Markov model with probabilistic sensitivity analysis of computer-assisted total knee replacement. *Int J Technol Assess Health Care*, 2006; **22**: 191–202.

Dutton AQ, Yeo SJ, Yang KY, Lo NN, Chia KU and Chong HC. Computer-assisted minimally invasive total knee arthroplasty compared with standard total knee arthroplasty. A prospective, randomized study. *J Bone Joint Surg Am*, 2008 Jan; **90**(1): 2–9.

Elfring R, de la Fuente M and Radermacher K. Assessment of optical localizer accuracy for computer aided surgery systems. *Comput Aided Surg*, 2010; **15**(1–3): 1–12.

Freeman MAR, Swanson SAVS, Todd RC. Total replacement of the knee using the Freeman/Swanson knee prosthesis. *Clin Orthop*, 1973; **94**: 153–170.

Fu CK, Wai J, Lee E, Hutchison C, Myden C, Batuyong E and Anglin C. Computer-assisted patellar resection system: development and insights. *J Orthop Res*, 2012 Apr; **30**(4): 535–40. doi: 10.1002/jor.21567.

Glossop ND. Advantages of optical compared with electromagnetic tracking. *J Bone Joint Surg Am*. 2009 Feb; **91**(Suppl 1): 23–8.

Gonzales FB, Engh CA Jr, Ammeen D and Hopper R. Accuracy of CT-based patient specific total knee arthroplasty instruments. *Annual Meeting of the American Association of Hip and Knee Surgeons*, 2010, Poster 7.

Gunston FH. Polycentric knee arthroplasty: prosthetic simulation of normal knee movement. *J Bone Joint Surg*, 1971; **53B**: 272–277.

Hofmann AA, Plaster RLvMurdock LE. Subvastus (Southern) approach for primary total knee arthroplasty. *Clin Orthop Relat Res*, 1991 Aug; **269**: 70–7.

Huddleston JI, Wiley JW and Scott RD. Zone 4 femoral radiolucent lines in hybrid versus cemented total knee arthroplasties: are they clinically significant? *Clin Orthop Relat Res*, 2005 Dec; **441**: 334–9.

Iorio R, Robb WJ, Healy WL, Berry DJ, Hozack WJ, Kyle RF, Lewallen DG, Trousdale RT, Jiranek WA, Stamos VP and Parsley BS. Orthopaedic surgeon workforce and volume assessment for total hip and knee replacement in the United States: preparing for an epidemic. *J Bone Joint Surg Am*, 2008 Jul; **90**(7): 1598–605.

Ishida K, Matsumoto T, Tsumura N, Kubo S, Kitagawa A, Chin T, Iguchi T, Kurosaka M and Kuroda R. Mid-term outcomes of computer-assisted total knee arthroplasty. *Knee Surg Sports Traumatol Arthrosc*, 2011 Jul; **19**(7): 1107–12. Epub 2011 Jan 14.

Jakopec MSH, Harris SJ Rodriguez Y Baena F Gomes P, Cobb J and Davies BL. The first clinical application of a 'hands-on' robotic knee surgery system. *Comput Aided Surg*, 2001; **6**: 329–39.

Klima S, Zeh A and Josten C. Comparison of operative time and accuracy using conventional fixed navigation cutting blocks and adjustable pivotal cutting blocks. *Comput Aided Surg*, 2008; **13**(4): 225–232.

Koenig JA and Plaskos C. Surgical accuracy and efficiency of computer-automated total knee arthroplasty: a report on the first 80 cases. 11th Annual Meeting of the International Society for Computer Assisted Orthopaedic Surgery London, UK, June 2011.

Koulalis D, O'Loughlin PF, Plaskos C, Kendoff D, Cross MB and Pearle AD (2010a) Sequential versus automated cutting guides in computer-assisted total knee arthroplasty. *Knee*, 2011 Dec; **18**(6): 436–42. Epub 2010 Sep 15. doi:10.1016/j.knee.2010.08.007.

Koulalis D, O'Loughlin PF, Plaskos C, Kendoff D and Pearle AD (2010b) Adjustable cutting blocks for computer-navigated total knee arthroplasty a cadaver study. *J Arthroplasty*, **25**(5): 807–811.

Lang JE, Mannava S, Floyd AJ, Goddard MS, Smith BP, Mofidi A, Seyler TM and Jinnah RH. Robotic systems in orthopaedic surgery. *J Bone Joint Surg Br*, 2011; **93**-B: 1296–9.

Laskin RS. Bone resection techniques in total knee replacement. p. 55–74. In Laskin RS (ed.): *Total knee replacement*. Springer-Verlag London Limited, 1991.

Laskin RS. New techniques and concepts in total knee replacement. *Clin Orthop*, 2003; **416**: 151.

Laskin RS, Beksac B, Phongjunakorn A, Pittors K, Davis J, Shim JC, Pavlov H and Petersen M. Minimally invasive total knee replacement through a mini-midvastus incision: an outcome study. *Clin Orthop Relat Res*, 2004 Nov; **428**: 74–81.

Lawrence RC, Helmick CG, Arnett FC, Deyo RA, Felson DT, Giannini EH, Heyse SP, Hirsch R, Hochberg MC, Hunder GG and Liang MH, Pillemer SR, Steen VD and Wolfe F. Estimates of the prevalence of arthritis and selected musculoskeletal disorders in the United States. *Arthritis Rheum*, 1998; **41**: 778–99.

Liau JJ, Cheng CK and Huang CH and Lo WH. The effect of malalignment on stresses in polyethylene component of total knee prostheses: a finite element analysis. *Clin Biomech (Bristol, Avon)*. 2002 Feb; **17**(2): 140–6.

Leitner F, Picard F and Minfeld R, *et al.* (1997) Computer-assisted knee surgical total replacement. In First Joint Conference of CVRMed and MRCAS, Grenoble, France Springer: 629–38.

Lennox DW, Cohn BT, and Eschenroeder HC Jr. The effects of inaccurate bone cuts on femoral component position in total knee arthroplasty. *Orthopedics*, 1988; **11**: 257.

Longstaff LM, Sloan K, Stamp N, Scaddan M and Beaver R. Good alignment after total knee arthroplasty leads to faster rehabilitation and better function. *J Arthroplasty*, 2009 Jun; **24**(4): 570–8. Epub 2008 May 19.

Lonner JH, John TK and Conditt MA. Robotic arm-assisted UKA improves tibial component alignment: a pilot study. *Clin Orthop Relat Res*, 2010; **468**(1): 141–6.

Mason JB, Fehring TK, Estok R, Banel D and Fahrbach K. Meta-analysis of alignment outcomes in computer-assisted total knee arthroplasty surgery. *J Arthroplasty*, 2007 Dec; **22**(8): 1097–106.

Matsen FA 3rd, Garbini JL, Sidles JA, Pratt B, Baumgarten D and Kaiura R. Robotic assistance in orthopaedic surgery. A proof of principle using distal femoral arthroplasty. *Clin Orthop Relat Res*, 1993 Nov; **296**: 178–86.

Mayman D, Plaskos C, Kendoff D, Wernecke G, Pearle AD and Laskin R. Ligament tension in the ACL-deficient knee: assessment of medial and lateral gaps. *Clin Orthop Relat Res*, 2009 Jun; **467**(6): 1621–8. Epub 2009 Feb 24.

Nam D, Dy CJ, Cross MB, Kang MN and Mayman DJ. Cadaveric results of an accelerometer based, extramedullary navigation system for the tibial resection in total knee arthroplasty. *Knee*, 2011 Oct 25. [Epub ahead of print]

Nam D, Jerabek SA, Haughom B, Cross MB, Reinhardt KR and Mayman DJ. Radiographic analysis of a hand-held surgical navigation system for tibial resection in total knee arthroplasty. *J Arthroplasty*, 2011 Dec; **26**(8): 1527–33. Epub 2011 Mar 11.

Ng VY, DeClaire JH, Berend KR, Gulick BC and Lombardi AV Jr. Improved accuracy of alignment with patient-specific positioning guides compared with manual instrumentation in TKA. Clin *Orthop Relat Res*, 2012 Jan; **470**(1): 99–107.

Novak E, Silverstein MD and Bozic KJ. The cost-effectiveness of computer-assisted navigation in total knee arthroplasty. *J Bone Joint Surg [Am]*, 2007; **89**(11): 2389–97.

Nunley RM, Ellison BS, Ruh EL, Williams BM, Foreman K, Ford AD and Barrack RL. Are patient-specific cutting blocks cost-effective for total knee arthroplasty? *Clin Orthop Relat Res*, 2012a Mar; **470**(3): 889–94. Epub 2011 Dec 20.

Nunley RM, Ellison BS, Zhu J, Ruh EL, Howell SM and Barrack RL. Do patient-specific guides improve coronal alignment in Total Knee Arthroplasty? *Clin Orthop Relat Res*, 2012b Mar; **470**(3): 895–902. Epub 2011 Dec 20.

Paul H, Bargar W and Mittlestadt B, Musits B, Taylor R and Kazanzides P, *et al.* Development of a surgical robot for cementless total hip arthroplasty. *Clin Orthop Relat Res*, 1992; **285**: 57.

Pearle AD, O'Loughlin PF and Kendoff DO. Robot-assisted unicompartmental knee arthroplasty. *J Arthroplasty*, 2010 Feb; **25**(2): 230–7.

Perrin N, Stindel E and Roux C. BoneMorphing versus freehand localization of anatomical landmarks: consequences for the reproducibility of implant positioning in total knee arthroplasty. *Comput Aided Surg*, 2005 Sep–Nov; **10**(5–6): 301–9.

Plaskos C, Cinquin P, Lavallée S and Hodgson AJ. Praxiteles: a miniature bone-mounted nobot for minimal access total knee arthroplasty. *Int J Med Robot*, 2005; **1**(4): 67–79.

Plaskos C, Hodgson AJ, Inkpen KB and McGraw RW. Bone cutting errors in total knee arthroplasty. *J Arthroplasty*, 2002; **17**(6): 698–705.

Radermacher K, Portheine F, Anton M, Zimolong A, Kaspers G, Rau G and Staudte H-W. Computer assisted orthopaedic surgery with image-based individual templates. *Clin Orthop Relat Res*, 1998; **354**: 28–38.

Ranawat CS, Insall JN and Shine J. Duo-condylar knee arthroplasty: hospital for special surgery design. *Clin Orthop*, 1976; **120**: 76–82.

Rasquinha VJ, Ranawat CS, Cervieri CL and Rodriguez JA. The press-fit condylar modular total knee system with a posterior cruciate-substituting design. A concise follow-up of a previous report. *J Bone Joint Surg Am*, 2006 May; **88**(5): 1006–10.

Ritschl P, Machacek J, Fuiko R, Zettl R and Kotte B. The Galileo system for implantation of total knee arthroplasty: an integrated solution comprising navigation, robotics and robot-assisted ligament balancing. In: *Navigation and robotics in total joint and spine surgery*. Eds: Stiehl, Konermann, Haaker. Springer-Verlag, 2004. pp. 281–361.

Ritter MA. Faris PM. Keating EM and Meding JB. Postoperative alignment of total knee replacement. Its effect on survival. *Clin Orthop*, 1994; **299**: 153.

Sastre S, Sanchez MD, Lozano L, Orient F, Fontg F and Nuñez M. Total knee arthroplasty: better short-term results after subvastus approach: a randomized, controlled study. *Knee Surg Sports Traumatol Arthrosc*, 2009 Oct; **17**(10): 1184–8. Epub 2009 Apr 18.

Schroer WC, Diesfeld PJ, Reedy ME and LeMarr AR. Mini-subvastus approach for total knee arthroplasty. *J Arthroplasty*, 2008 Jan; **23**(1): 19–25. Epub 2007 Sep 24.

Scuderi GR, Tenholder M and Capeci C. Surgical approaches in mini-incision total knee arthroplasty. *Clin Orthop Relat Res*, 2004; **428**: 61–7.

Scuderi GR, Bourne RB, Noble PC, Benjamin JB, Lonner JH and Scott WN. The new Knee Society Knee Scoring System. *Clin Orthop Relat Res*. 2012 Jan; **470**(1): 3–19.

Sharkey PF, Hozack WJ, Rothman RH, Shastri S and Jacoby SM. Insall Award paper. Why are total knee arthroplasties failing today? *Clin Orthop Relat Res*, 2002 Nov; (404): 7–13.

Siebert W, Mai S, Kober R and Heeckt PF. Technique and first clinical results of robot-assisted total knee replacement. *Knee*, 2002; **9**(3): 173–80.

Siston RA, Daub AC, Giori NJ, Goodman SB and Delp SL. Evaluation of methods that locate the center of the ankle for computer-assisted total knee arthroplasty. *Clin Orthop Relat Res*, 2005; **439**: 129–35.

Siston RA, Giori NJ, Goodman SB and Delp SL. Surgical navigation for total knee arthroplasty: a perspective. *J Biomech*, 2007; **40**(4): 728–35.

Slover JD, Tosteson AN, Bozic KJ, Rubash HE, and Malchau H. Impact of hospital volume on the economic value of computer navigation for total knee replacement. *J Bone Joint Surg [Am]*, 2008; **90**–A(7): 1492–1500.

Slover JD, Rubash HE, Malchau H and Bosco JA. Cost-effectiveness analysis of custom total knee cutting blocks. *J Arthroplasty*, 2012 Feb; **27**(2): 180–5. Epub 2011 Jun 14.

Smith TO, King JJ and Hing CB. A meta-analysis of randomised controlled trials comparing the clinical and radiological outcomes following minimally invasive to conventional exposure for total knee arthroplasty. *Knee*, 2012 Jan; **19**(1): 1–7. Epub 2010 Dec 31.

Stiehl JB, Jackson S and Szabo A. Multi-factorial analysis of time efficiency in total knee arthroplasty. *Comput Aided Surg*, 2009; **14**(1-3): 58–62.

Stindel E, Gil D, Briard JL, Merloz P, Dubrana F and Lefevre C. Detection of the center of the hip joint in computer-assisted surgery: an evaluation study of the surgetics algorithm. *Comput Aided Surg*, 2005 May; **10**(3): 133–9.

Stindel E, Briard JL, Merloz P, Plaweski S, Dubrana F, Lefevre C and Troccaz J. Bone morphing: 3D morphological data for total knee arthroplasty. *Comput Aided Surg*, 2002; **7**(3): 156–68.

Stulberg SD, Loan P and Sarin V. Computer-assisted navigation in total knee replacement: results of an initial experience in thirty-five patients. *J Bone Joint Surg Am*, 2002; **84**-A Suppl 2: 90–8.

Suero EM, Charles C, Citak M, Pearle AD and Plaskos C. Radiographic comparison of two different ankle registration techniques. *11th Annual Meeting of the International Society for Computer Assisted Orthopaedic Surgery*, London, UK, June 2011a.

Suero EM, Plaskos C, Dixon PL and Pearle AD. Adjustable cutting blocks improve alignment and surgical time in computer-assisted total knee replacement. *Knee Surg Sports Traumatol Arthrosc*, 2011b Nov 25. [Epub ahead of print] DOI: 10.1007/s00167-011-1752-1.

Swank ML, Alkire M, Conditt M and Lonner JH. Technology and cost-effectiveness in knee arthroplasty: computer navigation and robotics. *Am J Orthop (Belle Mead NJ)*. 2009 Feb; **38**(2 Suppl): 32–6.

Szeliski R and Lavallee S. Matching 3-D anatomical surfaces with non-rigid deformations using octree-splines. *Int J Comput Vision*, 1996; **18**(2): 171–86.

Takasaki M, Matsuda S, Fukagawa S, Mitsuyasu H, Miura H and Iwamoto Y. Accuracy of image-free navigation for severely deformed knees. *Knee Surg Sports Traumatol Arthrosc*, 2010; **18**: 763–8.

Tria AJ Jr, Coon TM: Minimal incision total knee arthroplasty: early experience. *Clin Orthop*, 2003; (416): 185–90.

Yen PL and Davies BL. Active constraint control for image-guided robotic surgery. *Proc Inst Mech Eng H*, 2010; **224**(5): 623–31.

Yaffe MA, Koo SS and Stulberg SD. Radiographic and navigation measurements of TKA limb alignment do not correlate. *Clin Orthop Relat Res*, 2008 Nov; **466**(11): 2736–44.

7
Robotics in ear, nose and throat (ENT) surgery

B. BELL, M. D. CAVERSACCIO and S. WEBER,
University of Bern, Switzerland

Abstract: The three main classes of robotics in ear, nose and throat (ENT) surgery (telemanipulation, image-guided functional servoing, and computer numerical control) are discussed and important examples of applications are described to show both technological and clinical developments. As access to many anatomical features of the head requires very small and compact tools to accurately perform procedures, examples are give in ear surgery where manipulation of the minute ossicles requires fine, dexterous movements.

Key words: minimally invasive sargery, ENT surgery, computer numerical control, telemanipulation, functional servoing.

7.1 Introduction

In this chapter, the general term robot refers to three specific classes which have found utility in ear nose and throat (ENT) surgery: telemanipulators, image-guided functional servoing systems and computer numerical controlled (CNC) manipulators. Because telemanipulators can be seen as an extension of, or mimicking of human movement, these interventions do not necessarily rely on image guidance, but are used in the more traditional way as master–slave devices. In contrast, image-guided functional servoing and CNC technologies rely entirely on two-dimentional (2D) or three-dimentional (3D) medical image data (and possibly additional functional information) to control the position, orientation, or functional state of the device.

7.1.1 Technology overview

Although the prevalence of robotic assistance in the operating room (OR) has increased steadily in recent years, such devices are slower in penetrating the ENT field owing to the small size and complicated layout of anatomical structures, which by their nature require a high technical accuracy. Thus, the implementation of robots in ENT is an important, yet challenging task. To illustrate this point, let us consider the small structures of the middle ear (ossicles), which have dimensions on the order of millimeters and can be potentially damaged with forces of a few newtons. The problem is further complicated by an extremely limited workspace and field of view. Thus, adapting industrial manipulators or other surgical robots to this application is to a large extent not feasible due to the relatively large size and shape of such manipulators.

It is generally held that the main objective of implementing surgical robots is to improve surgical outcome (Taylor, 1997). These improvements usually result in reduced invasiveness and/or refined, tremor-free manipulation of surgical tools leading to reduced trauma, blood loss, and recovery time. In addition, minimally invasive rhinological procedures also clearly benefit from minimal aesthetic impact as witnessed by the move to predominantly endoscopic procedures. Similarly, the precise manipulation of tools has particular importance in rhinology and the anterior skull base, where the size of the surgical access as well as the anatomical structures of interest can exceed the surgeon's visual perception and dexterity. Finally, such structures may have delicate mechanical properties which surpass normal haptic sensitivity. Thus, robotic technologies serve an important channel through which invasiveness can be reduced while simultaneously augmenting surgical skill. As previously mentioned, robotic devices in the field of ENT can be categorized as:

- telemanipulators, wherein the surgeon operates the robot in a master–slave configuration;
- image-guided functional servoing, wherein the functional state of a surgical tool is controlled based on real-time measurements of its location in or near the patient; and
- computer numerical control, wherein a robot performs a pre-planned move, or action automatically or semiautomatically, typically based on pre- or perioperative medical image data.

An excellent review of surgical robotics was conducted by Camarillo *et al.* (2004), the main points of which are summarized in Table 7.1. The following sections describe each of the interaction methods summarized above and the applicable research in each field.

7.2 Telemanipulators in ENT

Surgical applications of telemanipulators are described in the following sections.

7.2.1 Endoscope holders in functional endoscopic sinus surgery (FESS)

Functional endoscopic sinus surgery (FESS) has undergone the greatest increase in the use of telemanipulators in ENT surgery. Early developments

Table 7.1 Advantages and disadvantages of human and robot capabilities

	Surgeons	Robots
Advantages	Task versatility	Repeatability, stability and accuracy
	Judgment experience	Tolerant of ionizing radiation
	Hand-eye co-ordination	Optimized for particular environments
	Dexterity at millimeter-to-centimeter scale	Programmed hand–eye transformation
	Sensor input and data fusion	Multitasking
Drawbacks	Tremor	Expensive
	Fatigue	Cumbersome
	Imprecision	Large
	Variability in skill, age, state of mind	Inability to process qualitative information
	Inability to process quantitative information quickly	Not versatile
	Ineffective at submillimeter scale	Technology in its infancy

Source: adapted from Camarillo *et al.*, 2004.

in this field focused on endoscope holders for laparoscopic surgery and eventually culminated in the creation of the automated endoscope system for optimal positioning (AESOP) from Computer Motion, which first obtained FDA approval in 1994. Although initially developed for surgeries within the abdominal cavity, Obando and Payne (2003) used the device to treat five patients with nasal polyposis and concurrent sinusitis. The main advantage of the device is that it frees the surgeon's camera hand to perform other functions. In early models, the endoscope was positioned with hand and foot controls, but was later replaced with voice-activated commands. The primary advantages of this device are (Obando and Payne, 2003):

- the holder provides a steady view without unwanted movement and tremor which increases with fatigue;
- the assistant is available for other tasks;
- it allows two-handed operation of surgical instruments;
- the desired viewing field can be altered directly by the surgeon, thus decreasing latency and confusion associated with an assistant;
- favorable time expenditure (similar to manual endoscopy); and
- a more comfortable working situation for surgeon.

Similarly, Obando *et al.* (2004) also used the AESOP for seven transnasal hypophysectomies to treat pituitary tumors. A modified position of the device at the head of the surgical table allowed a more efficient use of the robotic arm and significant time savings compared with previous work in the paranasal sinuses. The most notable outcome reported was that the use of the robotic arm allowed two-handed manipulation of the microdebrider, which facilitated better, more precise control over the tool.

Although, several advantages of the AESOP were reported, disadvantages were also made apparent during the above studies. Foremost among these are the interruption of the normal workflow and the additional time needed to set up and use the device. Furthermore, cleaning the endoscope lens is much less efficient because it must be repetitively removed and inserted into the tool holder. This was also noted in our own tests with a custom-built otorinolaryngology (ORL) manipulator (Fig. 7.1). The necessity of uncoupling the endoscope from the robot for cleaning was very time consuming. An additional problem, not addressed by current instruments, is force monitoring and feedback, which can pose a significant risk to weak cranial bone structures if the endoscope is mistakenly driven into them. As a first step in addressing this problem, Wagner and coworkers measured and applied forces during normal FESS procedures and found an average of only 2.2 N and a maximum of 8 N was necessary to puncture many of the nasal bony structures (Eichhorn *et al.*, 2008). Similarly, the stiffness of several structures was also evaluated in a separate study which showed that stiffness and break strength are not necessarily correlated (Wagner *et al.*, 2008). Such data is vital in determining appropriate force thresholds for controlling endoscopic navigation devices.

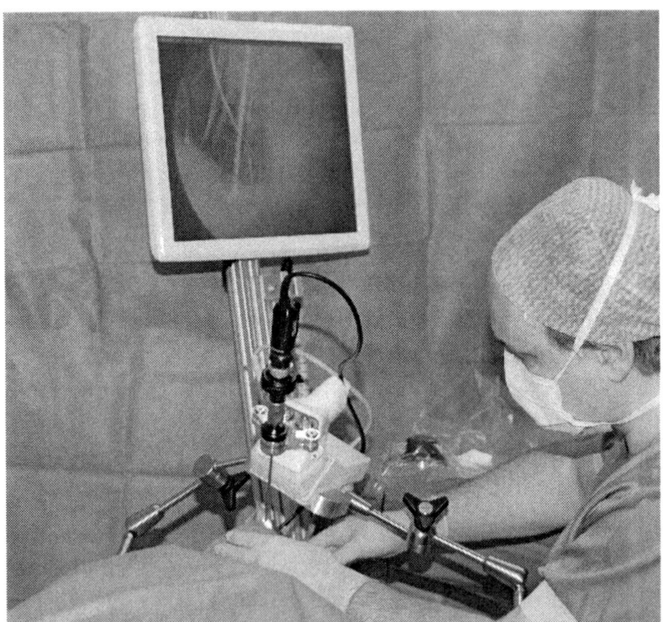

7.1 Testing a custom-built ORL robot with an endoscope attachment. This simple version uses a 6D input device to control the position of the endoscope.

7.2.2 Instrument manipulation

Tremor, fatigue, limited visibility and a small working-space make surgery in the middle and inner ear particularly difficult. For example, the non-ergonomic positioning of the hands when manipulating the ossicles or other middle ear structures during procedures such as the stapedectomy can increase the effects of tremor and increase the rate of fatigue. Additionally, instruments and the hands of the surgeon further restrict an already limited field of view. Mechanical manipulators offer attractive possibilities for overcoming these difficulties in otological surgery through tremor reduction, and reduced instrument size.

To date, two master–slave devices have been developed specifically for this field. The first, the 'MicroMan,' was developed at the Technical University of Munich (Fig. 7.2) with the objective of being small and compact in order to allow direct mounting of the device on the OR table in an unobtrusive way using a standard adjustable arm. The main purpose of the device is to assist the surgeon in performing tasks requiring fine motor skills in the tight quarters of the middle ear. Its utility was evaluated in this scenario by testing the accuracy of unassisted versus. robot-assisted tool placement. To this end, a middle-ear phantom was created by fixing a glass plate in the approximate location of the cochlea within a head dummy. A camera mounted behind this plate (triggered by a force sensor mounted on the plate) was then used to

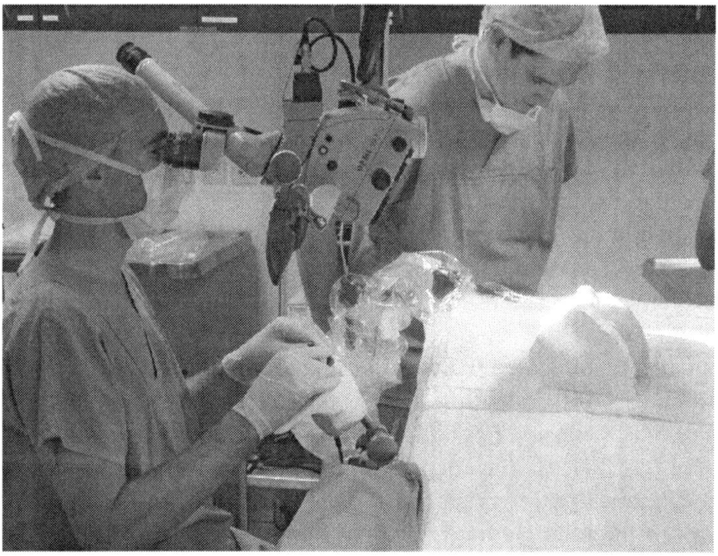

7.2 Testing the positioning accuracy of the MicroMan device in a technical phantom (image courtesy of Gero Strauss, Innovation Center Computer Assisted Surgery, University of Leipzig).

measure the tool positioning accuracy as the surgeon tried to touch a target painted on the glass surface in both assisted and unassisted scenarios.

Interestingly, the mean tool positioning error was higher for the manipulator assisted trials than for manual placement. This was true in spite of a significant improvement of positioning accuracy as the user became more familiar with the device. It is likely that a lack of correspondence between the input device and tool movement had a significant effect on the positioning accuracy. Thus, replacing the joystick input device used in this system with a haptic device which replicates the actual tool movement could improve eye-hand coordination and the final accuracy.

A second manipulator designed specifically for microsurgery in the ear is RobOtol, a device developed at the University of Paris (Miroir *et al.*, 2010). The main focus of this work was the optimization of the kinematic design which would enable the robot to respect the extracorporeal workspace (defined by the surgical microscope and patient anatomy) while minimizing obstruction of the microscope's field of view. The optimization procedure was based on a six degrees of freedom (DoF) arm which comprises three prismatic and three rotational axes. The translational axes are grouped in a base structure which is positioned next to the patient. The rotational DoF make up the remaining links of the arm, which enter into the surgical workspace and have a common center of rotation. The specific link dimensions were optimized by analyzing the theoretical field-of-view obstruction and distance to external obstacles. Once this optimization was completed, the design was implemented with three linear stages for the base structure, a harmonic drive for the first rotational joint, and two Bowden cable mechanisms for the final two joints to reduce the arm weight (Fig. 7.3).

Control of the tool pose is performed with a haptic input device (Phantom Omni, SensAble Technologies, USA) which is calibrated relative to the robot base. A velocity controller was implemented based on the haptic input where the movement is proportional to velocity. Furthermore, motion can be started or stopped at any point by engaging/disengaging an input button on the human–machine interface (HMI). The workspace of the manipulator was evaluated by accessing various anatomical locations within the middle ear with a micropick whereupon images from the microscope viewport were captured and compared with similar images recorded during normal surgical procedures. This evaluation showed that the robotic manipulator had better visibility of the surgical field in that only the tool was visible in all cases without occlusions due to the surgeon's hands. The robot was also able to reach more positions than is typically feasible during a normal surgery owing to the increased range of motion in the wrist of the robot. Finally, the combination of the device with endoscopic visualization was tested and showed that this could also be useful for reaching anatomies outside the normal sight path.

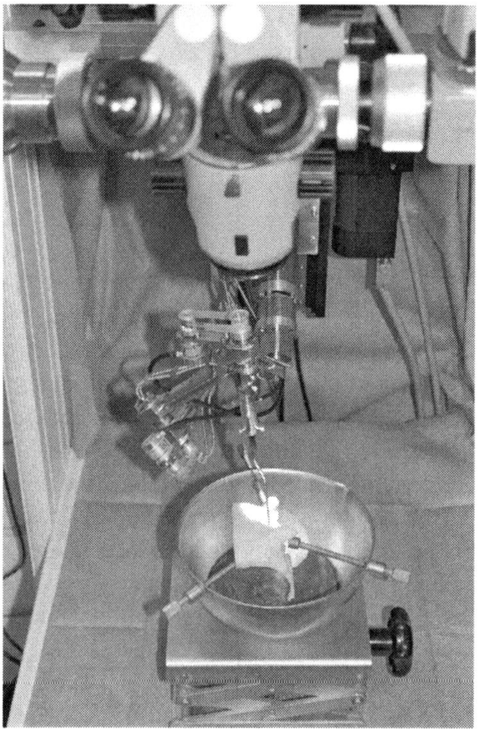

7.3 The kinematics of the RobOtol device were optimized to enable a clear field of view for the surgical microscope, the only obstruction being the tool itself (photo courtesy of Mathieu Miroir, INSERM, University of Paris, France).

7.2.3 Transnasal skull base access using the da Vinci telemanipulator

Despite being designed and optimized for use in visceral surgery, the da Vinci telemanipulator system has also been applied to ENT surgery. Strauss *et al.* (2005a) were among the first to attempt its use for paranasal sinus surgery by performing surgical procedures on cadaver specimens. From this study, the group defined four specific areas where the system should outperform conventional endoscopic instrumentation in order to prove useful:

- mechanical advantage, for example additional DoF, and motion scaling;
- enhanced visualization of the surgical field (stereoendoscopy);
- ergonomic positioning of hands, arms, head, etc.;
- integration, including scalability of motion, automatic trajectories from planned data, eye–hand co-ordination, and usability in the OR.

To evaluate the performance of the da Vinci surgical system in these four areas, the group undertook five different surgical procedures contralaterally on 14 cadaver preparations:

- anterior/posterior ethmoidectomy;
- orbital decompression;
- dissection of the frontal sinus;
- sphenoidectomy; and
- opening and dissection of the maxillary sinus.

In total, 140 surgical interventions were performed with the robotic manipulator which were followed by five conventional procedures for direct comparison. The results of their work confirmed that the da Vinci manipulator is useful for skull base surgery in that it outperformed conventional techniques in each of the four evaluation criteria. One significant drawback however, is that an additional 9 minutes are generally needed for setup of the device in the OR. The main advantage of the system is the increased dexterity afforded by the laparoscopic tools. For the majority of procedures (excluding maxillary sinus), full six DoF movement was possible with the surgeon seated in an ergonomic position. As a comparison, the conventional methods only facilitated 3–5 DoF.

Similar usability studies of the da Vinci system were performed by Hanna and coworkers (2007), who hypothesized that the surgical device could be used to meticulously suture dural defects following tumor excision. The inability to adequately close dural defects, leading to high cerebral spinal fluid leak rates, has deterred some surgeons from using a minimally invasive endoscopic approach and revert to a conventional open method. With this in mind, the da Vinci telemanipulator was evaluated in skull-base procedures with a focus on suture quality.

Hanna *et al.* (2007) used the telemanipulator on each of four cadaver specimens and reported that excellent access was granted to each of the following structures and regions: cribriform plate, fovea ethmoidalis, medial orbit, plenum sphenoidale, nasopharynx, and pterygopalatine fossa, clivus, sella turcica suprasellar and parasellar regions. Additionally, they reported that the increased dexterity of the robotic manipulators did indeed improve the ability to suture dural defects, and the 3D endoscope provided surgeons with increased depth perception. In summary, the authors were optimistic that this technique can provide clear benefits in terms of morbidity, and surgical outcome.

One universally reported disadvantage of the *da Vinci* telemanipulator is the lack of force feedback through the haptic interface. Without force feedback the surgeon must rely solely on visual cues to navigate and perform various tasks. In contrast, the addition of force feedback would enable the surgeon to detect collisions, and perhaps more importantly, control the level of force applied to tissues and sutures. This functionality is particularly important where visibility is poor or when working near delicate structures. Furthermore, force feedback could enable automatic collision detection and thus prevent collateral damage to surrounding structures.

7.2.4 Neck/larynx dissection

Similarly to sinus and transnasal skull-base procedures, transoral surgery could also benefit from laparoscopic surgery in that natural orifices can be used for surgical access. The main drawbacks, however, are limited dexterity and visibility. These limitations have stimulated the use of the da Vinci in neck and larynx surgeries with the hope that better visualization and dexterity may reduce the need for open surgeries in many cases. As in FESS surgery, the application of the da Vinci in neck surgery is also in an exploratory state and lacks standardized protocols. Thus, most studies have focused on the feasibility of using a telemanipulator trans-orally. To date, this has been attempted primarily for tumor resection (Park *et al.*, 2009; Solares and Strome, 2007), though one group also explored laryngeal cleft repair in children (Rahbar *et al.*, 2007). Each of these studies agrees that the increased dexterity afforded by the manipulator substantiates the additional cost in set-up time and effort. The major drawback, however, is the relative bulk or size of the manipulator components that often collide with each other when placed close together as is necessary for transoral procedures. For this reason, a large proportion of procedures were reverted to standard interventions owing to lack of adequate access, 3/5 (Rahbar *et al.*, 2007), 2/3 (Solares and Strome, 2007), whereas others report 100% success (Park *et al.*, 2009). In summary, although transoral interventions with the da Vinci may be feasible, they are not very attractive due to collisions occurring between the arms.

7.3 Image-guided interventions

Applications of navigation control are described in the following sections after an assessment of how accuracy is achieved.

7.3.1 The importance of accuracy

In contrast to telemanipulation, image-guided robotic surgeries leverage preoperative medical image data sets to compute and plan appropriate actions that are then precisely performed in the OR using a robotic system (possibly in conjunction with a stereotactic guidance system). This technique has the advantage of a high fidelity reproduction of the previously planned actions, critical for protecting sensitive anatomical structures through exact tool placement, and thus exact control of material removal. The actual procedure can be performed automatically such as in conventional CNC machining, or semiautomatically whereby the surgeon retains control of the drill position, but is restricted by the robot to a prescribed working volume. In each of these methods, it is possible to achieve much higher levels of accuracy than with free-handed techniques. This is especially true where complicated 3D geometries are concerned. Unfortunately, this process is at present limited to bony structures as adequate models of tissue deformation do not exist.

Because accuracy is of particular interest in image-guided robotic surgery, special care is required to minimize error in each step of the intervention as shown in Fig. 7.4. A major portion of the error occurs before the surgery even begins, and stems predominantly from imaging, image-based planning, and the subsequent registration of the digital dataset to the physical world. Additional errors are introduced from the tracking system (typical optical systems have RMS error of 0.25 mm) and instrument calibration.

New imaging technologies such as flat-panel cone-beam computerized tomography (CBCT) or digital volume tomography (DVT) are capable of simultaneously increasing image resolution and reducing radiation exposure. With these devices, isotropic voxel sizes down to 0.08 mm in each direction are possible, representing an increase in resolution along the imaging axis of 6–8 times compared with high-resolution CT data. This increase of spatial resolution does, however, come at the cost of image contrast which is significantly lower than conventional CT. In spite of this, CBCT still delivers clear benefits in terms of accuracy improvement in navigated surgery (Bartling *et al.*, 2007; Majdani *et al.*, 2008)

Final accuracy of the computer-aided plan is also a significant concern. The digitization of fiducial screws can, for example, directly influence the final registration accuracy. For this reason, we have developed a computer-aided design (CAD) based matching algorithm to identify screw locations with subpixel accuracy as seen in Fig. 7.5 (Zheng *et al.*, 2010).

Additionally, the accuracy of segmented structures is also important to properly reach target locations as well as avoid critical anatomy. Thus, significant effort is being expended in developing fast, accurate algorithms to

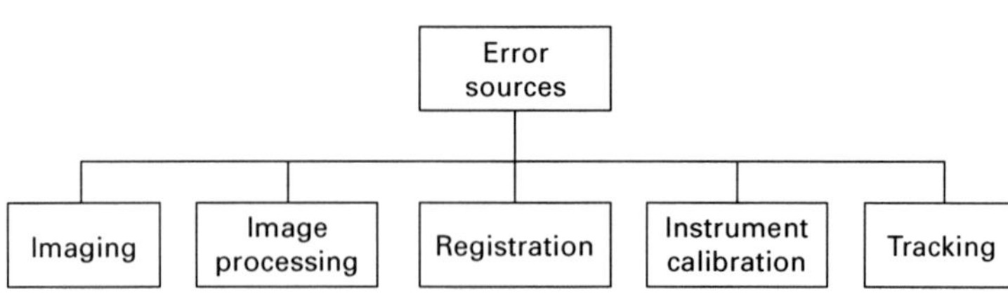

7.4 Summary of major error sources common to image-guided surgical procedures, the largest errors typically coming from imaging, registration, and tracking components.

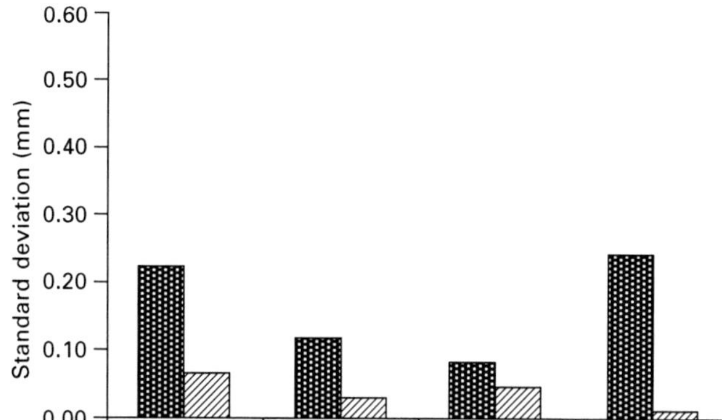

	Marker 1	Marker 2	Marker 3	Marker 4
Manual	0.22	0.12	0.08	0.24
Semiautomatic	0.07	0.03	0.05	0.01

7.5 Comparison of the variability of manual screw localization (black) and semiautomatic localization using the CAD model based matching algorithm.

segment structures in the ear (Noble *et al.*, 2007, 2010). Naturally, accurate registration methods are necessary to take advantage of an accurate plan. At present, point-based matching of bone-fixed fiducial markers represents the gold standard registration technique owing to its ability to accurately identify the center of the marker in the image and world co-ordinate systems. The cost of this accuracy, however, is a slight increase in invasiveness as the markers (typically titanium bone screws) must be implanted before image data is collected. Less invasive methods such as laser surface scanning are significantly less accurate, while methods such as dental splint-fixed references offer a non-invasive but relatively accurate referencing method (Wurm *et al.*, 2005).

One advantage robots provide is their capability to precisely reach and measure points in space. Force-based registration of screw fiducials was first documented as an improvement to the Robodoc orthopedic robot (Haidegger *et al.*, 2008). We also implemented this strategy in our robotic approach to minimally invasive ear surgery. Figure 7.6 shows the registration pointer nearing a fiducial screw, and the associated forces displayed on the user interface. Our tests indicate that the repeatability of the registration process using this type of geometry is less than 0.05 mm.

7.3.2 Navigated control

Navigated control is a method used to alter the active state of an instrument depending on its position and orientation (Strauss *et al.*, 2008). Thus, it is capable of preventing the accidental removal of tissue by a powered

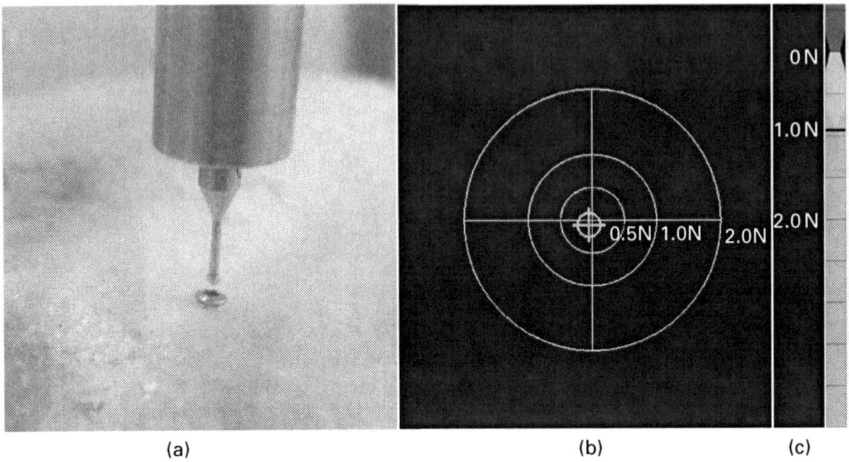

7.6 Illustration of the registration process: (a) the pointer of the robot approaching the fiducial screw on the bone surface; (b) a graphical representation of the lateral forces detected by the pointer, which are minimized to zero; and (c) forces along the axis of the tool. The registration algorithm is designed to achieve a threshold force (1 N) to ensure contact between the pointer and screw.

instrument such as a microdebrider or drill. Although this system does not fit into the traditional concept of a robotic system, it, nevertheless, incorporates important features common to medical robotics, particularly preplanned interventions.

This system consists of an optical navigation system (Karl Storz navigation panel unit, Tuttlingen, Germany), a powered tool with tracker (shaver, drill, etc.), and the control unit (navigated control unit, Karl Storz). The power to the tool is modulated by the control unit which receives a signal proportional to the distance from a risk structure (boundary) from the navigation panel. The accuracy and clinical applicability of this concept were demonstrated in a series of studies, which showed that the accuracy of shaved surfaces was 0.26 mm (standard deviation 0.58 mm) with errors up to 1.93 mm (Koulechov *et al.*, 2006).

7.3.3 Application of navigated control in FESS

On the head, navigated control was first implemented in functional endoscopic sinus surgery (FESS) procedures. Similar to other image-guided robotic interventions, the workflow of a procedure involving navigated control involves three basic steps: imaging, planning and surgical intervention assistance.

The imaging stage is performed using conventional CT or newer flat panel technologies. Importantly, the resolution of images should approximately match navigation accuracy. Furthermore, use of fiducial markers can be used to increase the navigation accuracy.

Following imaging, the preoperative planning stage can be performed. This involves the user definition (segmentation) of the tissues to be removed (active tool volume). Critical structures can be respected through conservative boundary definitions with larger safety margins.

During the actual navigated control procedure, the control functionality can be enabled or disabled at any time, thus allowing the surgeon to immediately override the system should the conditions warrant. Overall, the procedure differs very little from standard practice, yet provides greatly improved safety, which means that the system can be easily integrated into standard workflows with minimal training overhead.

The efficacy of the system was tested in a clinical trial of 10 patients diagnosed with sinusitis ethmoidalis (Hofer *et al.*, 2008). In this study, diseased tissue was removed with the shaver just as in normal FESS with the added benefit of the shaver stopping at the planned boundaries. This occurred on average 16.5 times per intervention. The authors placed great importance on the ability of the system to provide additional safety, which, in turn, improves surgeon confidence through reduced cognitive workload. Because the control unit is designed to stop the powered instrument before breaching a virtual boundary, the surgeon is able to focus on the endoscopic view rather than dividing his attention between the endoscope and navigation system.

7.3.4 Mastoidectomy

A further application of navigated control in ENT surgery is in drilling the mastoidectomy, which is the standard method used to gain access to the cochlea for electrode insertion. The mastoidectomy is created primarily because of the need to identify critical structures, such as the facial nerve, in an exploratory manner. In contrast to FESS, navigation is rarely used in the lateral skull base (owing largely to inadequate accuracy of navigation and manual manipulation) and the surgeon relies almost exclusively on visual (anatomical) cues.

Navigated control has been investigated in this application as a means of increasing the safety of the procedure, and thereby increasing efficiency of material removal. Just as in navigated control for FESS, the power to the drill is determined based on the spatial position of the tool tip relative to the patient anatomy. Thus, the mastoidectomy can be performed as usual with the addition of a safety layer which increases surgeon confidence and patient safety. This technique was tested by first comparing the size and shape of a pocket milled for implant electrodes in a phantom model (Strauss *et al.*, 2005b) and, second, by creating a mastoidectomy and allowing the drill to aid the surgeon in risk structure identification (Hofer *et al.*, 2008). Results of these studies suggest that the material removal can occur faster without damage to risk structures.

7.4 Computer numerical control (CNC)

Unlike telemanipulation and navigated control, computer numerical control (CNC) positions the tool automatically or semiautomatically according to a planned path or trajectory. Thus, a range of simple to complex shapes can be machined in an exact and efficient process. Because of this feature, robotic assisted surgery has the ability to not only ensure the accuracy of the procedure, but also to influence the way implants are introduced and fixed to bone.

7.4.1 Hearing aid implantations

The implantation of hearing devices consists of four basic steps. First, access to the middle ear is gained through a procedure known as the mastoidectomy. Once this access has been achieved, a cochleostomy is typically performed to provide entry to the cochlea. Finally, the electrode array is inserted and the accompanying electronics are fixed in a shallow bed milled into the cortical skull. Improvements are being developed for each of these steps and therefore, each will be treated separately.

Direct cochlear access (DCA)

As previously discussed, the mastoidectomy is performed to gain access to the cochlea for electrode insertion. The resulting cavity (mastoidectomy) is much larger than is necessary to complete the task of electrode insertion, owing simply to the fact that the surgeon typically locates the facial nerve in a proactive manner in order to avoid damage to this sensitive structure. This results in a significant comorbidity (damage to surrounding structures not directly involved in the pathology). Thus, several groups are actively researching methods of reducing the invasiveness of the procedure by creating a direct cochlear access (DCA). The objective of the DCA is to drill a small diameter tunnel (diameter 1.5–2.0 mm) directly to the cochlea based on an image-guided surgical plan. The subsequent steps of cochleostomy and array insertion can be performed through this small tunnel, thereby negating the necessity of the mastoidectomy.

The preferred drill path originates at the outer surface of the temporal bone just posterior to the auditory canal, passes through the facial recess and ends near the round window of the cochlea. The facial recess is an anatomical region with posterior and superior boundaries defined by the facial nerve, bounded anteriorly by the auditory canal, and inferiorly by the chorda tympani (Fig. 7.7). The main challenge of this procedure is placing the tunnel with sufficient accuracy such that these anatomical structures are not damaged (preference is given to the facial nerve). As part of an early attempt at this procedure, Schipper *et al.* (2004) determined that accuracies better

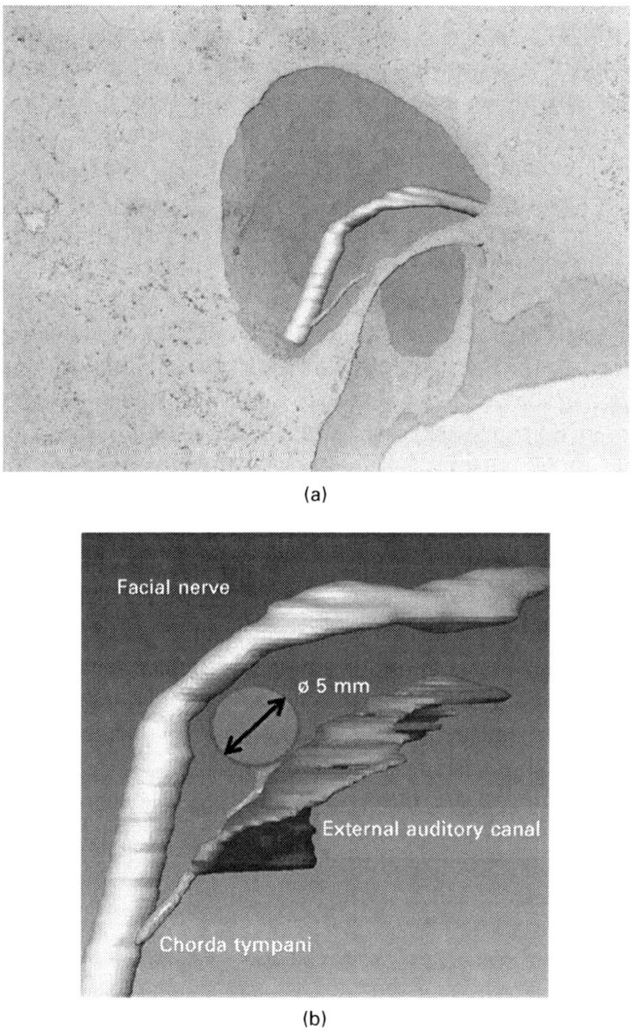

7.7 (a) Artistic rendering of the approximate location of the facial nerve and chorda tympani in the conventional mastoidectomy; (b) segmented anatomical structures of the facial recess as seen in the sagital view. The facial nerve is the most critical structure to avoid. It is estimated that an accuracy better than 0.5 mm is necessary to safely drill through this region.

than 0.5 mm are necessary. Although it is desirable that the chorda tympani remain whole, it is generally accepted that damage resulting in a change or partial loss in taste sensation is usually not perceived as a large problem, and diminishes over time. In contrast, damage to the facial nerve can lead to partial or full paralysis of the ipsilateral face. Therefore, although the facial nerve must be respected, more risk may be placed on the chorda tympani or external auditory canal since these structures are less important.

Owing to the small pathway through the facial recess, accuracy throughout the entire clinical workflow is paramount in ensuring a successful DCA surgery. As in any image-guided surgery, the total error is a sum of several sources. The main error sources are: imaging, segmentation and planning, patient-image registration, and navigation. Because the acceptable error level is lower than in conventional image-guided systems (IGS), care must be taken in order to ensure that errors from each stage are minimized. Table 7.2 summarizes the main error sources and compares values common in 'careful' IGS to levels expected to be necessary for DCA procedures.

The preoperative planning of minimally invasive DCA procedures closely matches that of normal IGS surgeries. The preoperative workflow is as follows: fiducial screw placement, image acquisition, and image-based planning. Bone-anchored fiducial screws are used because they represent the gold standard in terms of registration accuracy. Additionally, new flat-panel cone-beam imaging devices are being investigated for use in IGS because of the resolution advantages such devices offer (Bartling *et al.*, 2007). Once image data has been obtained, a surgical plan is finally created wherein anatomical structures of interest are segmented and represented in a 3D scene. A variety of methods are used to identify anatomy during the planning phase. These range from manual segmentation techniques using commercial software to automated processes in custom planning tools (Noble *et al.*, 2010; Zheng *et al.*, 2010). Additionally, automatic generation of optimal tunnel trajectories is also performed (Balachandran *et al.*, 2010).

Once the planning phase has been completed, the tunnel procedure is performed using assistive technologies to ensure optimal accuracy. The two leading techniques utilize either mechanical templates or CNC robots to provide the precise positioning that is required. Templates are typically

Table 7.2 Comparison of main error sources between standard IGS and the goal for DCA

Error source	Imaging	Planning	Registration	Navigation	Overall
Measurement	Voxel	Voxel	TFE	RMS	TRE
Unit	mm	mm	mm	mm	mm
IGS	0.50	0.25	0.76	0.25	1–2*
DCA	0.15	0.07	0.2–0.3	0.10	0.5–0.8

*(Li *et al.*, 2002; Haidegger *et al.*, 2009)

patient-specific (custom-machined) guides which constrain the drill axis according to the trajectory defined in the preoperative plan. Such templates are designed to mount directly to special bone-anchored fiducial marker screws which effectively provide automatic registration (Majdani *et al.*, 2009; Warren *et al.*, 2007). In contrast, CNC robots provide a more flexible alternative in terms of altering the drill trajectory, the ability to mill implant-specific cavities, or even drill multiple trajectories (multiple electrodes). To date, most research in this area has revolved around the use of industrial robots to accurately perform the drilling procedure. Baron *et al.* (2010) in Hannover were the first to attempt such a procedure and used a Kuka KR3 (Fig. 7.8) light industrial robot to drill a DCA in temporal bone specimens. Interestingly, this study used a basic visual servoing technique to correct the tool pose. The poses of the robot base, tool and patient were measured in the camera coordinate system. Next, an error signal calculated from the difference between the current tool pose and the desired tool pose is transformed to the robot base coordinate system and sent to the robot controller. The target accuracy of this system was reported as 0.78±0.29 mm. This group also performed a similar study in collaboration with Vanderbilt University, USA, with each site building their own robotic system for comparison of final accuracies (Baron *et al.*, 2010). The technical accuracy of these two systems was evaluated by drilling into a technical phantom which was registered and tracked automatically (based on predefined marker locations, which were verified with a caliper), thus effectively excluding errors owing to imaging and registration. Accuracies of the two systems were reported based on the

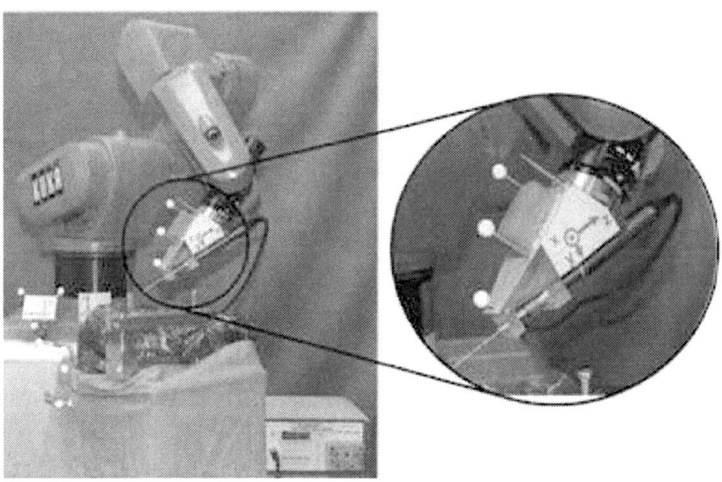

7.8 The Kuka KR3 robotic system for direct cochlear access uses optical navigation for correction of the tool tip position and achieves a target accuracy of 78±0.29 mm (photo courtesy of Dr Majdani, Medical University of Hannover).

spatial variation of the exit point (point where drill bit leaves the phantom) relative to the target point. The reported accuracy (maximum error for 99% confidence interval) of the Hannover device was 0.624 mm compared with 0.893 mm for the Vanderbilt system.

Although these studies show good technical accuracy, they are not well adapted to use in the OR owing to the bulky/heavy nature of the industrial devices. A purpose-built robot system developed recently at the University of Bern contrasts these systems with its smaller workspace and substantially reduced weight (Bell *et al.*, 2012). In addition to achieving the required technical accuracy, the secondary goal of this project was to create a robotic system that can be easily integrated into existing ORs and workflows in terms of setup, space requirements and interaction methodologies. The robot is designed to mount directly to the rails present on surgical tables, which reduces the possibility of motion between the robot and patient, as well as removing the need for a mounting platform, which would occupy additional floor space (Fig. 7.9).

Similarly to the Hannover and Vanderbilt systems, the Bern system also includes an optical tracking system. The high-precision optical camera (Cambar B1, Axios GmbH, Germany) measures marker positions with an accuracies up to 10–15 μm, depending on the hardware configuration and

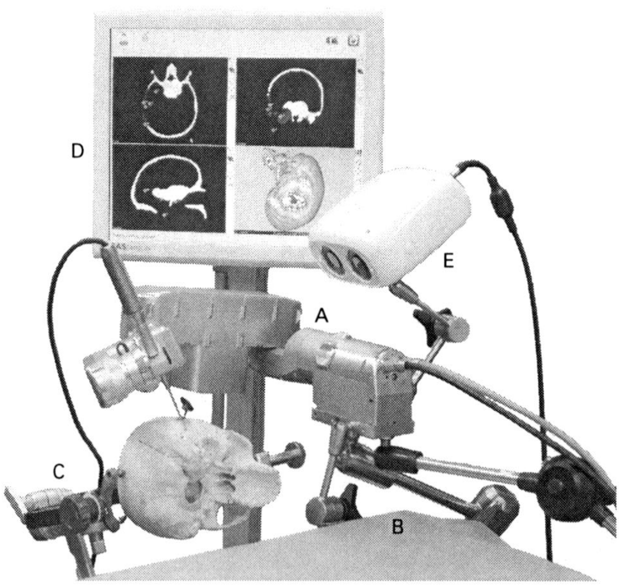

7.9 Mockup of the ENT robot system developed at the University of Bern showing the robot (A) mounted to the OR table (B) rails, the skull fixed in a Mayfield clamp (C), the navigation system user interface (D) and, finally, the high-precision optical tracking camera (E).

environmental variables. The small workspace (15 cm × 15 cm × 15 cm) and close working distance (15–30 cm) make mounting the camera directly to the robot base an ideal solution which prevents line-of-sight problems. Finally, the optical navigation system can function in either a supervisory role that only monitors the tool position, or it may provide the error signal for visual servoing. Figure 7.8 shows the proposed setup in the OR with the navigation system, DCA robot, and rigidly mounted skull model.

A lack of suitable clinically acceptable markers motivated the development of a new set of devices which can be used in the OR. In addition to the clinical practicality, the tracking accuracy, sensitivity, and camera refresh rate were also considered important factors. In the end, active LED trackers were chosen because of their faster tracking rate and superb accuracy (Fig. 7.10).

Testing of the Bern device was performed under 'clinic-like' conditions in order to account for all possible error sources. In this study, 15 DCAs were performed on whole head cadaver specimens. To begin, each case was fitted with four titanium fiducial screws and scanned using flat-panel CT. Next, a patient-specific drill trajectory was created, and the plan including digitized screw locations was transferred to the navigation platform, which guides the surgeon through the registration and drilling processes.

Following drilling, a postoperative DVT image was acquired and coregistered to the preoperative plan to enable direct comparison of planned and achieved trajectories. The results of this study showed that errors at the skull entry and target points were similar to previous results as shown in Table 7.3.

Milling of implant beds

An additional advantage of robotic devices in ORL surgery is the realization of implant-specific and exact milling operations. This ability is particularly useful for the direct acoustical cochlear stimulator (DACS), which is an electromechanical device that delivers a vibratory impulse directly to the intracochlear fluid. The placement of this device relative to the cochlea is important in order to ensure maximal signal conduction. This strict requirement of accurate placement further lengthens the implantation procedure up to 3 hours longer than the more common cochlear implant insertion. Thus, the ability to mill cavities into the bone in which an implant would fit perfectly would drastically reduce the time and effort needed for this procedure. The feasibility of this concept was evaluated by conducting all of the normal IGS planning steps on a plastic temporal bone model, and then milling an implant-specific geometry with the robot system as shown in Fig. 7.11. Though the cavity was successfully milled, one major problem with this approach was the poor performance of the milling burs, which are designed for manual

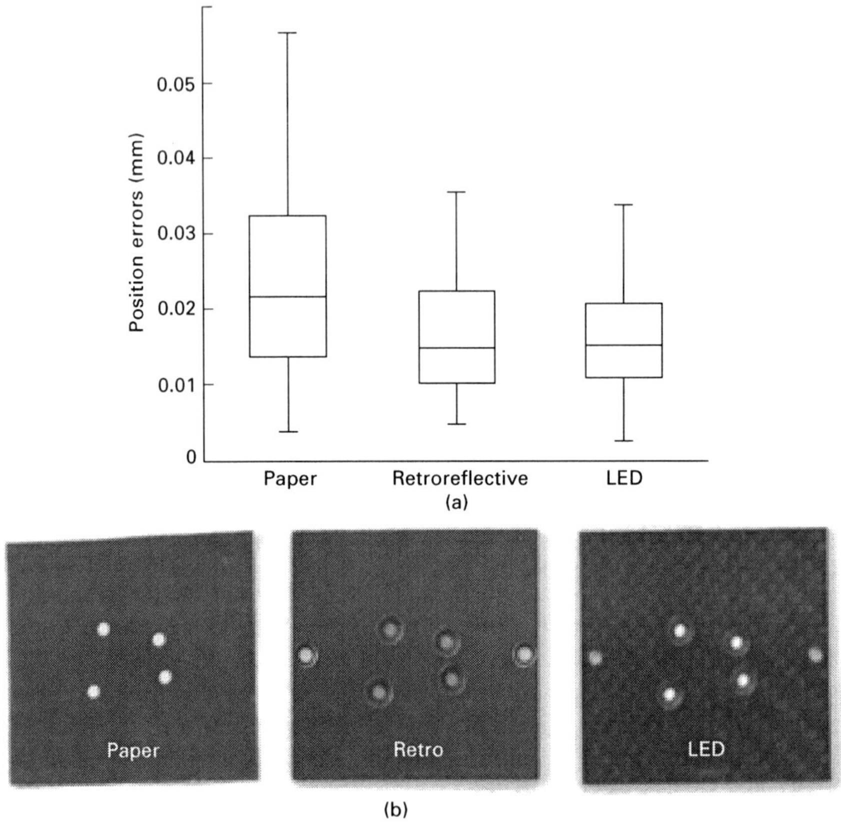

7.10 (a) The Euclidian distance errors of paper, retroreflective (retro) material, and active LED locators as measured by the Axios Cambar B1 camera. Though the absolute accuracy and variability of the retro and LED locators are similar, the acquisition rate is greatly improved for the active case. (b) Each locator has the same mask dimensions (2 mm diameter holes) for an unbiased accuracy measurement.

Table 7.3 Comparison of results from various attempts at direct cochlear access, including traditional IGS (hand-guided), template-based, and robot-assisted procedures

Author/year	Model	Error at target mm	Robot
Schipper *et al.* (2004)	Cadaver	1.6	Hand-guided
Labadie *et al.* (2005)	Temporal bone	Not reported	Hand-guided
Labadie *et al.* (2009)	Temporal bone	0.36±0.18	Template
Majdani *et al.* (2009)	Temporal bone	0.78±0.29	Kuka KR3
Klenzner *et al.* (2009)	Temporal bone	0.25 (virtual)	Staeubli RX90CR
Baron *et al.* (2010)	Phantom	0.62±0.25	Kuka KR3, MitsubishiRV-3S
Stieger *et al.* (2011)	Cadaver	2±0.64	Custom Built
Bell *et al.* (2012)	Cadaver	0.56±0.41	Custom Built

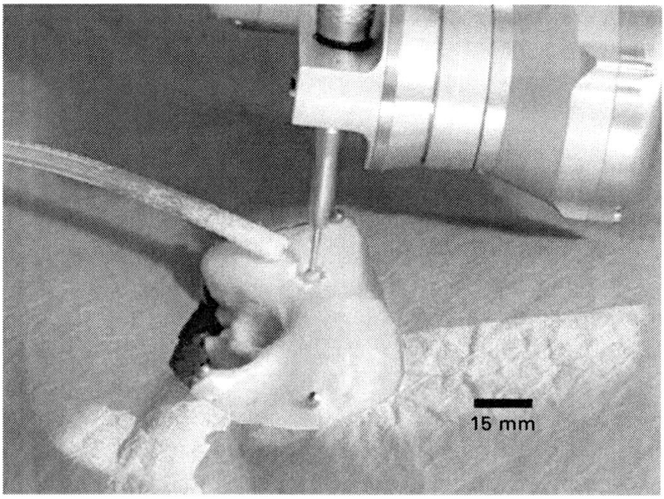

7.11 An implant cavity milled precisely by a robotic manipulator assists the surgeon in placing the implant in a predetermined location and orientation, thus reducing the overall surgical time, and improving surgical outcome.

use. Improved cutting geometries specific to bone and mechanical milling will certainly improve the outcome in terms of procedure time (40 minutes for milling at present).

Automated cochleostomy

Once a mastoidectomy (DCA) has been created, a cochlear implant is typically inserted through a cochleostomy, which is a small diameter hole drilled through the bony shell of the cochlea. It is thought that penetrating the underlying endosteum with a surgical drill can further damage sensitive hair cells, and have a significant impact on residual hearing. Thus, the goal of a study by Coulson *et al.* (2008) was to create an autonomous drill that could detect the breakthrough as the drill approaches the endosteum. In this study, a 1 DoF custom actuator simply advances the drill along its axis. The drill tool was mounted to the OR table via an adjustable arm. The position of the cochleostomy was adjusted by manually positioning the base of the drill actuator relative to the skull. The device also included a force–torque sensor, which measured axial and torsional forces as the drill is advanced to detect the breakthrough event. Specifically, as the drill approached the boundary of the bony shell, the axial portion of the cutting forces was reduced as the tip left the bone. A concomitant increase in torsion was also measured as the sides of the cutting tool removed more material. Of the five porcine cochleae drilled in this manner, all remained leak free and the endosteum was visible. These results indicated that tool forces can be used to accurately predict bony cavity penetration.

Array insertion

The final stage in the cochlear implantation procedure is the insertion of the electrode array through the cochleostomy into the cochlear space. This stage has the highest probability of damaging the internal structures of the cochlea and thus compromising residual hearing. Though most of the advancements in insertion technology have focused on optimizing the electrode design (advance off-stylet electrodes, steerable electrodes) to reduce insertion-induced trauma, additional effort is dedicated to automatic insertion tools. A robotic approach to electrode insertion developed by Zhang *et al.* (2010) combines linear actuation with a one DoF steerable electrode. With this device the group was able to show a reduction of insertion force of up to 20 g. A later version from the same group included two additional linear DoF and one rotational DoF to reduce the insertion force to less than 1 g (Hussong *et al.*, 2010).

In contrast to developing a steerable array, a second development created by Hussong *et al.* (2010) optimized the insertion of advance off-stylet electrodes. This device, Fig. 7.12, utilizes two linear actuators to control the insertion depth and stylet position independently during the insertion process. Rather than relying solely on force feedback data, this device controls the insertion depth and relative stylet position based on a mathematical model describing the internal shape of the cochlea in relation to the insertion point. Furthermore, the authors also indicate that the addition of force measurements would allow the process to be further optimized or aborted should the conditions warrant. Only intraoperative fluoroscopy and postoperative CT data were used to evaluate the effectiveness of the insertion device and the results indicated that 29/30 electrodes were successfully inserted 410° into a cochlea phantom, and a 17/20 success rate for a temporal bone specimen with an average insertion angle of 310°. Interestingly, such insertion tools could be integrated into robotic systems used for DCA drilling. This would benefit the surgeon by enabling high-precision placement and insertion for reduced trauma and increased residual hearing.

7.5 Conclusions

Though skull-base robot-assisted surgery is still in its infancy, significant progress has been made in determining its feasibility and identifying potential problems and drawbacks. As in all medicine, caution is certainly in order and a blind acceptance of new technology on grounds of 'progress' alone is foolhardy. Outside of technical feasibility, safety and overall improvement

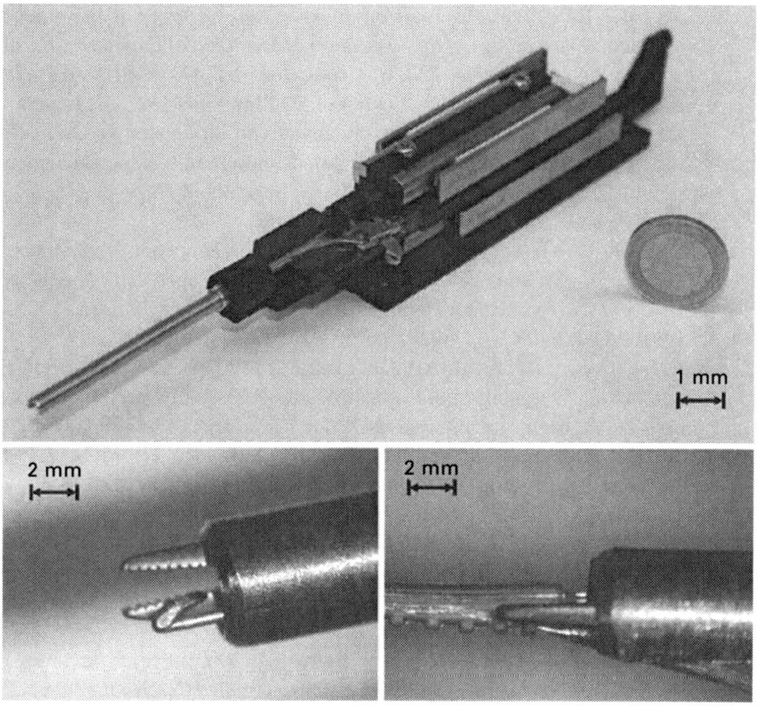

7.12 Automatic advance off-stylet electrode insertion tool (reprinted with permission from Hussong *et al.*, 2010).

of treatment costs in terms of time and equipment are also important issues to consider. The limited research to date suggests that robot-assisted interventions are likely to expend more time and capital, though they may improve outcomes to a degree that would justify the additional expenditure. Though a large portion of the research is focused on evaluating the currently most widely accepted robot, the da Vinci telemanipulator, more effort is being directed at procedure-specific devices (University of Bern DCA robot) which will ultimately be able to assist surgeons at a very high level. Finally, the absence of any commercially available robotic system specific to ENT surgery and the high accuracies needed to safely intervene in this region suggest that ample opportunities for further developments exist.

7.6 References

Balachandran, R, Mitchell, JE, Blachon, G, Noble, JH, Dawant, BM, Fitzpatrick, JM, and Labadie, RF (2010). Percutaneous cochlear implant drilling via customized frames: An in vitro study. *Otolaryngology – Head and Neck Surgery*, **142**, 421–426, doi:10.1016/j.otohns.2009.11.029.

Baron, S, Eilers, H, Munske, B, Toennies, J, Balachandran, R, Labadie, R, Ortmaier, T, and Webster, RT (2010). Percutaneous inner-ear access via an image-guided industrial robot system. *Proceedings of the Institution of Mechanical Engineers, Part H: Journal of Engineering in Medicine*, **224**, 633–649, doi:10.1243/09544119JEIM781.

Bartling, SH, Leinung, M, Graute, J, Rodt, T, Dullin, C, Becker, H, Lenarz, T, Stover, T, and Majdani, O (2007). Increase of accuracy in intraoperative navigation through high-resolution flat-panel volume computed tomography: experimental comparison with multislice computed tomography-based navigation. *Otology & Neurotology*, **28**, 129, doi:10.1097/01.mao.0000244364.16826.09.

Bell, B, Stieger, C, Gerber, N, Arnold, A, Nauer, C, Hamacher, V, Kompis, M, Nolte, L, Caoersaccio, M, and Weber, S (2012). A self-developed and constructed robot for minimally invasive cochlear implantation. *Acta Oto-laryngologica*, **132**, 355–360, d oi:10.3109/00016489.2011.642813.

Coulson, CJ, Taylor, RP, Reid, AP, Griffiths, MV, Proops, DW, and Brett, PN (2008). An autonomous surgical robot for drilling a cochleostomy: preliminary porcine trial. *Clinical Otolaryngology*, **33**, 343–347, doi:10.1111/j.1749-4486.2008.01703.x.

Camarillo, DB, Krummel, TM, and Salisbury, JK (2004). Robotic technology in surgery: past, present, and future. *The American Journal of Surgery*, **188**, 2–15, doi:S0002-9610(04)00375-7.

Eichhorn, KW, Tingelhoff, K, Wagner, I, Westphal, R, Rilk, M, Kunkel, M, Wahl, FM, and Bootz, F (2008). Evaluation of force data with a force/torque sensor during FESS. A step towards robot-assisted surgery. HNO, **56**, 789, doi:10.1007/s00106-007-1647-0.

Haidegger, T, Kovacs, L, Benyo, B, and Benyo, Z (2009). Spatial accuracy of surgical robots. *SACI'09. 5th International Symposium on Applied Computational Intelligence and Informatics*, pp. 133–138. Timisoara, Romania, doi:10.1109/SACI.2009.5136227.

Haidegger, T, Xia, T, and Kazanzides, P (2008). Accuracy improvement of a neurosurgical robot system. *2nd IEEE RAS & EMBS International Conference on Biomedical Robotics and Biomechatronics*, pp. 836–841, doi:10.1109/BIOROB.2008.4762912.

Hanna, EYEY, Holsinger, C, DeMonte, F, and Kupferman, M (2007). Robotic endoscopic surgery of the skull base: a novel surgical approach. *Archives of Otolaryngology – Head & Neck Surgery*, **133**, 1209–1214, doi:10.1001/archotol.133.12.1209

Hofer, M, Dittrich, E, Scholl, C, Neumuth, T, Strauss, M, Dietz, A, Lüth, T, Strauss, G (2008). First clinical evaluation of the navigated controlled drill at the lateral skull base. *Studies in Health Technology and Informatics*, **132**, 171–173.

Hussong, A, Rau, TS, Ortmaier, T, Heimann, B, Lenarz, T, and Majdani, O (2010). An automated insertion tool for cochlear implants: another step towards atraumatic cochlear implant surgery. *International Journal of Computer Assisted Radiology and Surgery*, **5**, 163–171, doi:10.1007/s11548-009-0368-0.

Klenzner, T, Ngan, CCC, Knapp, FBB, Knoop, H, Kromeier, J, Aschendorff, A, Papastathopoulos, E, Raczkowsky, J, Wörn, H, and Schipper, J (2009). New strategies for high precision surgery of the temporal bone using a robotic approach for cochlear implantation. *European Archives of Oto-Rhino-Laryngology*, **266**, 955–960, doi:10.1007/s00405-008-0825-3.

Koulechov, K, Strauss, G, Dietz, A, Strauss, M, Hofer, M, and Lueth, TC (2006). FESS control: realization and evaluation of navigated control for functional endoscopic sinus surgery. *Computer Aided Surgery: Official Journal of the International Society for Computer Aided Surgery*, **11**, 147–159, doi:10.3109/10929080600750789.

Labadie, RF, Mitchell, J, Balachandran, R, and Fitzpatrick, JM (2009). Customized, rapid-production microstereotactic table for surgical targeting: description of concept and in vitro validation. *International Journal of Computer Assisted Radiology and Surgery*, **4**, 273–280, doi:10.1007/s11548-009-0292-3.

Labadie, RF, Chodhury, P, Cetinkaya, E, Balachandran, R, Haynes, DS, Fenlon, MR, Jusczyzck, S, and Fitzpatrick, JM (2005). Minimally invasive, image-guided, facial-recess approach to the middle ear: demonstration of the concept of percutaneous cochlear access in vitro. *Otology & Neurotology*, **26**, 557–562.

Li, QH, Zamorano, L, Pandya, A, Perez, R, Gong, J, and Diaz, F (2002). The application accuracy of the NeuroMate robot. A quantitative comparison with frameless and frame-based surgical localization systems. *Computer Aided Surgery*, **7**, 90–98, doi:10.1002/igs.10035.

Majdani, O, Bartling, SH, Leinung, M, Stöver, T, Lenarz, M, Dullin, C, and Lenarz, T (2008). A true minimally invasive approach for cochlear implantation: high accuracy in cranial base navigation through flat-panel-based volume computed tomography. *Otology & Neurotology*, **29**, 120, doi:10.1097/mao.0b013e318157f7d8.

Majdani, O, Rau, TS, Baron, S, Eilers, H, Baier, C, Heimann, B, Ortmaier, T, Bartling, S, Lenarz, T, and Leinung, M (2009). A robot-guided minimally invasive approach for cochlear implant surgery: preliminary results of a temporal bone study. *International Journal of Computer Assisted Radiology and Surgery*, **4**, 475–486, doi:10.1007/s11548-009-0360-8.

Miroir, M, Nguyen, Y, Şzewczyk, J, Mazalaigue, S, Ferrary, E, Sterkers, O, and Grayeli, AB (2010). RobOtol: from design to evaluation of a robot for middle ear surgery. *Design*, 850–856, doi: 10.1109/IROS.2010.5650390.

Noble, JH, Majdani, O, Labadie, RF, Dawant, B, and Fitzpatrick, JM (2010). Automatic determination of optimal linear drilling trajectories for cochlear access accounting for drill-positioning error. *The International Journal of Medical Robotics and Computer Assisted Surgery*, **6**, 281–290, doi:10.1002/rcs.330.

Noble, JH, Warren, FM, Labadie, RF, Dawant, B, and Fitzpatrick, JM (2007). Determination of drill paths for percutaneous cochlear access accounting for target positioning error. *Proceedings of SPIE*, 650925-650925-10. doi:10.1117/12.709605.

Obando, MA, and Payne, JH (2003). The future application of the robotic arm (automatic endoscopic system for optimal positioning or AESOP) with voice recognition in sinus endoscopic surgery. *IX World Congress of Rhinology, Washington, DC* (Vol. **14**, pp. 55–57), Washington DC: Elsevier. doi:10.1016/S1043-1810(03)90043-1.

Obando, M, Liem, L, Madauss, W, Morita, M, and Robinson, B (2004). Robotic surgery in pituitary tumors. *Operative Techniques in Otolaryngology – Head and Neck Surgery*, **15**, 147–149, doi:10.1016/j.otot.2004.02.009.

Park, YM, Lee, WJ, Lee, JG, Lee, WS, Choi, EC, Chung, SM, and Kim, S-H (2009). Transoral robotic surgery (TORS) in laryngeal and hypopharyngeal cancer. *Journal of Laparoendoscopic & Advanced Surgical Techniques. Part A*, **19**, 361–368, doi:10.1089/lap.2008.0320.

Rahbar, R, Ferrari, LR, Borer, JG, and Peters, CA (2007). Robotic surgery in the pediatric airway: application and safety. *Archives of Otolaryngology Head Neck Surgery*, **133**, 46–50; discussion 50.

Schipper, J, Aschendorff, A, Arapakis, I, Klenzner, T, Teszler, CB, Ridder, GJ, and Laszig, R (2004). Navigation as a quality management tool in cochlear implant surgery. *The Journal of Laryngology and Otology*, **118**, 764–770, doi:10.1258/0022215042450643.

Solares, CA, and Strome, M (2007). Transoral robot-assisted CO_2 laser supraglottic laryngectomy: experimental and clinical data. *The Laryngoscope*, **117**, 817–820, doi:10.1097/MLG.0b013e31803330b7.

Stieger, C, Caversaccio, M, Arnold, A, Zheng, G, Salzmann, J, Widmer, D, Gerber, N, Thurner, M, Nauer, C, Mussard, Y, Kompis, M, Nolte, LP, Häusler, R, and Weber, S (2011). Development of an auditory implant manipulator for minimally invasive surgical insertion of implantable hearing devices. *The Journal of Laryngology and Otology*, **125**, 1–9, doi:10.1017/S0022215110002185.

Strauss, G, Dittrich, E., Baumberger, C., Hofer, M, Strauss, M, Stopp, S, Koulechov, K, Dietz, A and Luth, T (2008). [Improvement of registration accuracy for navigated-control drill in mastoidectomy (autopilot)]. *Laryngo- rhino- otologie*, **87**, 560–564, doi:10.1055/s-2007-995629.

Strauss, G, Winkler, D, Jacobs, S, Trantakis, C, Dietz, A, Bootz, F, Meixensberger, J and Falk, V (2005a). [Mechatronic in functional endoscopic sinus surgery. First experiences with the daVinci Telemanipulatory System]. *HNO*, **53**, 623–630, doi:10.1007/s00106-005-1242-1.

Strauss, M, Olze, H, and Lueth, T (2005b). Accuracy analysis of cavities for cochlea implants milled conventionally and manually with navigated control. *International Congress Series*, **1281**, 553–558, doi:10.1016/j.ics.2005.03.168.

Taylor, R (1997). Robots as surgical assistants: where we are, wither we are tending, and how to get there. In Keraunou, E, Garbay, C, Baud, R, and Wyatt, J (Eds), *Artificial intelligence in medicine*, **1211**, pp. 1–11, Springer Berlin/Heidelberg.

Wagner, I, Tingelhoff, K, Westphal, R, Kunkel, ME, Wahl, F, Bootz, F, and Eichhorn, K (2008). Ex vivo evaluation of force data and tissue elasticity for robot-assisted FESS. *European Archives of Otorhinolaryngology*, **265**, 1335–1339, doi: 10.1007/s00405-008-0644-6.

Warren, FM, Balachandran, R, Fitzpatrick, JM, and Labadie, RF (2007). Percutaneous cochlear access using bone-mounted, customized drill guides: demonstration of concept in vitro. *Otology & Neurotology*, **28**, 325–329, doi:10.1097/01.mao.0000253287.86737.2e.

Wurm, J, Dannenmann, T, Bohr, C, Iro, H, and Bumm, K (2005). Increased safety in robotic paranasal sinus and skull base surgery with redundant navigation and automated registration. *The International Journal of Medical Robotics Computer Assisted Surgery MRCAS*, **1**, 42–48.

Zhang, J, Wei, W, Ding, J, Roland, JT, Manolidis, S, and Simaan, N (2010). Inroads toward robot-assisted cochlear implant surgery using steerable electrode arrays. *Otology & neurotology*, 31, 1199–206, doi:10.1097/MAO.0b013e3181e7117e.

Zheng, G, Gerber, N, Widmer, D, Stieger, C, Caversaccio, M, Nolte, L-P, and Weber, S (2010). Automated detection of fiducial screws from CT/DVT volume data for image-guided ENT surgery. *IEEE Engineering in Medicine and Biology Society Conference*, **1**, 2325-2328, doi:10.1109/IEMBS.2010.5627459.

8
Robot-assisted vitreoretinal surgery

H. C. M. MEENINK, R. HENDRIX, G. J. L. NAUS, M. J. BEELEN, H. NIJMEIJER and M. STEINBUCH, Eindhoven University of Technology, The Netherlands, E. J. G. M. VAN OOSTERHOUT, Catherina Hospital Eindhoven, The Netherlands and M. D. DE SMET, Montchoisi Clinic, Switzerland and University of Amsterdam, The Netherlands

Abstract: To improve the time efficiency of current vitreoretinal surgical procedures and to enable new procedures demanding increased accuracy, a robotic system to assist in vitreoretinal procedures has been developed, extending human capabilities beyond current limitations. The robotic master–slave system is compact, lightweight and easy to set up. A combination of high-precision mechanical design and high-performance controller synthesis facilitates high accuracy down to 10 μm, tremor filtering, motion scaling, automated instrument changing an ergonomic body posture for the surgeon and haptic feedback. First functional tests with the demonstrator system show a short setup time, an intuitive usage and good ergonomics. With a knife and a pick, a successful peel of the inner shell membrane of the chorioallantoic membrane of a chicken egg has been achieved.

Key words: eye surgery, vitreoretinal surgery, robot-assisted surgery, master–slave system, haptic feedback.

8.1 Introduction

Currently, approximately 37 million people in the world are completely blind and a further 124 million have some sort of visual impairment. Reduced vision substantially impacts the quality of life of patients because it can severely limit their participation in society, ability to work and mobility, imposing a huge burden on society (Langelaan *et al.*, 2007). For many diseases of the eye, surgery is the only adequate treatment to improve vision or to prevent further decline in visual acuity and blindness. In eye surgery, the accuracy required to perform the procedures is particularly challenging. It is close to or even beyond what humans can achieve. This is especially true for vitreoretinal surgery that involves the manipulation of tissues in the back of the eye, with a required accuracy smaller than 0.1 mm or 100 μm. These problems can be overcome by introducing robot assistance to vitreoretinal surgery.

The surgical management of the vitreous humour, the retina, and the underlying structures is grouped under the heading vitreoretinal surgery. An estimated 900 000 vitreoretinal procedures are performed worldwide each year, treating diseases such as retinal detachments, vitreous hemorrhages, and a variety of retinal pathologies such as epiretinal membrane, macular hole and vitreomacular traction. Human manual accuracy, which is of the order of 125 μm, is limiting further exploration of vitreoretinal treatments (Riviere *et al.*, 1997). Surgical treatment of common conditions such as retinal vein occlusion (RVO), which is among the major causes of visual impairment and blindness (Berker and Batman, 2009; Ueta *et al.*, 2009), requires an accuracy of the order of 10 μm. For a human surgeon, this is practically impossible at this time. Robot-assisted surgery can reduce the incidence of complications and, hence, enhance treatment outcomes for all established vitreoretinal surgical procedures, while enabling new procedures.

Currently, there is no robotic solution commercially available that meets the accuracy and dexterity required for vitreoretinal surgery. There are a few scientific initiatives addressing this topic, coming from the University of Tokyo (Ueta *et al.*, 2009), Johns Hopkins University (Mitchell, 2007) and Columbia University (Fine, 2010). An overview of the identified initiatives is given in Table 8.1. All initiatives claim micrometer accuracy and most of them incorporate force feedback in their system. The project at the University

Table 8.1 Initiatives on robot-assisted vitreoretinal eye surgery

Institute	System	Force feedback	Accuracy (μm)	Operating region	Status
Eindhoven University of Technology	Master and slave robot	Yes	<10	90° × 90°	Starting validation and user tests
University of Tokyo	Master and slave robot	Scaling 40×	30	90° × 40°	Focus is on brain surgery rather than eye surgery
Johns Hopkins University and Carnegie Mellon	Handheld tool for tremor filtering, and slave robot	Scaling 10–100×	5	60° × 60° 3.0 mm × 3.0 mm × 0.8 mm	*Ex vivo* cannulation on chicken egg chorioallantoic membranes; *ex vivo* artificial membrane peeling (robot controlled)
Columbia University	Slave robot	No	<5	40° × 40°	No public test results
KAIST	Slave robot	Yes	50	20 mm × 20 mm × 20 mm	Current status unknown

Source: Meenink, 2011.

of Tokyo focuses on microsurgery in general rather than eye surgery; the resulting instrument manipulating slave robot measures 1.0 × 0.5 × 0.4 m, which is relatively large. The Johns Hopkins University project, dedicated to vitreoretinal eye surgery, progressed rapidly and achieved several milestones, having performed multiple *ex vivo* tests. The developments were partitioned into two separate projects; first a manually held instrument with built-in actuators and sensors compensating hand tremor, initially developed by Carnegie Mellon and, second, a computer-controlled instrument manipulator, which can also be used as a supporting arm, allowing instruments to be kept in a fixed position.

In close collaboration with several vitreoretinal surgeons, a robotic system that is dedicated to vitreoretinal surgery has been designed by Eindhoven University of Technology (TU/e), Control Systems Technology group and Dynamics and Control group, supported by University of Amsterdam's Academic Medical Centre (AMC), Department of Ophthalmology, and TNO (Hendrix, 2011; Meenink, 2011). The vitreoretinal surgical system has been realized as a proof-of-concept demonstrator, which is depicted in Fig. 8.1. As per January 2012, integration of the demonstrator systems as depicted is being completed, including electronics and software functionality.

The main advantage of the developments at the TU/e compared with the other initiatives in Table 8.1 are the combination of both a dedicated master and slave robot, the integrated solution for mounting the system to the operating table, including compactness, ease of installation and integrated electronics. Additional advantages include the possibility of performing an entire vitreoretinal intervention as opposed to only sections, and the availability of an automated instrument-changing system.

In Section 8.2, the requirements for robot-assisted vitreoretinal surgery are discussed, leading to the design of the master console (Section 8.3) and the slave manipulator (Section 8.4) of which proof-of-concept demonstrators have been realised. In Section 8.5, integration of the demonstrator system and the first functional tests are discussed. The chapter closes with conclusions and future work (Section 8.7).

8.2 Requirements for vitreoretinal surgery

The characteristics of vitreoretinal surgery are now described followed by an examination of user needs and an overview of the robotic system.

8.2.1 Vitreoretinal surgery

Vitreoretinal surgery is a form of minimally invasive surgery (MIS), which is widely used in abdominal and thoracic surgery as an alternative to traditional open surgery because it minimizes trauma and facilitates fast recovery.

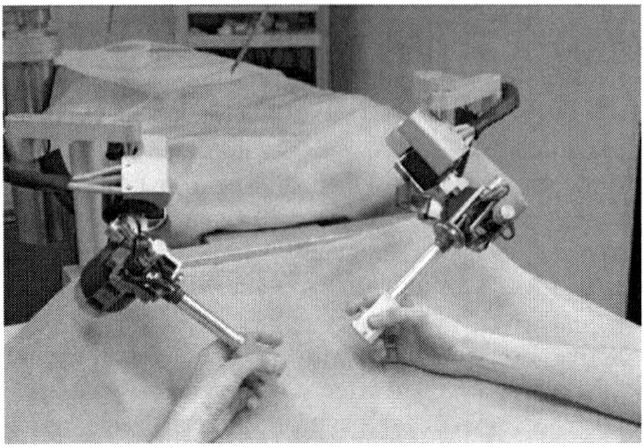

(a)

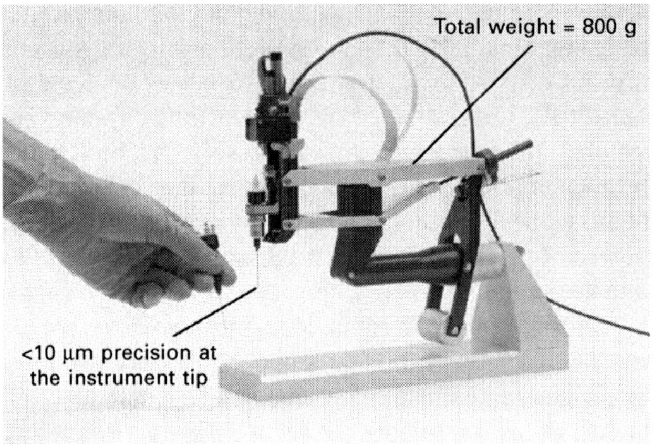

(b)

8.1 Master control interface operated by (a) the surgeon and (b) the robotic slave instrument manipulator.

The instruments are introduced into the eye through surgeon-made scleral openings, often fitted with a cannula. The instruments are about 30 mm in length, with a diameter of 27 to 20 gauge (0.41 to 0.91 mm, respectively). The small scleral openings induce only a small amount of trauma, resulting in a short recovery time and minimizing the chance of infection (Raja *et al.*, 2010; Rizzo *et al.*, 2006, 2009). By using instruments with a diameter smaller than 23 gauge (0.64 mm) and using specific incision techniques (Rizzo *et al.*, 2009), postoperative suturing becomes superfluous.

To fully benefit from the advantages of this type of surgery, it is preferred to apply the least amount of force on the scleral openings during surgery and thus, minimize the stress on the sclera. Therefore, instruments must

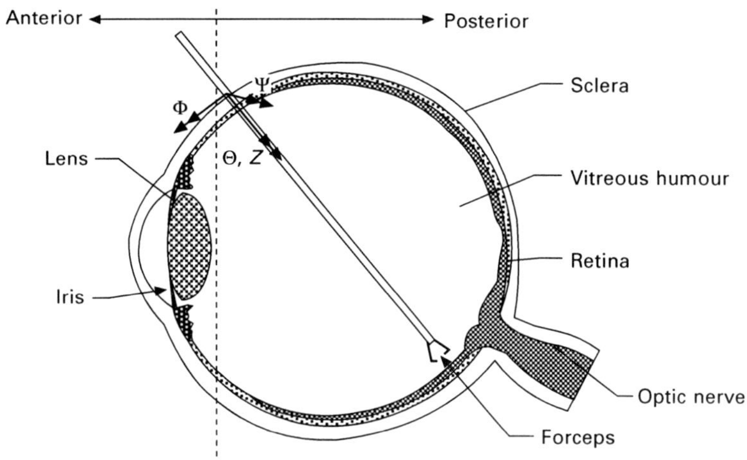

8.2 Anatomy of the human eye and a vitreoretinal instrument. Surgery can be performed to the anterior as well as the posterior side of the eye. An instrument can be manipulated in four degrees of freedom through the surgeon-made scleral opening: three rotations Φ, Ψ and Θ, and one translation in axial direction *Z*. The closing of a forceps is an additional degree of freedom.

be manipulated about the scleral openings, which act as pivoting points where all axes of rotation/translation intersect. This leaves four degrees of freedom (DoFs) to manipulate, three rotations (Φ, Ψ and Θ) and one translation in axial direction (*Z*), Fig. 8.2. The manipulation of the instrument tip, e.g. a gripping motion, can be considered as an additional degree of freedom. As instruments are manipulated on the outside of the eye, the pivoting insertion point inverts lateral movements (Φ and Ψ rotation) and it scales the movements proportional to the insertion depth Z of the instrument.

In conventional vitreoretinal surgery, the surgeon is sitting at the top end of the surgical table in line with the patient's head, Fig. 8.3. A microscope provides stereoscopic visual feedback, which gives a 5 to 25 × magnification of the operation area. Characteristically, the manipulation of delicate intraocular tissue is required. By resting the hands on the patient's forehead, the shortest eye–instrument–hand force loop and the highest accuracy is achieved. The surgeon can only use two instruments at any given time, of which one position is usually occupied by an illumination probe, leaving only one instrument for tissue manipulation. Forces are below the human detection limit of 0.06 N, which means that surgeons must rely on visual feedback only. The use of a microscope is of great importance, but it forces the surgeon into a static and non-ergonomic body posture.

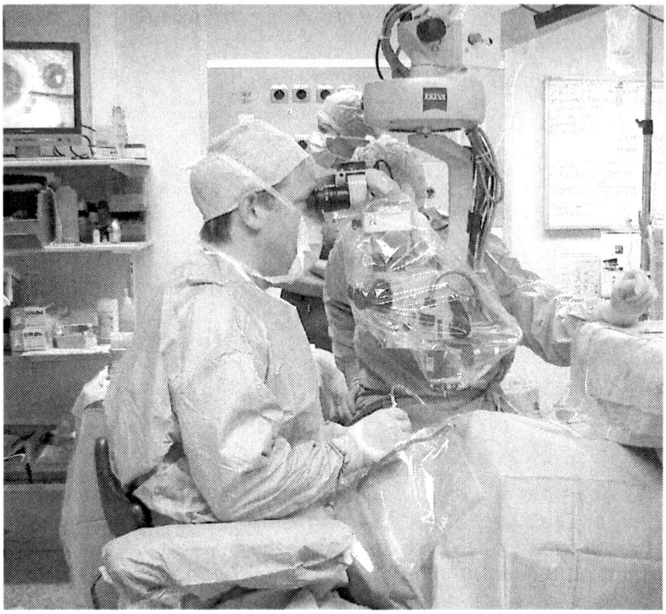

8.3 Surgeon M. D. de Smet performing vitreoretinal surgery. The surgeon is sitting at the top end of the patient (covered by sterile drapes). The microscope gives a magnified, stereoscopic view of the operation area.

Summarizing, vitreoretinal surgery is characterized by:

- small and inverted instrument movements, depending on the *Z*-insertion depth;
- manipulation of delicate, intraocular tissues with micrometer thickness;
- instrument forces below the human detection limit (visual feedback only);
- a maximum number of two instruments simultaneously used;
- a static and non-ergonomic body posture.

8.2.2 User needs

The small scale and the delicacy of structures in the eye require the highest possible accuracy to prevent any collateral damage. However, accuracy, inherent to manual operation, is very dependent on experience and can decrease over time owing to aging or fatigue. Surgeons are further challenged in their accuracy by the poor ergonomics inherent to current day vitreoretinal surgery. These limitations can have a negative impact on the outcome of the procedure. For the patient, this can mean suboptimal restoration of their visual acuity. Human manual accuracy (c. 125 µm) is also a limiting factor for surgical treatment of common conditions such as retinal vein occlusion (RVO). Robotic assistance can solve these problems by improving upon human capabilities.

RVO is a retinal vascular disorder and the third most common cause of severe visual impairment in the westernized world (Klein *et al.*, 2008; Weiss and Bynoe, 2001). Although various pharmaceutical and surgical approaches have been suggested, no effective medical treatment is currently available. Cannulation of the retinal veins requires the insertion of a microcannula in the vein that measures about 20–200 μm in diameter. As the maximum tremor of a vitreoretinal surgeon during an intraocular procedure reportedly exceeds 125 μm, this cannot be performed manually (Riviere *et al.*, 1997; Ueta *et al.*, 2009). Such accuracy is well within the range of a robotic system.

An epiretinal membrane comprises a contractile membrane formed on the retinal surface in response to mechanical stimulation, inflammation or injury. It is commonly seen in diabetic retinopathy. Vitreoretinal surgeons can treat the disease by membrane peeling, a delicate procedure that involves the separation of the epiretinal membrane from the retinal surface. Similarly, repairing a retinal detachment, as a result of which the retina disconnects from its underlying layer of supporting tissue, involves delicate manipulation. Any distortion in the movement or excessive forces applied by the surgeon can cause functional and mechanical damage to the retina and vasculature, e.g., bleeding (Terasaki *et al.*, 2001; Uemoto *et al.*, 2002; Uemura *et al.*, 2003). To prevent damage, micrometer accuracy is required when manipulating the instruments. Furthermore, haptic feedback, when employed, can help surgeons to optimally distinguish between an epiretinal membrane and the retina, enabling them to feel tissues beyond human capabilities. Decreasing the procedure time can reduce the risks for infection and light toxicity.

8.2.3 System overview

The developed system consists of a master console operated by the surgeon that controls two robotic arms (slave) that, in practice, perform the surgery (Hendrix, 2011; Meenink, 2011). A schematic overview of the various elements in the system is depicted in Fig. 8.4. The master console provides the motion reference for the instrument manipulators of the slave system. The slave system performs the actual surgery by controlling instrument manipulators that directly handle the instruments. Control comprises the electronics and software between the master and slave hardware. To improve the surgeon's ergonomy, an alternative system for the visual feedback is required.

In Fig. 8.5, an artist's impression of an optimal system is shown. As in manually performed surgery, the surgeon is sitting at the top end of the surgical table. The system is table-mounted. For bimanual operation, at least two instrument manipulators are used. Additional instrument manipulators

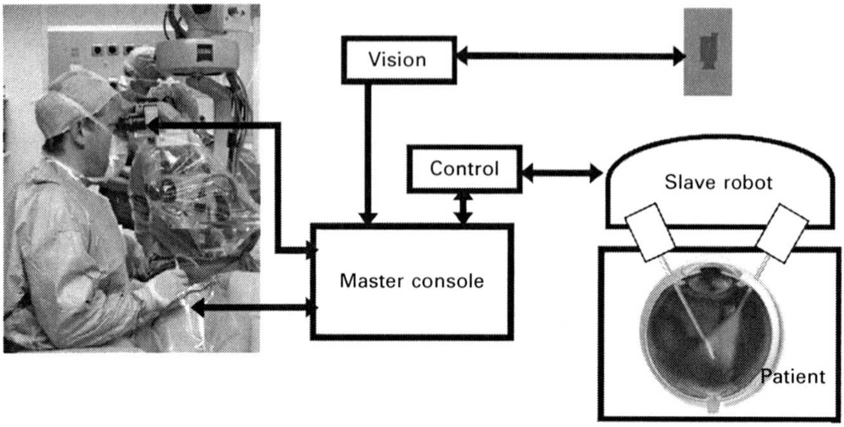

8.4 Schematic representation of the developed system.

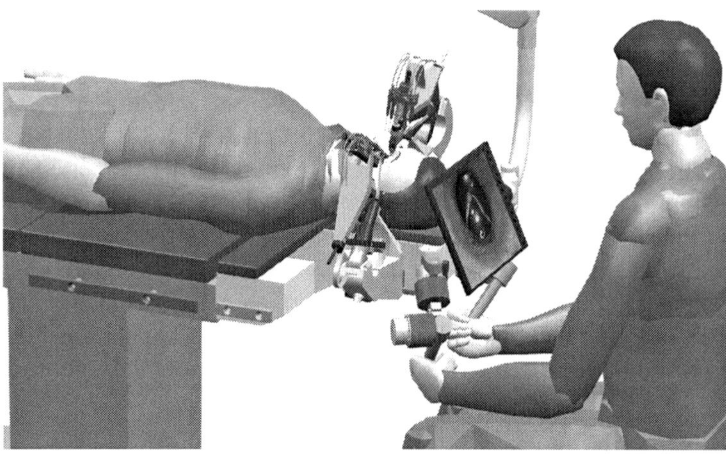

8.5 Schematic representation of a master–slave setup for vitreoretinal eye surgery. The instrument manipulators handle the instruments and are controlled by the surgeon via haptic interfaces. The passive support provides a stiff connection between the instrument manipulator, patient and surgical table.

can be used for non-active tools, e.g. an illumination probe or an endoscope. During surgery, various instruments are used interchangeably, requiring a system facilitating easy and fast instrument changes.

Presurgical adjustments are required to position the instrument manipulators over the eye. These adjustments are integrated in a support system, which is an integral part of the patient's head rest. On either the left or right side, two exchangeable manipulators can be installed onto the support system, depending on the eye being operated upon. A compact, lightweight and easy to install design allows for a short setup time and quick removal in case of a complication. The compact and table-mounted design also allows direct patient access, leaves legroom for the surgeon and allows foot switches to be used as desired.

Integrated into the support system is the master console. The main components of the master console are two haptic interfaces controlled by the surgeon and a vision system, e.g. a three-dimensional (3D) display for visual feedback. A comfortable and intuitive working environment is realized by simulating manipulation of the instrument tip inside the eye. All degrees of freedom in the master are equipped with a DC motor and an encoder/measurement system to provide accurate force feedback and position input for the instrument manipulators.

The design of the master and the slave robots are discussed in the following sections. Requirements and user needs that have been taken into account in the system design include:

- hand tremor filtering;
- filtering of sudden movements (shock, such as a shiver or cold);
- scaling and mirroring of movements;
- measurement and scaling of forces to enable force feedback;
- stand-by functionality;
- high accuracy to enable new interventions; and
- automatic instrument changing.

8.3 Master console

The master console provides an ergonomic and intuitive working environment for the surgeon. It consists of a frame with arm rest, a screen and two haptic interfaces. The console is mounted to the patient's head rest. A table-mounted device with a screen, as opposed to a microscope system, is compact, easy to place and allows the surgeon to have a direct view on and physical contact with the patient. Furthermore, the surgeon is not forced to work in a static body posture.

8.3.1 System layout

The surgeon uses the haptic interfaces for bimanual control of the instruments. As indicated in Fig. 8.2, each instrument has to be manipulated in four DoFs about the entry point and is operated by an additional DoF, e.g., for a forceps. The haptic interface must provide force feedback on all of these five DoFs. Mode switching allows the control of three or more instrument manipulators (in Fig. 8.5, only two instrument manipulators are shown) with only two haptic interfaces. As a vitrectomy procedure requires the largest range of motion, these values are taken as a design requirement for the interface.

Various haptic interfaces are commercially available, for example the Phantom© product line of SensAble Technologies (http://www.sensable.com) and the Omega and Delta devices of Force Dimension (http://www.forcedimension.com). Owing to the overall size of these devices, it is not possible to integrate them into the setup depicted in Fig. 8.5. Therefore, a dedicated and compact, stylus-based 5-DoF haptic interface was designed. Compared to commercially-available 6- or 7-DoF devices, it has fewer mechanical links and pivot points. This provides a higher stiffness and better system performance is ensured. Furthermore, it is not necessary to constrain any unused degrees of freedom.

Figure 8.6 gives a schematic representation of the stylus-based interface. It has the same degrees of freedom as the instrument inside the eye. Together with the visual feedback from the captured microscopic or endoscopic images, the surgeon perceives the action as if he/she were grasping the instrument near its tip within the eye. The similarity between the hand motion (Fig. 8.6b) and the motion of the instrument tip (Fig. 8.6a), which is shown to the surgeon on a display, results in an intuitive manipulation. The most comfortable operation is obtained when the rotation point of the stylus is placed above the surgeon's wrist. This results in a stylus length of 150–175 mm and a geometric scaling of 1:7 in lateral direction when working in the direct neighborhood of the retina.

8.3.2 Force feedback

The stylus-based interfaces of the master console are designed as haptic devices, facilitating the feedback of forces that are measured at the instrument's

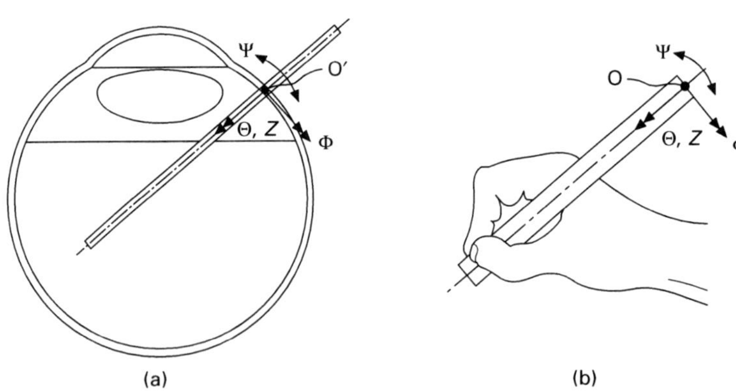

8.6 (a, b) An intuitive working environment is created by placing the hand of the surgeon virtually inside the eye. The rotation point O is placed above the surgeon's wrist and represents the entry point O′ of the instrument.

tip back to the surgeon. There are two distinct classes of haptic devices; impedance-controlled devices and admittance-controlled devices (Linde *et al.*, 2003; Hannaford and Okamura, 2008). For impedance control, a movement of the master devices is detected, e.g., via an encoder on the force feedback motor. The controller uses the positional information for a correct representation of the force and contact stiffness. For admittance control, a force sensor at the end effector tip of the haptic device measures the forces that are executed by the surgeon and a controller makes a correct movement at the end effector tip. The choice of impedance or admittance architecture influences the design requirements. In this case, an impedance-controlled device is chosen, preventing the need for expensive force and torque sensors.

Extended lists of design requirements for impedance controlled devices have been compiled (Fisher *et al.*, 1990; Hayward, 1995; Millman and Colgate, 1991; Stocco *et al.*, 2001). The five most important characteristics to be taken into account in the design are now described.

Low inertia and moving mass

A high inertia makes it more difficult for the operator to perform a specific task and can result in fatigue. System performance decreases as a function of inertia, owing to lower eigenfrequencies. This makes it, for example, more difficult to represent the high-frequency content of the force feedback.

High stiffness

The stiffness of the device is higher than the maximum tissue stiffness expected during surgery, as required for appropriate force feedback. Furthermore, it results in higher eigenfrequencies and a higher control bandwidth. Most ideal, but not pursued in this case for reasons of feasibility, is a bandwidth that equals the 1 kHz perceptual bandwidth for vibrotactile stimuli.

Low friction

Friction results in a lower force resolution because it directly interferes with the feedback of the forces as measured at the instrument. A lower friction allows a more precise manipulation of the instrument.

Backdrivability

A device without force measurement at the end effector must be backdrivable. This means that the drive train must employ relatively low gear ratios.

Zero backlash

Backlash results in control instabilities. Furthermore, it has a negative effect on performance as the slave does not instantaneously follow when the master device changes direction of movement. A direct drive or a preloaded transmission avoids backlash.

8.3.3 Mechanical design

The haptic interface consists of four modules by which the surgeon manipulates the stylus: a Φ housing, a Ψ housing, a Z–Θ module and a button part (Fig. 8.7). The allocation of the different DoFs is according to the instrument movements during surgery. For example, the Z movement and the Θ rotation are always along the centerline of the instrument. Therefore, they are placed after the Φ and the Ψ rotation in the kinematic chain (Fig. 8.7). Actuation of the Z and the Θ DoF is done in a parallel way. The other three DoFs are placed in a serial kinematic layout. Although it is not strictly necessary, this layout complies with the kinematic layout of the slave robot, which simplifies the master–slave control algorithms.

The mechanical design of the Φ and the Ψ module is almost identical. The core of each of these modules is a frameless and brushless DC motor, which is glued inside a compact housing. The brushless motors are placed in the direct neighborhood of the rotation point to have the lowest contribution to the system inertia. An analog current amplifier with sinusoidal commutation prevents any torque ripple. Each housing is fitted with two deep grove ball bearings to support the motor shaft. A spring pre-tensions the bearings to

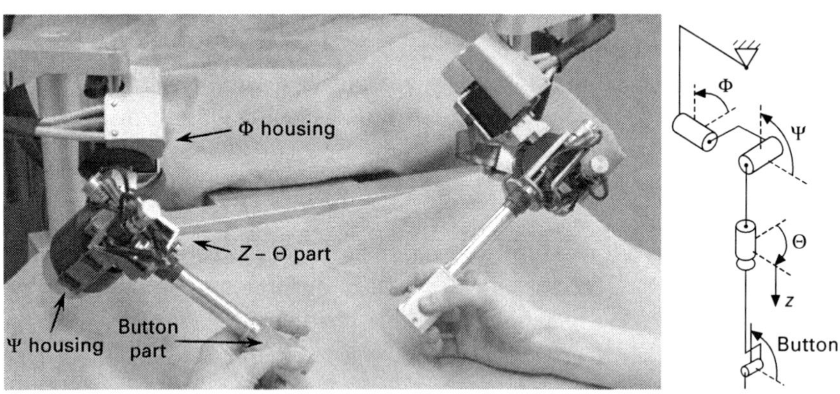

8.7 (a) The two 5-DoF haptic interfaces with temporary supporting frame. The operator can manipulate two instruments simultaneously; (b) a schematic layout of the kinematic chain.

achieve an O arrangement, increasing the stiffness and eliminating play. The Φ and the Ψ rotation are ±90° and –45°/+88°, respectively (Fig. 8.8).

The *Z*–Θ module is placed on top of the Ψ shaft. It has a hand-held stylus which is guided by two bearing bushes. These bushes leave two DoF: the desired *Z*–Θ motion, each driven by a DC motor which facilitates force feedback. The motors are also placed in the direct neighborhood of the rotation point. Low geared, backdrivable transmissions are applied for a compact layout and to reduce motor weight.

The button part is mounted at the bottom side of the hand-held stylus. It offers two parallel surfaces for a tight grasp between thumb and middle finger, necessary to guarantee a precise manipulation of, for example, a forceps during the peeling of a membrane. The surgeon operates the forceps (or another instrument) by pushing the button with his/her index finger.

Finally, the electronic wiring, which is routed internally by two flexible printed circuits, results in a disturbance force of only 10 mN at the button of

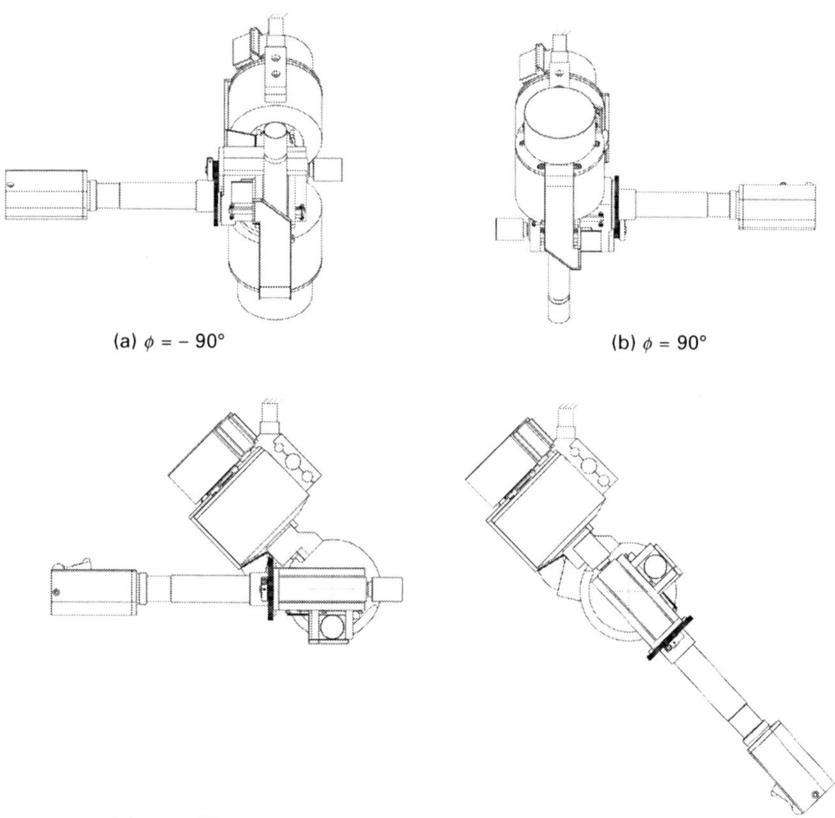

(a) $\phi = -90°$ (b) $\phi = 90°$

(c) $\psi = -45°$ (d) $\psi = 88°$

8.8 (a–d) Range of motion of the Φ and the Ψ DoF.

the interface. Table 8.2 gives an overview of the haptic interface characteristics. The Z stroke is kept smaller than specified for a vitrectomy procedure, as a stylus length >175 mm gives a forced and uncomfortable Φ and Ψ rotation of the button part between the fingertips. A combination of velocity and position control is used to control the instrument in its whole range. This algorithm is also implemented for the Θ rotation of the instrument, as the human hand does not allow for larger rotations than approximately 180°.

8.4 Slave robot

The slave robot consists of two active robotic arms, viz the instrument manipulators, and a passive support or presurgical adjustment system, supporting both the patient's head and the instrument manipulators. The instrument manipulators are designed for system performance, allowing precise movements and time-efficient surgery, whereas the passive support system provides a rigid support, as well as easy installation and presurgical preparation. The design provides an optimal balance between the support system and the instrument manipulators, both contributing to usability and performance of the system.

8.4.1 Instrument manipulator

The instrument manipulator is designed for high system performance (Rosielle and Reker, 2004). Advanced mechanical design principles are employed, resulting in a statically determined design with high stiffness, low weight, low inertia, and low friction and free of play and/or backlash for reasons specified in Section 8.3.2. These characteristics allow fast and accurate movements and they provide system safety. With smartly designed actuators, equipped with high-resolution encoders, micrometer resolution is achieved at the instrument tip at the maximum insertion depth of 25 mm.

The instrument manipulator has a serial layout, grouping the manipulated DoFs into a Z–Θ manipulator and a Φ–Ψ manipulator. The Z–Θ manipulator

Table 8.2 Characteristics of the haptic interface, measured at the tip in its nominal position

Characteristics	Φ	Ψ	Z	Θ	Button
Continuous force/torque	3 N	3 N	2.4 N	0.05 N m	1.9 N
Maximum force/torque	9.5 N	9.5 N	32 N*	0.65 N m*	3.9 N
Range	180°	133°	16 mm	340°	5 mm
Resolution	37 μm	37 μm	1.8 μm	0.1 mrad	25 μm
Moving mass/inertia	0.17 kg	0.11 kg	0.16 kg	2.2×10^{-5} kg m^2	0.04 kg

*limited for safety.

relies on linear guides, ball bearings and rotary DC motors to be actuated. It is stacked to and manipulated along with the Φ–Ψ manipulator for which a double parallelogram mechanism is chosen. The parallelogram mechanism kinematically constrains the pivoting access point to the eye, while manipulating the instrument in the Φ and Ψ directions. Figure 8.9 shows the design of the instrument manipulator.

The instrument manipulator is about 270 mm in length, 65 mm wide and from the Φ-axis to the top of the Θ–*Z* manipulator 175 mm in height. For overall safety, all DoFs are backdrivable, allowing the surgeon or surgical assistant to overrule the actuator. To minimize the required actuator torques and to further improve inherent safety of the system, a counterweight is added, by which the center of gravity is brought to the Φ-axis, Fig. 8.9. As a result, the weight of the manipulator is balanced when electronics or software fails, regardless of the orientation of the manipulator. The instrument manipulator weighs about 800 g, of which 480 g is contributed by the counterweight.

Table 8.3 summarizes the design characteristics of the manipulator. The design is optimized to emulate manually performed surgery, considering three typical interventions: vitrectomy, membrane peeling and repair of retinal detachment (Section 8.2.2). Vitrectomy is performed to remove and replace the vitreous humor e.g. in case of a vitreous hemorrhage, which causes the vitreous humor to turn opaque. The vitrectome is an instrument to remove the vitreous humor, which requires a reach covering the entire posterior cavity.

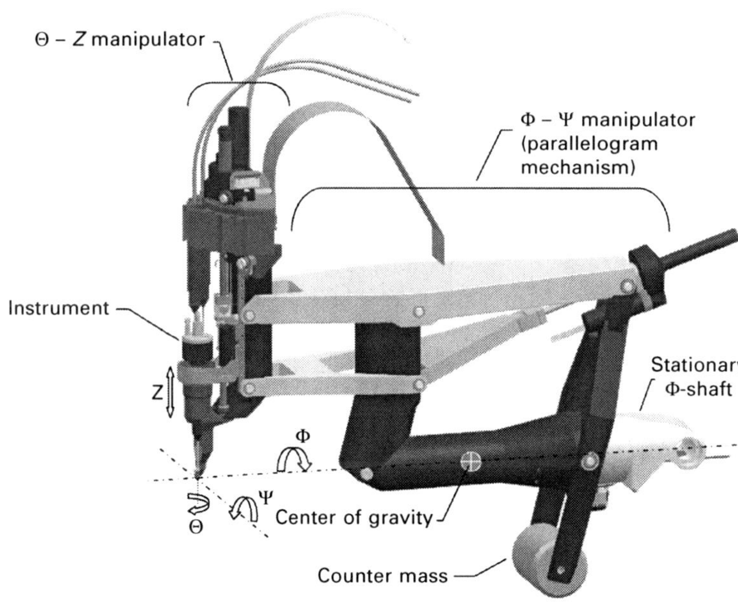

8.9 The instrument manipulator.

Table 8.3 Instrument manipulator design characteristics

Characteristics	Φ	Ψ	*Z*	Θ
Sensor force range	±2 N	±2 N	±2 N	0.05 N m
Sensor force resolution	1 mN	1 mN	1 mN	0.025 mN
Range	±45°	±45°	30 mm	>360°
Resolution	4 µrad	4 µrad	1 µm	20 mrad
Actuator force/torque	12.5 mN m	12.5 mN m	6 N	0.2 mN m

For two instruments accessing the eye on opposite sides from the cornea, this requires an instrument reach of: Φ, $\Psi = \pm 45°$ and $Z = 25$ to 30 mm. An epiretinal membrane, a scar tissue that forms over the retina, is mostly treated in the macula region. With a micro forceps, a membrane is peeled off the delicate retina. Membrane peeling does not require a large reach, but membranes have a thickness of the order of 35 to 125 µm (Wilkins *et al.*, 1996), prescribing the required positioning accuracy. Finally, to enable force feedback, it is required to measure forces down to 1 mN, which is significantly below the human detection limit.

8.4.2 Features of the instrument manipulator

The design of the instrument manipulator guarantees maximum accessibility to the eye. All mechanics are placed towards one side, away from the instruments and the eye to achieve a slender front-end of the manipulator. Except for the clamp enclosing the instrument, no mechanics are placed in front of or at the side of the instrument. The design targets are:

- maximizing accessibility to the eye for the surgeon and assistants;
- the use of multiple instrument manipulators;
- maximizing accessibility for peripheral surgical instrumentation;
- minimizing obstruction of the light envelope of the microscope.

In bimanual surgery, the instrument tips are always pointing towards each other. As movements are inverted by the entry point to the eye, the instrument's axes and, consequently, the instrument manipulators are orientated away from each other. This contributes to the accessibility to the eye and leaves room for the light envelope of the microscope, Fig. 8.10.

Changing instruments is a time-consuming activity in manually performed eye surgery. It requires various steps, including the removal of the instrument, flipping away part of the microscope to choose the desired instrument and introducing the desired instrument. The focus of the surgeon is diverted from the surgical area when introducing an instrument. The entry points of the instruments are well defined by using cannulas. However, the instruments have a typical diameter of only 0.5 mm, complicating the introduction of an

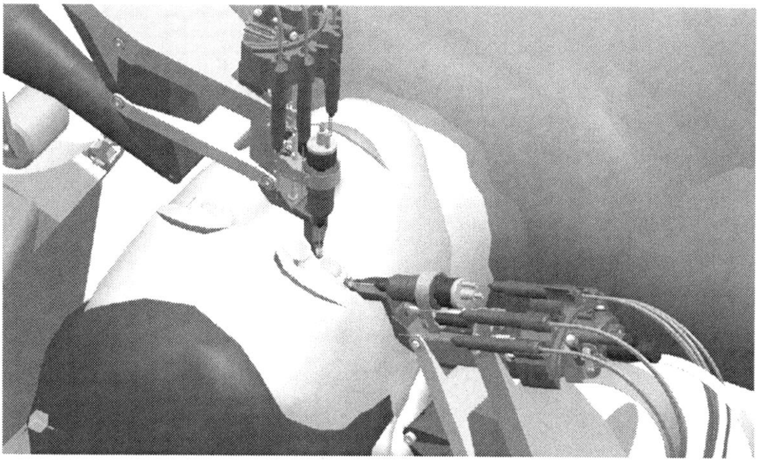

8.10 The slender instrument manipulator design leaves room around the eye for the use of a microscope or peripheral equipment. Here, two instrument manipulators are used.

instrument. For safety, often both instruments are withdrawn simultaneously from the eye. To decrease surgery time and minimize light toxicity, the instrument manipulators are equipped with an automated instrument changing system. Up to five instruments are available in a container, from which an instrument can be taken. An instrument can be changed in seconds at a single command, by automating all the steps.

The instrument manipulator allows for measurement of the forces and torques that are applied to the instrument. The most accurate commercially available 6-DoF force/torque sensor ATI-AI Nano17 is built into the manipulator. The sensor has milliNewton and Newton millimeter accuracy at an operating range of –12 to 12 N and –120 to 120 N mm, respectively (ATI Industrial Automation, NC, USA; http://www.ati-ia.com).

8.4.3 Support system

The support system allows presurgical adjustments of the instrument manipulators, positioning the manipulators exactly onto the patient's eye. Taking into account anatomical diversity of the human head and eye, three DoF are adjustable, Fig. 8.11. A lightweight, compact, modular and easy to install design is pursued, allowing efficient use for the surgical staff, including maneuverability, installation and adjustment.

Figure 8.11 shows an exploded view of the passive support system with presurgical adjustments. It is a table-mounted design with the headrest as a part of the support system. The system facilitates presurgical adjustments of the instrument manipulators in the *X* and *Y* direction. The *Y*-stage is located

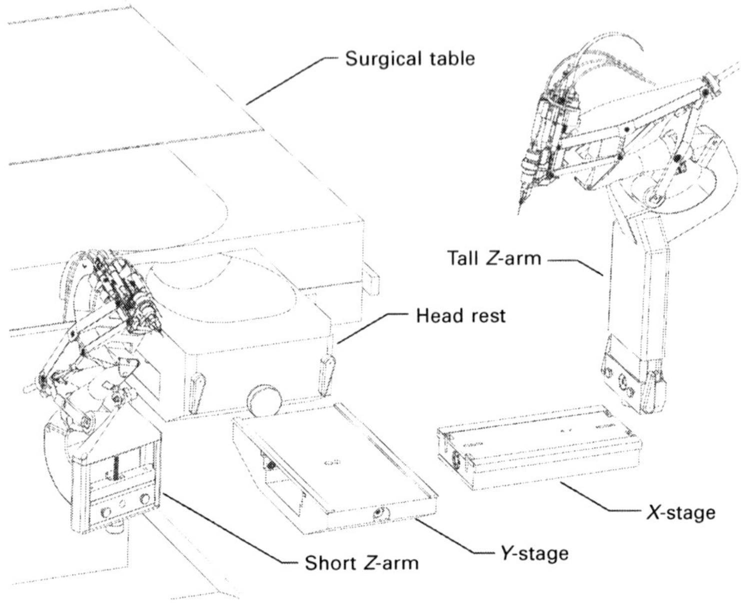

8.11 Exploded view of the modular support or presurgical adjustment system with three DoFs, *X*, *Y* and *Z*, respectively.

completely inside the head rest, whereas the *X*-stage is guided through the *Y*-stage. The instrument manipulators are supported by two support arms (or *Z*-arms). The tall *Z*-arm standing over the patient's head (on the right in Fig. 8.11) and the short *Z*-arm for the instrument manipulator standing beside the patient's head (on the left in Fig. 8.11), are attached to the ends of the *X*-stage that extend from the headrest. They can be interchanged for surgery on either the left or the right eye. Furthermore, the arms are modular and easy to install, remove and exchange. As a result, they allow fast removal in case of an emergency.

The total width of the system nearly fits within the typical width of a surgical table, i.e., 580 mm. The compact design leaves room for the surgeon to approach as close as desired and allows the operating room to be arranged as preferred. Furthermore, it allows the master console to be attached to the top end of the headrest. The total weight of the slave robot is about 8 kg, including the headrest (1.5 kg) and built-in electronics. Both *Z*-arms have a similar weight of about 1.9 kg in total. When the operating room is prepared from non-eye surgery to eye surgery, the heaviest part to install is the headrest assembly of about 3.8 kg.

For the design of the presurgical adjustment system similarity of actuation, guidance and fixation is applied. All presurgical adjustments are made manually by the use of positioning screws. Guide rollers combined with sliding surfaces are used for guidance of the degrees of freedom. Fixation is realized by levers, pressing the sliding surfaces together with preloaded springs.

8.5 Results

A demonstrator setup of the robotic master–slave system described in the previous sections has been realized, including a temporary vision solution, electronics, and the first version of control software. The integration of the system and the first functional tests with the system are described in this section.

8.5.1 System integration

Figure 8.12 is a picture of the total system with Professor M. D. de Smet, one of the ophthalmic surgeons that is actively involved in the project, controlling the right haptic interface and the right instrument manipulator to perform surgical tasks on the chorioallantoic membrane of a chicken egg. In this experimental setup, the master console (Section 8.3) is mounted to a frame and situated on a table alongside the slave (Section 8.4.1), which is attached to the operating table via a support system as described in Section 8.4.3. Eventually, the master console is integrated with the slave robot, as illustrated in Fig. 8.5. Until now, visual feedback has been obtained using a HD video camera and a 24″ HD monitor, with a magnification factor of 20.

In Fig. 8.13, a schematic overview of the system integration is shown, including the controller PC with software, the electronics, the hardware devices, the vision system, the surgeon and the patient. The EtherCAT protocol is adopted for communication between the hardware devices and the controller

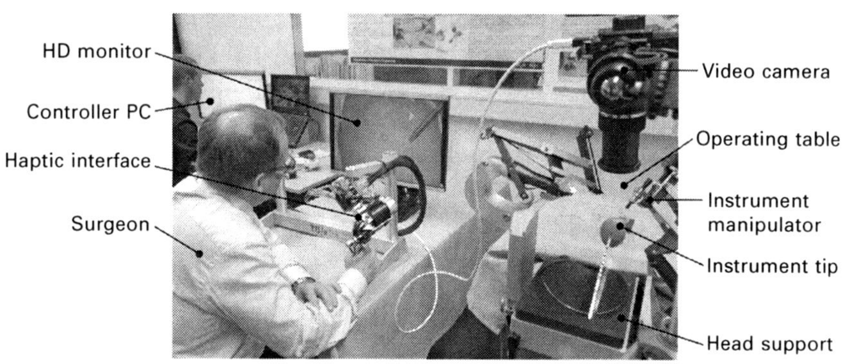

8.12 Ophthalmic surgeon M. D. de Smet performing a task using the robotic surgical system, while looking at the HD monitor.

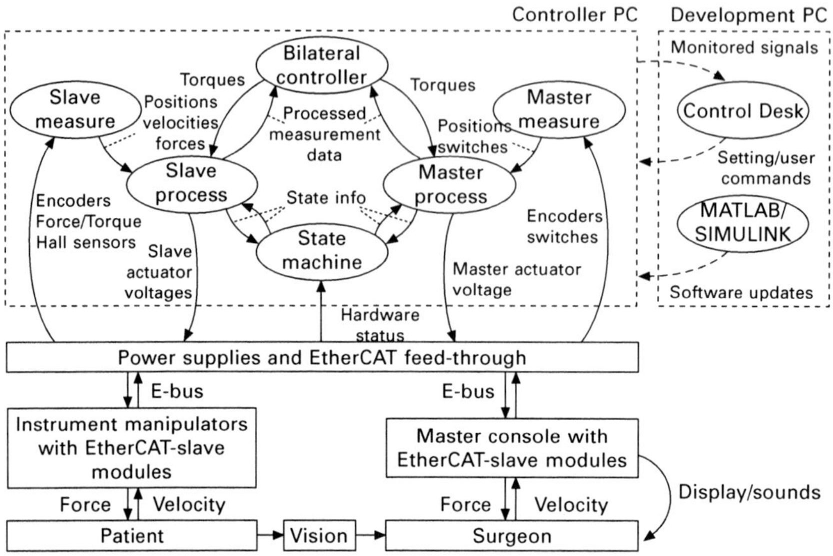

8.13 Schematic overview of the system integration.

PC (Janssen and Büttner, 2004). The electronic modules of the slave robot are integrated in the instrument manipulators and the support system. The modules include signal pre- and postprocessing and motor amplifiers. Hence, control of the slave robot actuators is decentralized and power amplification is performed locally, which has several advantages over a centralized control architecture. First, the combination of local signal processing and actuator control minimizes wiring length, thus preventing the transmission of analog signals over long distances with the potential of signal loss. Second, the number of signals that has to be included in the wiring is minimized to four signals only, including power supply and EtherCat data transfer.

The controller PC (Fig. 8.12) is used as a rapid control prototyping platform, running in real time at 1 kHz using MATLAB/Simulink in a Linux environment. A separate development PC is available for signal monitoring, logging and parameter adjustment, e.g., to change user settings during execution. Figure 8.13 illustrates the control software architecture on the controller PC. Measurements are postprocessed (slave measure and master measure) and converted to SI units. A safety level monitors the measured signals, checking, e.g., the motor currents, the velocities and the supplied voltages (slave process and master process). The state machine combines all information, including a heartbeat signal from the EtherCAT slaves that are integrated in the master and slave hardware. Error handling and safety procedures in case of failure are included in the state machine, ensuring safe operation of the system at all time. A manually operated switch is used to couple the master and the slave devices. When the master and the slave devices are decoupled, the instrument manipulators are put in stand-by mode.

A bilateral controller ensures accurate position tracking of the instrument manipulators and force feedback to the surgeon at the master console. Furthermore, the controller includes a weight-compensation algorithm for the master console, force and position scaling and hand tremor filtering. Both measured and virtual force feedback are implemented, using forces measured with a force/torque transducer, and virtually generated forces based on position constraints. For example, a force signal based on a virtual spring is transmitted through the master to alert the user when the instrument manipulator reaches the boundaries of its workspace. Finally, a ballistics algorithm increases the position scaling when the user makes a fast movement and decreases the scaling for low velocities. The algorithm is based on the consensus that the user wants to move a large distance when moving at high speed, whereas accuracy has priority at low velocities.

8.5.2 Experimental results

The system accuracy was validated by measuring both the repeatability and the smallest step size. Validation measurements were performed at the instrument tip with an insertion depth of 25 mm. The displacement was measured contactless, using a Laservibrometer (Polytec OVF-5000 with OVF-552, at 500 μm V^{-1}). The result was an intrinsic accuracy of 2 μm for the Z and the Ψ DoF and 10 μm for the Φ DoF, which corresponds to the requirements (see sections 8.2 and 8.4).

The first user tests included a training program with simple tasks on paper and more advanced surgical tasks on a chicken egg chorioallantoic membrane (Leng *et al.*, 2004). The simple tasks on paper included following a predefined path with the tip of a pinching instrument and pointing/pinching tasks on marked spots (Fig. 8.14). The tests show an intuitive usage combined with good ergonomics and satisfactory instrument reach and accuracy. User tremor is effectively filtered and a motion scaling of 20 to 40 times was considered adequate. The intuitive usage resulted in a short learning curve; users adapt in minutes and are able to perform surgical tasks successfully within an hour of first usage. Pointing tasks on squared millimeter paper show an accuracy down to 38 ±28 μm (Fig. 8.14a left image). Accuracy of these tasks is limited by the magnification of the currently implemented visualization system, which will be addressed in future developments.

The chorioallantoic membrane (CAM) of chicken eggs is used as a model to practice surgical tasks, the transparent membrane shown in Fig. 8.14b. The CAM of chicken eggs is commonly used as a model for the retina as the membrane has similar characteristics as the retina (Leng *et al.*, 2004). The first task involved peeling of the white inner shell membrane from the underlying

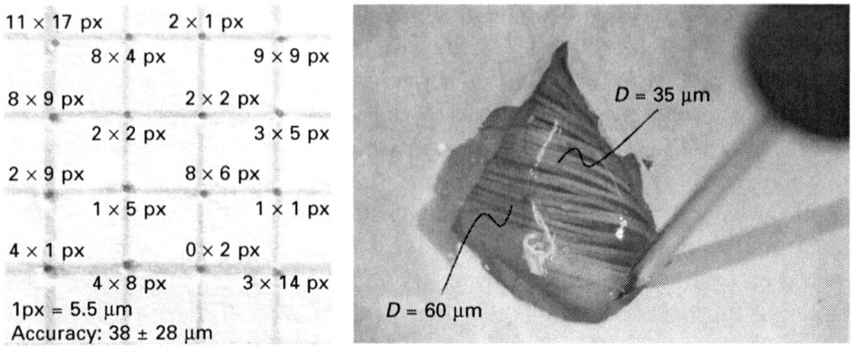

(a) (b)

8.14 (a) User accuracy experiment by pinching intersections of squared millimeter paper; (b) hemorrhage caused by pinching veins with a diameter down to 35 μm on the chorioallantoic membrane of a chicken egg.

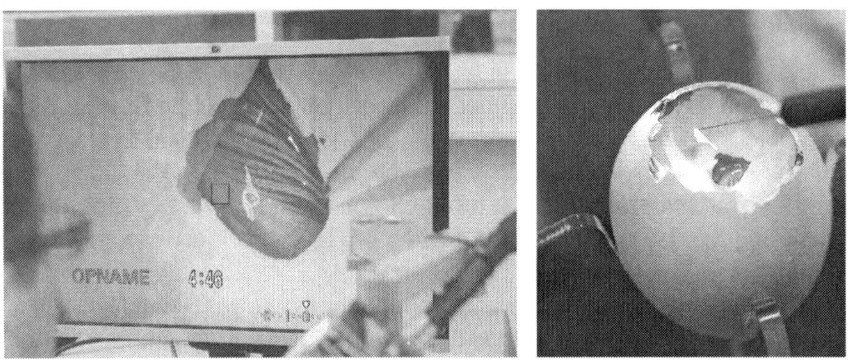

8.15 Surgical tasks performed on the chorioallantoic membrane of a chicken egg.

CAM. With a knife and pick, the peel was successfully executed on the first attempt. It was performed within 2 min and without any complications such as bleeding (Fig. 8.15). After removing a piece of the inner shell membrane and exposing the CAM, retinal vein cannulation was simulated successfully by inducing bleedings in the veins on the CAM, having a diameter down to 35 μm (Fig. 8.14b). The outcome of these surgical tasks were consistent in subsequent experiments with various users.

8.6 Conclusions and future trends

To improve the time efficiency of current vitreoretinal surgical procedures and to enable new procedures demanding improved accuracy, a robotic system has been developed, extending human capabilities beyond current limitations. The system is developed in close collaboration with several vitreoretinal surgeons by Eindhoven University of Technology (TU/e), Control Systems Technology group and Dynamics and Control group, supported by Academic Medical Centre Amsterdam (AMC), Department of Ophthalmology, and TNO Science and Industry. Currently, the system has been realized as a demonstrator prototype. As per January 2012, integration of the demonstrator system is being completed, including electronics and software functionality.

The result is a compact, lightweight and easy to set up robotic master–slave system. The demonstrator that has been realized can reach all major areas within the vitreous cavity, including the periphery. A combination of advanced mechanical and control design facilitates high accuracy, tremor filtering, automated instrument changing and an ergonomic body posture for the surgeon. Appropriate translation of user needs into a high-precision design, thereby employing advanced constructions and mechanism concepts, is key in achieving the required accuracy. The haptic interface as part of the master console allows the surgeon to manipulate a surgical instrument in an intuitive and comfortable way. Special attention is paid to minimize any disturbance forces, such as friction, as they interfere with the force feedback.

First functional tests with the demonstrator system show a short setup time of less than 2 min, an intuitive usage in combination with good ergonomics and satisfactory instrument reach and accuracy. The system has an intrinsic accuracy of 10 μm. Pointing tasks show accuracy down to 38 ±28 μm, which is restricted by the current visualization system. User tremor is effectively filtered and a motion scaling of 20 to 40 times is considered convenient. The intuitive usage results in a short learning curve; users adapt in minutes and are able to perform surgical tasks successfully within an hour of first usage. With a knife and a pick, a successful peel of the inner shell membrane of the chorioallantoic membrane of a chicken egg is made on the first attempt.

The developed system promises to improve current vitreoretinal surgical procedures in time-efficiency and accuracy, and to enable new, high-precision procedures. The focus of future research is on preclinical validation of the robotic system as a valuable tool for vitreoretinal surgeons to improve the outcome of vitreoretinal surgery. Furthermore, the demonstrator proof-of-concept system requires a redesign to arrive at a prototype that can be employed for regulatory approval; safety, sterilizability and manufacturability of the system are amongst the topics that are addressed.

8.7 Acknowledgments

The authors gratefully acknowledge the Equipment and Prototyping Centre at Eindhoven University of Technology for their assistance in realising the mechanical hardware. This research was financially supported by the IOP Precision Technology program of the Dutch Ministry of Economic Affairs.

8.8 References

Berker, N. and Batman, C. (2009), Surgical treatment of central retinal vein occlusion, *Acta Ophthalmologica*, **86**(3): 245–252.

Fine, H. Wei, W. Goldman, R.E. and Simaan, N. (2010), Robot-assisted ophthalmic surgery, *Canadian Journal of Ophthalmology*, **45**: 581–584.

Fischer, P. Daniel, R. and Siva, K.V. (1990), Specification and design of input devices for teleoperation, *IEEE International Conference on Robotics and Automation* (ICRA), **1**: 540–545.

Hannaford, B. and Okamura, A.M. (2008), Haptics, in *Handbook of robotics*, Siciliano, B. and Khatib, O. (eds), Springer, Berlin, Heidelberg, pp. 719–739.

Hayward, V. (1995), Toward a seven axis haptic device, *IEEE/RSJ International Conference on Intelligent Robots and Systems (IROS)*, **3**: 133–139.

Hendrix, R. (2011), Robotically assisted eye surgery: A haptic master console, PhD thesis (supervisors: Nijmeijer H., Steinbuch, M.), Eindhoven University of Technology, Eindhoven, the Netherlands.

Janssen, D. and Büttner, H. (2004), Real-time Ethernet: the EtherCAT solution, *Computing & Control Engineering Journal*, **15**: 16–21.

Klein, R. Moss, S.E. Meuer, S.M. and Klein, B.E.K. (2008), The 15-year cumulative incidence of retinal vein occlusion, *Archives of Ophthalmology*, **126**(4): 513–518.

Langelaan, M. de Boer, M.R. van Nispen R.M. Wouters, B. Moll, A.C. and van Rens, G.H. (2007), Impact of visual impairment on quality of life: a comparison with quality of life in the general population and with other chronic conditions, *Ophthalmic Epidemiology*, **14**(3): 119–126.

Leng, T. Miller, J.M. Bilbao, K.V. Palanker, D.V. Huie, P. and Blumenkranz, M.S. (2004), The chick chorioallantoic membrane as a model tissue for surgical retinal research and simulation, **24**(3): 427–434.

Linde, R.Q. van der, and Lammertse, P. (2003), Haptic master – a generic force controlled robot for human interaction, *Industrial Robot: An International Journal*, **30**(6): 515–524.

Meenink, H.C.M. (2011), Vitreo-retinal eye surgery robot: sustainable precision, PhD thesis (supervisors: Steinbuch, M., De Smet, M.D.), Eindhoven University of Technology, Eindhoven, the Netherlands.

Millman, P.A. and Colgate, J.E. (1991), Design of a four degree-of-freedom force-reflecting anipulandum with a specified force/torque workspace, *IEEE International Conference on Robotics and Automation* (ICRA), pp. 1488–1493.

Mitchell, B. Koo, J. Iordachita, M. Kazanzides, P. Kapoor, A. Handa, J. Hagar, G. and Taylor, R. (2007), Development and application of a new steady-hand manipulator for retinal surgery, IEEE International Conference on Robotics and Automation, pp. 623–629.

Raja, M. Anshuman, S. Rajeev, R. Sannapaneni, K. and Baruch, K. (2010), Faster visual recovery after 23-gauge vitrectomy compared with 20-gauge vitrectomy, *Retina*, **30**: 1511–1514.

Riviere C.N. Rader R.S. and Khosla P. (1997), Characteristics of hand motion of eye surgeons, *19th Annual Conference of the IEEE Engineering in Medicine and Biology Society*, pp. 1690–1693.

Rizzo, S. Patelli, F. and Chow, D.R. (2009), *Essentials in ophthalmology: vitreoretinal surgery, progress III*, Springer-Verlag Berlin Heidelberg, ISBN 978-3-540-69461-8.

Rizzo, S. Genovesi–Ebert, F. Murri, S. Belting, C. Vento, A. Cresti, F. Palla, M. and Di Bartol, E. (2006), 25 gauge sutureless vitrectomy and standard 20 gauge pars plana vitrectomy in idiopathic epiretinal membrane surgery: a comparative study, *Graefe's Archive for Clinical and Experimental Ophthalmology*, **244**(4): 472–479.

Rizzo, S. Genovesi-Ebert, F. and Augustin, A.J. (2009), Small-gauge incision techniques: the art of wound construction, *Retina Today*, Jan/Feb 2009.

Rosielle, P.C.J.N. and Reker, E.A.G. (2004), Constructieprincipes 1, Eindhoven University of Technology, Lecture notes.

Stocco, L.J. Salcudean, S.E. and Sassani, F. (2001), Optimal kinematic design of a haptic pen, *IEEE/ASME Transactions on Mechatronics*, **6**(3): 210–220.

Terasaki, H. Miyake, Y. Nomura, R. Piao, C.H. Hori, K. Niwa, T. and Kondo, M. (2001), Focal macular ERGs in eyes after removal of macular ILM during macular hole surgery, *Investigative Ophthalmology & Visual Science*, **42**: 229–234.

Uemoto, R. Yamamoto, S. Aoki, T. Tsukahara, I. Yamamoto, T. and Takeuchi, S. (2002), Macular configuration determined by optical coherence tomography after idiopathic macular hole surgery with or without internal limiting membrane peeling, *British Journal of Ophthalmology*, **86**: 1240–1242.

Uemura, A. Kanda, S. Sakamoto, Y. and Kita H. (2003), Visual field defects after uneventful vitrectomy for epiretinal membrane with indocyanine green-assisted internal limiting membrane peeling, *American Journal of Ophthalmology*, **136**: 252–257.

Ueta, T. Yamaguchi, Y. Shirakawa, Y. Nakano, T. Ideta, R. Noda, Y. Morita, A. Mochizuki, R. Sugita, N. Mitsuishi, M. and Tamaki, Y. (2009), Robot-assisted vitreoretinal surgery: development of a prototype and feasibility studies in an animal model, *Ophthalmology*, **116**(8): 1538–1543.

Weiss, J.N. and Bynoe, L.A. (2001), Injection of tissue plasminogen activator into a branch retinal vein in eyes with central retinal vein occlusion, *Ophthalmology*, **108**(2): 2249–2257.

Wilkins, J.R, Puliafito C.A., Hee, M.R. Duker, J.S. Reichel, E. Coker, J.G. Schuman, J.S. Swarson, E.A. and Fujimoto, J.G. (1996), Characterization of epiretinal membranes using optical coherence tomography. *Ophthalmology*, **103**: 2142–2152.

9
Robotics for minimally invasive surgery (MIS) and natural orifice transluminal endoscopic surgery (NOTES)

J. REYNOSO, A. MEYER, J. UNNIREVI and D. OLEYNIKOV, University of Nebraska Medical Center, USA

Abstract: The development of single-incision and robotic procedures to decrease the invasiveness of surgery is reviewed. In particular, natural orifice transluminal endoscopic surgery (NOTES), which is a minimally invasive surgical (MIS) procedure that eliminates incisions altogether, is discussed in detail and current research being conducted to develop robotic and endoscopic technology to expand its clinical applications are described.

Key words: minimally invasive surgery, natural orifice transluminal endoscopic surgery, single incision laparoscopic surgery, surgical robot.

9.1 Introduction

Minimally invasive surgery (MIS) aims to reduce patient morbidity by decreasing the incision length needed for access. The advent of laparoscopic techniques and instrumentation brought about a change in surgical proficiency and a significant improvement in patient outcomes, by way of decreased pain, decreased convalescence, improved cosmesis, and decreased hernia formation. As surgeons moved from direct vision of the operative field and manual manipulation of tissue to videoimaging and indirect instrument actuated tissue manipulation, new technology was required to ensure patient safety. Laparoscopic suturing devices, improved optics, laparoscopic gastrointestinal anastomosis staplers, and laparoscopic surgical energy devices are examples of new technology developed to overcome the limitations imposed by the minimally invasive technique. Traditional laparoscopic technique inherently includes a decrease in dexterity, loss of tactile sensation, restriction in entry points, decrease in depth perception, and decrease in degrees of freedom. The development of surgical robotics has aimed to overcome these constraints while continuing to decrease the length of the incision.

The quest for further refinement in MIS procedures led to the advancement of robotic surgical technology, foremost of which is the da Vinci robotic system (dVSS; Intuitive Surgical, Sunnyvale, CA). This surgical robot offers motion scaling, which electronically enhances resolution of the human hand and eliminates tremor. The three-dimensional (3D) vision allows for improved depth perception. EndoWrist™ technology increases degrees of freedom in movement and improves dexterity.

Single incision laparoscopic surgery (SILS™) and natural orifice transluminal surgery (NOTES) are a continuation of the trend of decreasing surgical incision length and number of incisions. SILS aims to reduce the amount of abdominal wall incisions to one small port through which all instruments are passed. To avoid an abdominal incision altogether, the NOTES technique utilizes a natural orifice to access the peritoneal cavity. The evolution of each of these techniques presents new limitations to overcome. New surgical robot prototypes and technology are currently under development to continue the progression of MIS.

9.2 Minimally invasive surgery (MIS)

Traditional open surgery with a large incision provides the most natural operative feel. A surgeon's stereovision is naturally aligned with their hands which, in turn, directly manipulate and palpate tissue. Manual dexterity is only limited by a surgeon's innate ability. However, the price for this optimal surgical exposure is increased morbidity for the patient. In order to reduce operative risk for the patient, the paradigm of MIS has developed.

Conventional MIS involves the use of multiple ports placed through incisions that are approximately 1 cm in length. In an attempt to recreate the natural alignment of the eyes with the hands, the laparoscopic surgeon triangulates his instruments. To accomplish this, the camera should be in line with the target tissue and centered between the surgeon's right and left hands. These working trocars should be placed so that the instruments pass through these ports and meet at 90° at the target tissue with 50% of the instrument in the abdominal cavity. Often the function of retraction is now performed by gravity with the patient placed in steep Trendelenburg, reverse Trendelenburg, or rotated to the right or left. Retraction may also be performed laparoscopically by an assistant or by specialized laparoscopic instrumentation, such as the Nathanson liver retractor (Cook Medical, Bloomington, IN, USA).

These innovations in surgical technique, instrumentation and technology have allowed laparoscopic surgery to become the gold standard for several procedures. The laparoscopic cholecystectomy is the classic example of this change. Additionally, the fields of bariatric surgery, antireflux surgery, urology, gynecology, and colorectal surgery have all demonstrated significantly improved patient outcomes. Several studies have demonstrated the safety and efficacy of laparoscopic surgery, and patients are afforded the benefits of earlier return to activity, decreased hospital stay, improved cosmesis, decreased pain and decreased incisional hernia formation.

However, laparoscopic technique still presents limitations of decreased dexterity, poor ergonomics, and two-dimensional (2D) imaging. Laparoscopic instruments normally provide four degrees of freedom, which include rotation and movement along *x*, *y* and *z* axes. The abdominal wall becomes the fulcrum with the instrument acting as the lever. The tip of the instrument moves exactly opposite in relation to the hands in the *x* and *y* axis; this means that as the hand moves down, the tip goes up, and as the hand goes right, the tip goes left. In and out movement and rotation of the instrument directly correlate to the movement of the hands. Laparoscopic surgeons must learn to overcome this inconstancy in instrument maneuvering. This can become problematic when the camera is not centered between the instruments, especially when the camera is directly opposite the surgeon. Surgical robotic technology aims to decrease the technical difficulties associated with conventional laparoscopic surgeries.

9.2.1 MIS and da Vinci

Currently, the da Vinci surgical system (dVSS; Intuitive Surgical, Sunnyvale, CA) is the most widely utilized surgical robot. The initial research for this device was performed in the late 1980s by the non-profit organization SRI International in Menlo Park, CA. The National Institutes of Health and the Defense Advanced Research Projects Administration (DARPA) also provided funding for this research, the latter of these groups being interested in remotely controlled robots performing operations in a battlefield setting. In the mid-1990s, Intuitive Surgical devices built on this previous research would eventually become the dVSS. This surgical robot was approved by the Food and Drug Administration for use in the United States in 2000 (Palep, 2009).

To create a more natural feel, the human wrist was used as a model for the function of this surgical robot. The four degrees of freedom of conventional laparoscopic surgery are increased to seven with this system. The surgeon sits at a console, which is designed for ergonomic comfort and controls the robot using the thumb and a finger. The surgeon's hand and wrist may move naturally and the robotic end effectors precisely mirror their movement. When the hand moves right, the instrument tip moves right, and when the hand moves up, the instrument tip moves up, removing the counterintuitive maneuvering present in laparoscopic surgery. Additionally, hand tremor is eliminated and motion-scaling electronically enhances the resolution of the human hand. In addition, the concept of triangulation is utilized with the camera centered between the right and left robotic arms. This camera provides 3D stereovision which allows for depth perception. At the operating console, the surgeon rests his or her head comfortably against an eyepiece that provides the high-definition imaging. Several options for end effectors are available in the Endowrist™ catalog, including a cautery hook, several types of forceps, needle drivers and clip appliers.

The dVSS has been utilized for several clinical applications. It is now commonly used for nerve-sparing prostatectomy, hysterectomy and low anterior resection. Additionally, this surgical robot has been used for Heller myotomy, adrenalectomy, gastric bypass, mitral valve replacement, internal mammary artery mobilization, transaxillary thyroidectomy, pancreatectomy and nephrectomy. It has been proven safe and efficacious and shown to confer a reduction in morbidity similar to the laparoscopic technique. Newer versions of the operating console have a second station to facilitate surgical training. The mentor and the trainee can rapidly transfer control of the system while performing these robotic procedures.

However, widespread use of the dVSS has been limited by the large size and the high cost of the robot. The most recent version can cost up to \$1.75 million for initial purchase and several thousand dollars a month for replacement parts and maintenance. The console and the robot are large and bulky, taking up a considerable portion of operating room space. The robotic arms do not provide haptic or tactile feedback. The surgeon must use visual feedback to avoid placing excessive force on tissue. Additional steps of docking and sterilely draping the robot can add to the total operative time. In spite of these constraints the dVSS is widely utilized, and many hospitals have invested in this technology to ensure their facility can offer this state of the art MIS.

9.2.2 Single-incision surgery

The trend of MIS has been towards decreasing the length and number of incisions with the goal of decreasing morbidity and improving cosmesis. Most recently, surgeons have been performing laparoscopic procedures through a single small incision, usually hidden in the umbilicus. This technique has been given several names, including the commonly used single-incision laparoscopic surgery (SILS) and laparoendoscopic single-site surgery (LESS).

The initial single-incision procedure was a cholecystectomy described by Navarra *et al.* (1997). Their approach included two 10 mm trocars placed through the umbilicus. Transabdominal sutures for retraction were placed in the gallbladder fundus, neck and infundibulum. This single-incision surgical approach has since been applied to additional procedures, including colectomy, gastric banding, nephrectomy, appendectomy, adrenalectomy, splenectomy, total extraperitoneal inguinal hernia repair, and hysterectomy. Improved cosmesis is demonstrated, and the scar may be completely hidden in the umbilicus. Further studies are underway to investigate possible reduction in pain and decreased recovery time for patients (Joseph *et al.*, 2011; Tsimoyiannis *et al.*, 2010).

Operating through a single incision with multiple instruments presents a new set of surgical limitations. Instruments are all placed in line with the camera and are predisposed to collide. Several companies have created novel ports that allow several instruments to be passed through a single fascial incision. The SILS Port (Covidien) is a foam product that can accommodate three trocars and has tubing for insufflation. An hourglass shape allows for the waist of this port to fit easily though a 2 cm incision. The ACS TriPort system (Advanced Surgical Concepts, Wicklow, Ireland) also accommodates three trocars through a 1.2 to 2.5 cm incision. This port has an adjustable length plastic sheath with a plastic ring which is inserted through the incision with the assistance of a soft plastic introducer.

The GelPoint access port (Applied Medical, Rancho Santa Margarita, CA, USA) consists of two parts. The GelSeal Cap accepts three ports and allows for insufflation and smoke evacuation. It uses an Alexis Wound Retractor, which is a plastic sheath with two plastic rings on either end. Once the Wound Retractor is placed through a 1.5 to 7 cm incision, the GelSeal Cap is attached to its top.

Another approach to single-incision surgery includes one skin incision with multiple ports placed through their own small fascial defect, the so-called 'Swiss cheese' technique. As the camera is also in line with the instruments, the view of the operative field may be obstructed. Endoscopic cameras with flexible tips allow for imaging with less collision. Articulating instruments with a flexible tip also help to avoid collision, but require the application of off-axis forces. Additionally, these instruments are often crossed at the abdominal wall. With this technique the function of the right and left hands are reversed, which is counterintuitive.

The dVSS can be set to reverse the function of the right and left robotic arms. This allows for the arms to be crossed without the surgeon having to reverse their control from right to left. The feasibility of this 'chopstick' technique was initially proven in animal studies. One such study used a GelPort access port (Applied Medical, Rancho Santa Margarita, CA, USA), a porcine cholecystectomy and lateral segmentectomy of the liver were performed. In these animal studies, a 2.5 cm single incision was used to place a GelPort with a 12 mm camera port, a 5 mm assistant port and two 8 mm ports for the robotic arms. In an additional effort to avoid clashing of robotic arms in single-incision robotic surgery, Intuitive Surgical has designed novel robotic instruments. Named VeSPA, this line of products include curved cannulae and semirigid instruments specifically designed for introduction through a single fascial incision. In porcine nephrectomy, partial nephrectomy and pyeloplasty, these instruments have been demonstrated to improve ergonomics and decrease instrument collision.

The clinical application of robotic single-incision surgery has been demonstrated in urologic case series. Nephrectomy, prostatectomy and pyeloplasty procedures have been safely performed in humans using surgical robot single-incision technique. In a recent series of robotic laparoscopic single-site (R-LESS) radical nephrectomies both the SILS port (Covidien, Mansfield, MA, USA) and the GelPOINT port (Applied Medical) were employed in a intraumbilical incision (White *et al.*, 2011). No changes from the traditional robotic nephrectomy setup were made. The dVSS was similarly docked. The robotic arms were not crossed as in the previously described 'chopstick' technique. When using the SILS port, the robotic arm trocars were placed laterally along the outside of the port with the camera placed through the specialized SILS port. All trocars were placed through the GelPOINT platform. In this series of ten cases, no additional transabdominal ports were needed to complete the procedure; no conversions to open or traditional laparoscopic surgery were made. Preliminary results from this retrospective series demonstrate significant decrease in length of hospital stay and narcotic requirement in the R-LESS group compared with the conventional laparoscopic group (White *et al.*, 2011).

Currently new surgical robot prototypes are under development to perform single-incision robotic surgery (Wortman *et al.*, 2011). The *in vivo* dexterous robot developed by Olcynikov and Farritor at the University of Nebraska Medical Center (Fig. 9.1) was demonstrated to be feasible in several porcine procedures, including cholecystectomy, colectomy, and tissue biopsy. Additional surgical maneuvers demonstrated include intracorporeal suturing,

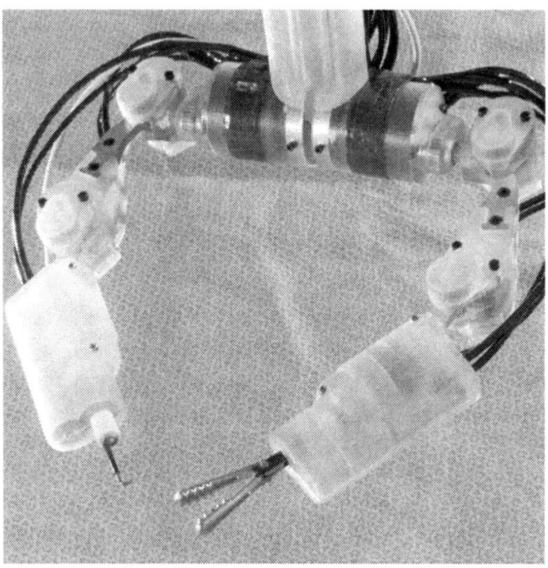

9.1 Prototype of SILS robot.

tissue manipulation, bowel manipulation, cautery hemostasis and intestinal mesentery dissection. This multifunctional miniature robot consists of two arms, each with six degrees of freedom. Currently available interchangeable end effectors for these robotic arms include monopolar cautery, graspers and needle drivers. This surgical robot is controlled by a prototype interface with videoimaging, two controllers and a foot pedal. The movements of the surgeon's hands on the interface are directly mirrored by the robot. Imaging modalities utilized include standard 2D laparoscopic as well as a prototype 3D camera. These images are clearly visualized at a remote console where the surgeon can manipulate the robot (Fig. 9.2).

Triangulation is achieved with the imaging source centered between the robotic arms. Each arm of the dexterous robot is inserted separately through the small, single incision. These arms are then assembled through the incision and securely attached to a post. Currently, a gelport is utilized to assist in maintaining pneumoperitoneum. The motors that power movement are located in the robotic arm joints, which allows for significant reduction in the size of the robot. This is in contrast to the dVSS in which the robotic arms are externally driven by large motors.

9.3 Natural orifice transluminal endoscopic surgery (NOTES)

Natural orifice transluminal endoscopic surgery (NOTES) utilizes natural orifices to access the peritoneal cavity. The feasibility of the NOTES technique

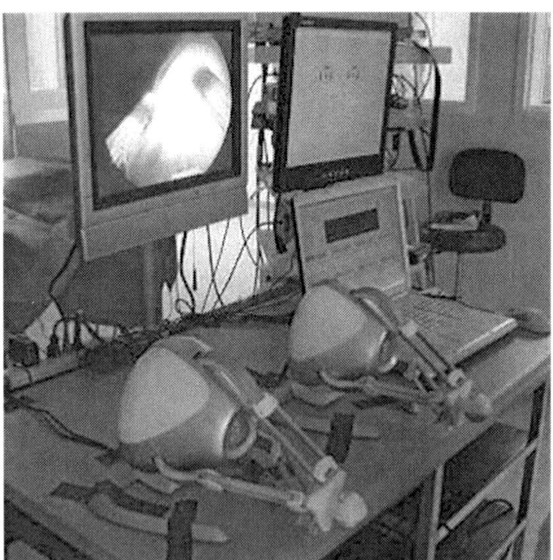

9.2 Prototype surgical console for robotic SILS.

was demonstrated in animal studies utilizing peroral gastrotomy, transurethral cystotomy, transvaginal and transcolonic approaches. Several procedures including organ resection, gastrojejunostomy, gastrojejunal anastomosis, oopherectomy, salpingectomy, cholecystectomy and appendectomy have been performed in animal studies. NOTES cholecystectomy, appendectomy and nephrectomy have since been performed in humans (Santos and Hungness, 2011).

Initially, a standard flexible endoscope was introduced through a NOTES incision, to visualize the intraperitoneal cavity. This approach has several inherent limitations when compared with open or laparoscopic surgery. Triangulation is lost when the standard endoscopic channels are used, as the instruments passed though these ports are in line with the videoimaging. In this configuration, forces must be applied off-axis in order to combat this limitation. One is also limited by the available instruments that may pass through the endoscope. Dexterity is significantly decreased owing to the constraints of this platform. To overcome these constraints, prototypes such as the EndoSAMURAI (Olympus Corp., Tokyo, Japan) have been developed. This endoscopic platform has two independent end effectors with five degrees-of-freedom, as well as a standard endoscopic channel. The operator interface includes controllers which are very similar in design to standard laparoscopic handles. An overtube has been used with this device to increase stability. The EndoSAMURAI has been used in NOTES porcine cholecystectomy via the transgastric approach and has been demonstrated in benchtop experiments to be able to perform surgical tasks such as suturing and knot-tying (Spaun *et al.*, 2009). The TransPort multichannel access device (USGI Medical, San Clemente, CA, USA) is an endoscope with four ports (6, 6, 4 and 4 mm) available for passing flexible instruments. This device has been used in clinical studies to perform transgastric appendectomy, transumbilical appendectomy and endoluminal pouch and stoma reduction (Horgan *et al.*, 2011). The Anubiscope (Karl-Storz, Tuttlingen, Germany) is a flexible endoscopic platform for NOTES that has a light and video source. The articulating head contains two opposing movable arms, capable of triangulation, that contain two 4.2 mm working channels. The distal head has jaws that open to reveal the functioning arms but when closed serve as a blunt tipped trocar during insertion (Dallemagne and Marescaux, 2010). The Direct-Drive Endoscopic System (Boston Scientific, Natick, MA, USA) has three lumens through which interchangeable 4 mm flexible instruments can be inserted. Available flexible instruments include graspers, scissors, needle drivers and cautery. This flexible laparoscopic multitasking platform is capable of seven degrees of freedom. This device is controlled by rail-guided drive handles and has a sheath that can lock into position (Shaikh and Thompson, 2010).

The master and slave translumenal endoscopic robot (MASTER) developed by Phee *et al.* (2010) at the National University of Singapore represents another novel solution to the decreased dexterity inherently found in the endoscopic NOTES platform. It is similar to the EndoSAMURAI in that it has two robotic arms which cap the end of an endoscope. However, with the MASTER, any standard upper endoscope may be outfitted with these robotic arms that are capable of tissue manipulation, triangulation, off-axis forces and monopolar cautery. Mechanical forces are applied to the end effectors through a tendon-sheath power transmission mechanism which allows for nine degrees of freedom. The surgical interface is a 'passive, steerable, motion-sensing exoskeleton with two articulating arms'. The surgeon's hand and wrist movements are directly mirrored by the robotic grasper and cautery end effectors. In a porcine animal study, this system was able to perform a transgastric hepatic wedge resection with minimal bleeding. All imaging and lighting was provided by a standard upper endoscope. A sterile endotube was placed through the esophagus. The gastrotomy was created using the monopolar cautery of the robotic arm. The standard upper endoscope was retroflexed in the peritoneal cavity to provide the surgical robot access to the liver. Tissue retraction provided access for the robotic cautery arm to excise a suitable liver sample. The specimen was then extracted though the mouth. The gastrotomy was not closed in this non-survivable animal study (Phee *et al.*, 2010).

The standard NOTES flexible endoscope platform is unstable, and forces applied to the target organ are transmitted to the endoscope. This results in a need to continually reposition the endoscope. To overcome the instability produced by flexible endoscopes passed through a hollow lumen, fixation and stiffening of the endoscope has been employed. A flexible robotics platform aims to drive a stiffened endoscope through a 3D space with computer assistance. At the Stanford University School of Medicine, a prototype has been demonstrated by Eisenberg *et al.* (2010) to be feasible in cadaver studies in which a multichannel flexible robotic endoscope was navigated using a joystick interface. Transgastric intraperitoneal access was achieved, and the platform was able to tolerate forces generated by tissue manipulation and endoclipping. Imaging was provided by the endoscope for this study. Additionally, the endoscope was repositioned without difficulty for access to different target organs.

The dVSS has been used to perform a robot-assisted NOTES nephrectomy in a porcine model, although an additional transabdominal port was placed for laparoscopic visualization. Intraperitoneal access was achieved via transvaginal and transcolonic placement of the robotic arms. The renal artery and vein were dissected using the robot and then transected using standard vascular endoscopic staplers through the vaginal port. The kidney was removed through the vagina. The NOTES technique with the dVSS was also utilized for a porcine pyeloplasty.

Use of the dVSS for NOTES has been confined to animal study and has not been used to date in humans. Although the surgical system provides several advantages, such as multiple degrees of freedom, increased dexterity and stereovision, its size has precluded a widespread application of the dVSS for NOTES. Additionally, the robotic arms are prone to collide and do not conform to the geometry of the intraperitoneal space. For this reason, novel prototypes, as described below, have been created to further develop a robotic platform for NOTES.

9.3.1 Miniature surgical robots for NOTES

Miniature *in vivo* surgical robots offer an alternative solution to the inherent limitations of NOTES. As previously mentioned, the flexible endoscopic and flexible robotics platform for NOTES are constrained by the distribution of instruments through a hollow visceral lumen into the abdominal cavity while still coupled to external control. Multiple miniature robots may be serially deployed through a single transvisceral access, allowing for a virtually unlimited number of surgical instruments. In this paradigm each miniature robot can serve a separate function, a distinct advantage over any single instrument that must provide all functionality. Separate robots may provide imaging, lighting, tissue manipulation, and mobility. A family of these robots can co-operate to perform a NOTES procedure, and have done so in experimental models (Tiwari *et al.*, 2010). Standard upper endoscopes have been used to place an esophageal overtube through which these miniature robots have been sequentially placed in the stomach and then into the abdominal cavity. The gastrotomy is created with a standard endoscopic needle knife.

Initial prototypes of *in vivo* miniature robots for NOTES included a fixed-base imaging robot meaning, once placed, it was unable to self navigate to an alternative intraperitoneal position. The creation and use of the pan and tilt camera has resolved this navigational barrier. This 15 mm metallic cylinder has three retractable legs, which provide stability when this device is placed on its end. Two independent motors afforded 360° panning and 45° tilting capability. However, the motor originally used for the panning mechanism was later employed for image focusing. Visual feedback from this instrument was used in a porcine cholecystectomy.

Advancing this technology further are self navigating, mobile robots powered by two helical-profiled wheels. Each wheel moves independently, allowing for forward, reverse and turning motions. Initial prototypes included a cylindrical robot that measured 15 mm in diameter and 75 mm in length (Fig. 9.3). The small diameter allows this mobile imaging robot to be easily deployed through a transgastric incision or a small abdominal incision. The safety and feasibility of this design was demonstrated in animal studies. The next prototype of this design included a camera, and the diameter was

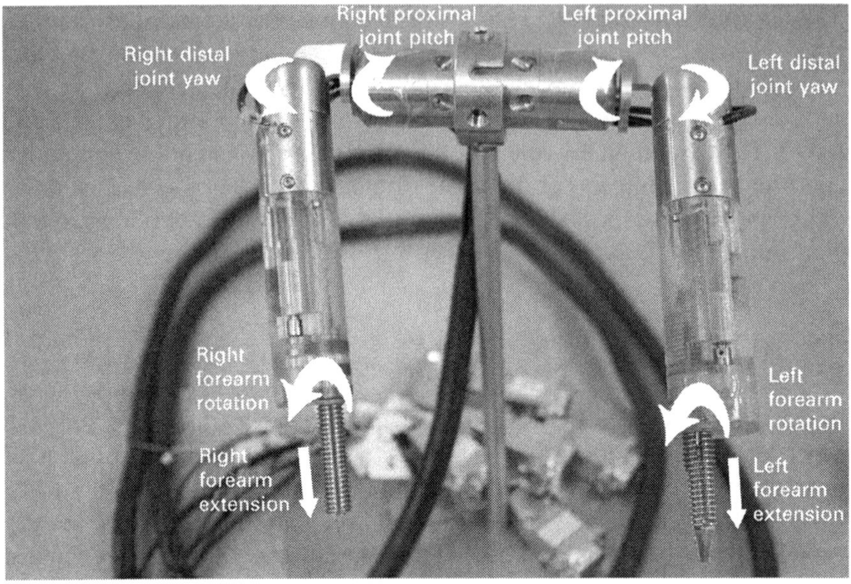

9.3 In vivo miniature robot for NOTES.

increased to 20 mm. The mobile adjustable-focus robotic camera (MARC) was able to transverse the deformable intraperitoneal cavity utilizing the dual helical-profiled wheel design. During a porcine cholecystectomy, this miniature imaging robot supplied the sole video required to complete the procedure.

In a subsequent prototype, the mobile *in vivo* surgical imaging robot was augmented with a 2.4 mm wide robotic grasper. All of the imaging and mobility capabilities inherent in previous designs were present in this design. The force generated from powered wheels was sufficient to procure a tissue biopsy. The camera on this miniature robot was used for visual feedback while selecting a porcine hepatic biopsy site. This robot was deployed in animal studies through the abdominal wall and demonstrated self navigation, imaging and tissue biopsy capability.

The mobile endoluminal robot was the first *in vivo* miniature surgical robot to be used in a NOTES procedure. In a porcine study, a standard upper endoscope was introduced per ora into the stomach, and a sterile esophageal overtube was placed with direct visualization. The 12 mm (diameter) and 75 mm (length) miniature robot explored the gastric cavity under endoscopic imaging. A gastrotomy was created with an endoscopic needle-knife and this robot was placed into the intraperitoneal space. Utilizing the same helical-profiled wheels design, the robot was able to self navigate over the liver and the deformable territory of the porcine intestines. Visualization was provided via the endoscope. After this robot was retracted back into the stomach, the gastrotomy was closed with two standard endoclips and one endoloop.

In vivo co-operative robots represent the next step in NOTES prototypes. In this concept, the functions of imaging, lighting and tissue manipulation are executed separately by a family of robots. As previously demonstrated, these miniature robots were deployed into the porcine intraperitoneal space through a sterile esophageal overtube. A standard upper endoscope was used to create a gastrotomy using a needle-knife. The lighting, imaging and retraction robots were serially placed into the abdominal cavity and held in place against the abdominal wall using magnets. Using this technique, the family of co-operative robots was able to manipulate tissue under their own lighted imaging. These initial prototypes were tethered by wires for both power source and control. Currently in development at the University of Nebraska are *in vivo* miniature robots, powered by on-board batteries and radio-controlled.

These initial NOTES porcine experiments included miniature robots with minimal ability to manipulate tissue. The *in vivo* dexterous robot was designed to improve dexterity. Six degrees of freedom were achieved with two arms attached to a central body. One arm was fitted with monopolar cautery and the other a grasper. Triangulation is made possible by stereovision cameras placed on the body of the robot between the two arms. A lower arm telescopes in and out of the upper arm, which is attached to the body via a rotational shoulder joint. Robotic arms were remotely controlled at a surgical console consisting of two analog joysticks and a foot pedal that controlled the monopolar cautery. The feasibility of NOTES cholecystectomy was demonstrated over several animal studies. Transabdominal and transgastric placement were both employed. Using the onboard imaging, the porcine gallbladder was dissected free from its hepatic attachments and the cystic duct was severed. Transabdominal magnets were used to maintain the robot's position. The ability to triangulate, apply off-axis forces, provide visualization and dexterously manipulate tissue was demonstrated in these *in vivo* dexterous robot animal studies.

As previously mentioned, in current prototypes of this multifunctional dexterous robot, the SILS technique has been employed. The proficiency of both the surgical robot and the surgical console has increased significantly, and complex tasks such as intracorporeal suturing are now possible. Continuing design of this robot includes decreasing size, increasing the capability of the surgical interface, and expanding the surgical applications to more complex procedures such as colectomy.

9.4 Future trends and conclusions

The future of MIS depends on the continued development of novel technology and robotics able to safely perform surgery with the least amount of trauma and morbidity. The success of SILS and NOTES will be determined by the advancement of robotic prototypes proven in benchtop and animal studies. Once proven in animal studies, this technology must be safely translated to human use. Currently, the clinically available flexible endoscopy platform for NOTES requires great skill and has limited utilization to specific centers worldwide. Problems with instrument triangulation, platform instability and off-axis forces continue to place constraints on surgical dexterity. A robotic platform for NOTES aims to decrease these limitations and novel prototypes continue to be developed. The utilization of this platform will ultimately be a function of demonstrated clinical safety and controlled cost. For widespread acceptance of a robotic NOTES platform, it must contain a skill set that is easily transferable to most surgeons and demonstrates advantage over currently available laparoscopic and robotic techniques. At a reasonable cost, the safety, clinical benefits, and cost effectiveness of NOTES needs to be demonstrated in research trials in order to be accepted for clinical use. Overall, NOTES represents a great paradigm shift from conventional open or laparoscopic surgery and will necessitate a great advancement in clinically available technology before it is widely available. Novel surgical robotics with increased miniaturization, dexterity, maneuverability and visualization may allow for additional clinical utilization in the future. Also needed for NOTES to continue advancement is an endoscopically deployable tissue sealing device capable of sealing lymphatics, blood vessels, ducts and tissue. Additionally, the morbidity of transvisceral access to the peritoneum is still under investigation, and a standard access closure device with proven safety and efficacy will need to be verified and implemented.

Single-incision surgery represents less of a paradigm shift away from conventional surgery than NOTES. Consequently, presently available technology has been more readily transferable to clinical use. Indeed, single incision surgery is widely available to the general public. Although the dVSS has had a minimal role in NOTES, and only then in animal studies, it has been proven to be safe and efficacious in single-incision clinical studies. The current dVSS may be modified to facilitate robotic single incision surgery, and novel instrumentation for this robotic surgical system promises to increase its ease of use. Additionally, novel robotic prototypes, including the multifunctional dexterous robot, are being developed specifically for single-incision deployment. The feasibility of this SILS robot has been demonstrated in several animal studies, and clinical studies proving safety and efficacy of this novel robotic system may allow further adoption of the robotic single-incision approach. As with every aspect of academic medicine, the future of minimally invasive robotic surgery should be based on evidenced-based medicine and increased benefit to patients.

9.5 References

Dallemagne, B. and Marescaux, J. 2010 Notes: past, present an future. *Asian J Endosc Surg*, **3**, 115–21.

Eisenberg, D., Storne, E. and Belson, A. 2010. Use of a flexible robotic transgastric natural orifice translumenal endoscopic surgery (NOTES) platform in a cadaver to test access, navigation, maneuverability, and stability. *Surg Endosc*, **24**, 2323.

Horgan, S., Thompson, K., Talamini, M., Ferreres, A., Jacobsen, G., Spaun, G., Cullen, J. and Swanstrom, L. 2011. Clinical experience with a multifunctional, flexible surgery system for endolumenal, single-port, and NOTES procedures. *Surg Endosc*, **25**, 586–92.

Joseph, S., Moore, B. T., Sorensen, G. B., Earley, J. W., Tang, F., Jones, P. and Brown, K. M. 2011. Single-incision laparoscopic cholecystectomy: a comparison with the gold standard. *Surg Endosc*, **25**, 3008–15.

Navarra, G., Pozza, E., Occhionorelli, S., Carcoforo, P. and Donini, I. 1997. One-wound laparoscopic cholecystectomy. *Br J Surg*, **84**, 695.

Palep, J. H. 2009. Robotic assisted minimally invasive surgery. *J Minim Access Surg*, **5**, 1–7.

Phee, S. J., Ho, K. Y., Lomanto, D., Low, S. C., Huynh, V. A., Kencana, A. P., Yang, K., Sun, Z. L. and Chung, S. C. 2010. Natural orifice transgastric endoscopic wedge hepatic resection in an experimental model using an intuitively controlled master and slave transluminal endoscopic robot (MASTER). *Surg Endosc*, **24**, 2293–8.

Santos, B. F. and Hungness, E. S. 2011. Natural orifice translumenal endoscopic surgery: progress in humans since white paper. *World J Gastroenterol*, **17**, 1655–65.

Shaikh, S. N. and Thompson, C. C. 2010. Natural orifice translumenal surgery: Flexible platform review. *World J Gastrointest Surg*, **2**, 210–16.

Spaun, G. O., Zheng, B. and Swanstrom, L. L. 2009. A multitasking platform for natural orifice translumenal endoscopic surgery (NOTES): a benchtop comparison of a new device for flexible endoscopic surgery and a standard dual-channel endoscope. *Surg Endosc*, Apr 10 2009, DOI 10.1007/s00464-009-0476-5.

Tiwari, M. M., Reynoso, J. F., Lehman, A. C., Tsang, A. W., Farritor, S. M. and Oleynikov, D. 2010. In vivo miniature robots for natural orifice surgery: state of the art and future perspectives. *World J Gastrointest Surg*, **2**, 217–23.

Tsimoyiannis, E. C., Tsimogiannis, K. E., Pappas-Gogos, G., Farantos, C., Benetatos, N., Mavridou, P. and Manataki, A. 2010. Different pain scores in single transumbilical incision laparoscopic cholecystectomy versus classic laparoscopic cholecystectomy: a randomized controlled trial. *Surg Endosc*, **24**, 1842–8.

White, M. A., Autorino, R., Spana, G., Laydner, H., Hillyer, S. P., Khanna, R., Yang, B., Altunrende, F., Isac, W., Stein, R. J., Haber, G. P. and Kaouk, J. H. 2011. Robotic laparoendoscopic single-site radical nephrectomy: surgical technique and comparative outcomes. *Eur Urol*, **59**, 815–22.

Wortman, T. D., Strabala, K. W., Lehman, A. C., Farritor, S. M. and Oleynikov, D. 2011. Laparoendoscopic single-site surgery using a multi-functional miniature in vivo robot. *Int J Med Robot, Comput Assist Surg*, **7**(1), 17–21.

10
Mesoscale mobile robots for gastrointestinal minimally invasive surgery (MIS)

J. L. GORLEWICZ, R. J. WEBSTER III and
P. VALDASTRI, Vanderbilt University, USA

Abstract: Wireless capsule endoscopes, swallowable devices such as commercial pill cameras designed for minimally invasive surgery of the gastrointestinal tract, are reviewed, and the basic modules of robotic capsules are described. Latest research results in the development of robotic capsules are presented, and a perspective on the future prospects for clinical implementation of wireless robotic capsule-based surgical systems is presented.

Key words: wireless capsule endoscopy, robotic capsules, swallowable devices, surgical endoscopy, minimally invasive surgery.

10.1 Introduction

As discussed in previous chapters of this book, robotic systems have been applied to a wide range of surgical procedures including abdominal surgery, neurosurgery, cardiac surgery, otolaryngology, and urology, among many others. In the future, one can expect to see many more customized robotic systems, purposely designed for specific clinical needs in specific surgical procedures.

From a technical perspective, future robots will become smaller and increasingly less invasive in their approach to the surgical site. One way to achieve this using endoscope-like tools is to move toward natural orifice surgery, as reviewed in Chapter 9. An alternate paradigm is to 'cut the cord', making the robot completely untethered and mobile within the body. This enables the robot to enter the body though either a natural orifice or a very small incision, and then maneuver itself to a surgical site that need not be in close proximity to the point of entry.

Such mobile medical robot systems may be created on a variety of scales including the micro- and nanoscales, as discussed in chapters 8, 9 and 11. Unlike micro- and nanoscale robots which are useful in areas such as the eye (Ergeneman *et al.*, 2008) or the capillaries (Martel *et al.*, 2009) where larger robots are precluded by anatomical constraints, mesoscale robots are ideal for areas like the gastrointestinal (GI) tract and abdomen where their larger payload capacity is advantageous. The mesoscale (broadly defined as

1–100 mm) includes robots that are small, but easily visible and manipulable by unaided human eyes and hands. Although there do exist some robots in this category designed to be inserted through incisions (Lehman *et al.*, 2009; Patronik *et al.*, 2009; Platt *et al.*, 2009; Rentschler *et al.*, 2006; Simi *et al.*, 2012), many more robots in this category are designed to be swallowable.

Because it provides a natural means of robot locomotion and is difficult to access any other way, the GI tract has been the proving ground for the vast majority of mesoscale mobile robots developed to date. For this reason, and because the basic modules in mesoscale mobile robots are similar regardless of method of entry into the body, in this chapter we will focus on swallowable capsule robots intended for the GI tract. As an emerging technology, many of these robots are still in the research and development phase and have not yet been clinically implemented, although an increasing number have been applied in animal studies. Combined with the commercial and clinical success enjoyed by camera pills, the future of mesoscale mobile robots as platforms for surgical interventions is bright.

10.2 Commercial gastrointestinal wireless capsule endoscopes

The first wireless capsule endoscopes (WCEs) were pills containing cameras, which captured images deep within the GI tract. The first commercial WCE, the PillCam (Given Imaging) and other commercial capsules (Fig. 10.1) have been used to diagnose diseases such as obscure gastrointestinal bleeding (OGIB), cancer, celiac disease, and Crohn's disease, all of which occur in the small intestine (Moglia *et al.*, 2009). In addition to becoming the preferred method of diagnosis within the small intestine, commercial WCEs have recently been developed for other parts of the GI tract. The GI tract consists of the esophagus, stomach, small intestine, and large intestine (colon), which vary in size and shape, creating many different challenges for WCEs.

The esophagus, a hollow muscular tube approximately 25 cm long and 1.5–2 cm in diameter (Brittannica, 2009) is the first area a capsule reaches after being swallowed. Because a capsule passes through the esophagus in approximately 10 s, images must be rapidly acquired. For this reason, commercial esophageal capsules (PillCam ESO and ESO2 by Given Imaging, Inc.) have dual cameras and capture images at higher frame rates than the capsules used in the small and large intestine (Moglia *et al.*, 2007).

Studies with these esophageal capsules show that they can achieve very high accuracies in diagnosing Barrett esophagus and portal hypertension, but are not sensitive enough to diagnose neoplastic lesions (Heresbach *et al.*, 2010). Gastro esophageal reflux disease (GERD) requires long-term

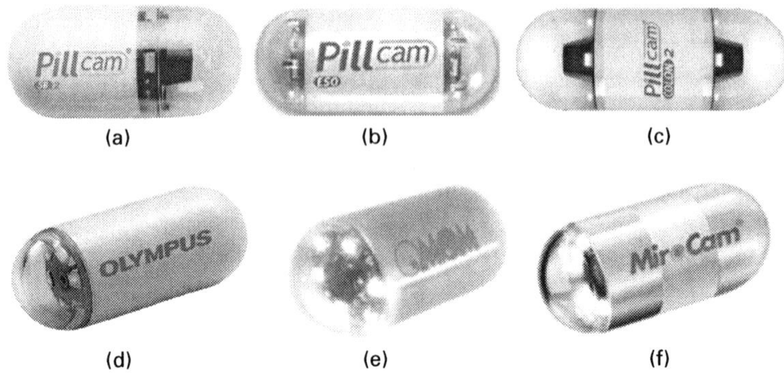

10.1 Current commercial camera capsules include: (a) PillCam SB2, (b) PillCam ESO (and ESO2), (c) PillCam Colon2 (and Colon), all by Given Imaging, Inc. and (d) EndoCapsule by Olympus, Inc., (e) OMOM by Jinshan Science and Technology Group, and (f) MiroCam by Intromedic, Co. Most of the capsules above are used for diagnosis within the small intestine, but the PillCam ESO and ESO2 target the esophagus, and the PillCam Colon and Colon2 target the large intestine. All capsules are 11 mm in diameter × 26 mm in length except for OMOM (13 mm × 27.9 mm), MiroCam (10.8 mm × 24 mm), and PillCam Colon2 (11 mm × 31 mm).

pH monitoring (generally at least 24 h) for diagnosis. The Bravo capsule (Given Imaging, Inc.) is designed for this purpose but requires fixation to the esophageal wall via an endoscopic procedure (Kwiatek and Pandolfino, 2008). A clinical capsule that can stop and anchor itself on the esophageal wall has yet to be realized, though several research capsules have been developed which include braking or anchoring mechanisms such as legs (Glass *et al.*, 2008; Tognarelli *et al.*, 2009) or magnets (Gonzalez-Guillaumin *et al.*, 2007), which are discussed further in Section 10.3.4.

A capsule exits the esophagus into the stomach, a large, typically deflated, elastic sac. The stomach is lined with a thick mucous membrane which makes it difficult for capsules to achieve traction on the stomach wall. As a result, no clinical capsules for the stomach have yet been developed. Research prototypes include a 'swimming' capsule (Tortora *et al.*, 2009) and a multimodule robotic system consisting of several units that are independently swallowed and then assemble within the stomach (Nagy *et al.*, 2009).

Just beyond the stomach, the capsule reaches the small intestine, where WCEs have made their most significant clinical impact. The small intestine is an elastic lumen (3 to 4 cm in diameter) and is the longest part of the GI tract (approximately 670 to 760 cm) (Britannica, 2009). Capsules move through the many curves and folds within the intestine via natural muscle contractions known as peristalsis. Commercial capsules designed for the small intestine (Fig. 10.1) include the PillCam SB and SB2 and Agile Patency System (a dissolvable pill) by Given Imaging, Inc., the EndoCapsule by

Olympus, Inc., the OMOM capsule by the Jinshan Science and Technology Group Co., Ltd., and the MiroCam capsule by Intromedic Co. The Agile capsule, an accessory to the PillCam, can be used before the ingestion of the PillCam SB to verify adequate capsule passage through the GI tract in patients with known or suspected strictures. This capsule assists in detecting the problem of capsule retention, which occurs in 0.75% of OGIB cases, but may occur at a rate of up to 6.7% in patients with Crohn's disease (Moglia *et al.*, 2007). These commercial capsules designed for use in the small intestine vary slightly in size, optical sensors such as complementary metal oxide semiconductor (CMOS) or change coupled device (CCD), and frame rate (Cavallotti *et al.*, 2009).

A capsule generally takes approximately 8–10 h to pass through the entire GI tract, with the majority of the time spent in the small and large intestines (Drossman *et al.*, 2005). The large intestine or colon, which is about 150 cm in length and 6 cm in diameter, is the last region a capsule encounters before exiting the body. Because of the larger lumen diameter, it is almost impossible for capsules to view the entire surface area of the internal intestinal wall. Furthermore, because the capsules are much smaller in size than the lumen itself, they tend to tumble within the lumen, making visualization even more difficult. To address this, the PillCam Colon and Colon2, the only commercially available capsules for the colon, are longer in length than the other commercial capsules and contain two on board cameras. In a multicenter performance study, the PillCam Colon2 achieved a sensitivity of 89% and a specificity of 76% in detecting colonic polyps ≥ 6 mm, suggesting that it is a safe and effective method for visualization in the colon and for detecting lesions (Eliakim *et al.*, 2009). It is not yet clear what clinical impact these colon capsules have as neither the Colon or Colon2 have received Food and Drug Administration (FDA) Approval yet.

10.3 Robotic capsule modules

Although the above camera capsules have made a significant impact on minimally invasive diagnoses within the GI tract, they are passive devices that lack the ability to accomplish definitive (e.g. biopsy) diagnosis or enable direct surgical intervention. In addressing these issues, a great deal of recent research has focused on developing robotic capsules to enhance diagnosis and provide treatment within the GI tract (Toennies *et al.*, 2010). Active robotic capsules that can see, diagnose, and treat within the GI tract require a variety of possible modules (Fig. 10.2), each of which pose a number of engineering challenges. The major modules of a robotic capsule include vision, telemetry, localization, locomotion, non-visual sensors, interventional systems, and power. Integrating two or more of these in the very limited space on board a capsule is also challenging, as underscored by the many

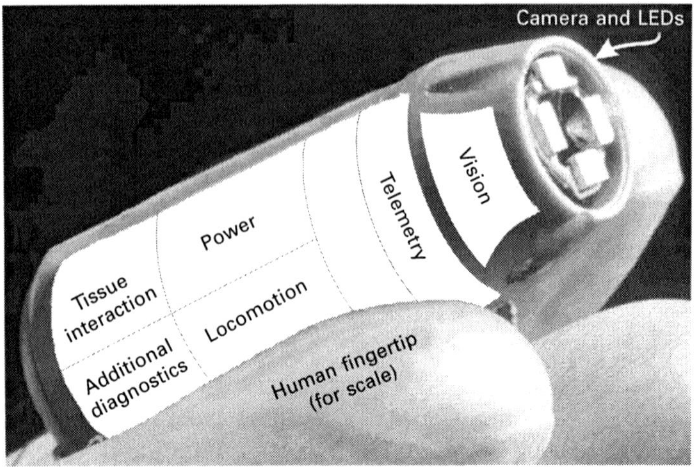

10.2 Potential modules required for a wireless robotic capsule include vision, telemetry, localization, locomotion, sensing, intervention, and power.

prototype capsules built to date that only contain a subset of these modules. Whether all of these modules can be integrated into one capsule that can perform all tasks or whether a cooperative multicapsule approach will be required is not yet known, though a large number of robotic modules will be needed in either case. The current technical progress of each of these modules is discussed in detail in the following sections.

10.3.1 Vision

The very existence of WCEs can be attributed to the development of miniature camera(s) integrated within swallowable pills (Swain, 2008). Typical images obtained from a camera pill are shown in Fig. 10.3. The primary goal of all vision systems is to provide clear, high resolution internal images of the GI tract. In order to do this, a number of hardware components are required on board a capsule including a vision sensor, a lens, an illumination source, and a compression chip. The primary image acquisition chip used by most capsules, including the PillCam (Given Imaging, Inc.), OMOM (Jinshan Science and Technology Group, Ltd., Co.), and MiroCam (Bang *et al.*, 2009), is based on CMOS technology, though the Olympus EndoCapsule (Olympus, Inc.) relies on a CCD. Although both imaging chips provide similar diagnostic performance, recent studies have shown that the EndoCapsule generally scores higher in image quality and resolution than the PillCam SB (Cave *et al.*, 2007; Metzger *et al.*, 2009). A detailed review of the vision capabilities associated with each technology is available in (Moglia *et al.*, 2009).

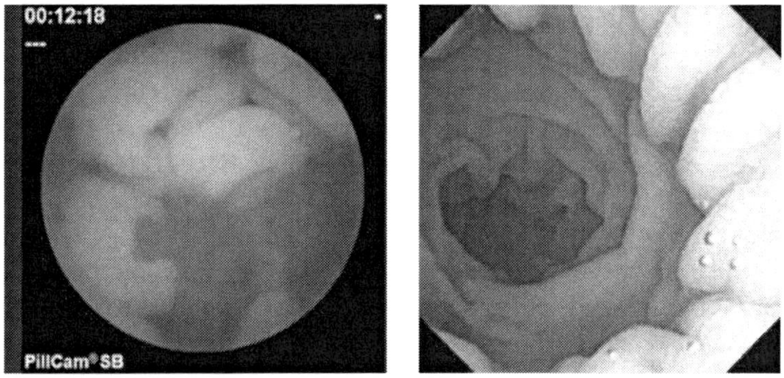

(a) (b)

10.3 (a) A typical image showing a bleeding lesion obtained from a PillCamSB, (Image courtesy of Rajesh Kumar, Johns Hopkins University). (b) An image of the gastric cavity with the pylorus seen distally from an Olympus capsule endoscope (© 2010 Georg Thieme Verlag KG, reprinted with permission, Rey *et al.* 2010).

Current commercial imaging chips must compromise between image quality and power consumption (Vatteroni *et al.*, 2010). Several researchers have been working to develop smaller, more efficient image acquisition chips. For example, CMOS technology has been used to develop a monolithic 320 × 240 active-pixel red, green, blue (RGB) or gray level camera-on-a-chip sensor to improve imaging sensitivity while decreasing the power consumption of the chip (Vatteroni *et al.*, 2010). This imaging chip has been tested in an *ex vivo* setting, and preliminary results suggest low noise and good image uniformity (Vatteroni *et al.*, 2010). Further, toward developing a high dynamic range vision system, a linear–logarithmic CMOS pixel with a programmable dynamic range extendable beyond 110 dB was developed and integrated in a 100 × 100 array within a monochrome imager (Vatteroni *et al.*, 2011). An integrated three-dimensional (3D) sensor which uses a multispectral CMOS sensor and a pulsed pattern projector for 3D reconstruction of images has been demonstrated on a large-scale by (Kolar *et al.*, 2009). There has also been some work in combining technologies from both CMOS and CCD to develop an improved hybrid camera (Swain, 2008).

The type of optics, including both the lens and illumination source, is also important in obtaining quality images from a capsule platform. To date, all available WCEs have a fixed focal length lens (Cavallotti *et al.*, 2009). Although this is acceptable for passive capsules, because the lumen is almost always collapsed around the capsule keeping the distance from the camera to the lumen wall constant, it would not be ideal for capsules that can actively locomote or distend tissue. To this end, Cavallotti *et al.* (2009) developed a prototype system that uses a liquid lens actuated by a pulse width modulated signal to adjust the focal length from 15 to 100 mm. Good illumination is also necessary for obtaining high-quality images from a capsule. Current commercial capsules use anywhere from 4–6 light-emitting diodes (LEDs). Beyond this, new image-enhanced technologies have been developed that allow physicians to view the GI tract in much greater detail than ever before, even on a cellular level (Hasan and Wallace, 2009). A few of these techniques include chromoendoscopy and autofluoresence (light working in conjunction with dyes applied to the GI mucosa or with chemicals in the tissue that fluoresce, respectively), confocal laser endomicroscopy (for real-time histology), and spectroscopy (which has been used to detect dysplasia) (Hasan and Wallace, 2009). These technologies may be integrated into future robotic capsules, enabling optical diagnoses deep within the GI tract.

A second, yet equally important, goal of a capsule vision system is the transmission of acquired images to an offline receiver. Because thousands of images are captured by the capsule, each containing a large amount of information, these images must be compressed in order to transmit them over the relatively low data rate telemetry links currently available (see Section 10.3.2). Image compression is challenging, as it requires retaining sufficient image information while keeping power consumption and transmission time low. The optimal level of compression is dependent upon the medical objective of the capsule. Current capsules for the small intestine, which have frame rates ranging from 2–3 Hz (Cavallotti *et al.* 2009), produce diagnostically useful results, though there is little doubt that higher frame rates would be desirable.

When higher frame rates are achieved, such as in the PillCam ESO and ESO2, which acquire images at a rate of 14–18 frames per second (fps), the battery life of the capsule is significantly reduced. Fortunately, because esophageal capsules only need to function for a few minutes at most, battery life is not as much of a concern for these capsules (Moglia *et al.*, 2007). For active robotic capsules that may be teleoperated by a surgeon, it is expected that frame rates of 20 fps or more will be required (Turgis and Puers, 2005). Several researchers have worked on developing efficient compression algorithms and low-power compression chips (Lin *et al.*, 2006; Turcza *et al.*, 2008; Turgis and Puers, 2005). Toward addressing power consumption, Chen *et al.* (2009) developed a system that can reduce average power consumption by 45% using a power efficient image compression module, a power management unit, and a novel wireless wake-up subsystem with zero stand-by current. A versatile field-programmable gate array (FPGA)-based system has been developed by Cavallotti *et al.* (2011) which enables testing of different configurations of the submodules that compose the entire vision system, including the camera, illumination, image compression, and telemetry. The optimal configuration that was found for endoscopic capsules attained an average frame rate of 19 fps over a transmission channel of 1.5 Mbit s^{-1} (Cavallotti *et al.*, 2011).

Once the images have been compressed and transmitted, they must be analyzed either manually by a physician or automatically by computer algorithms. This external post-processing of images is very useful, as a typical small intestine capsule returns approximately 50 000 images from a single use (Bejakovic *et al.*, 2009), but only a few contain useful diagnostic information. To alleviate physicians from the task of manually sorting through these images, algorithms are being developed to automatically guide the physician to the most important images (Bejakovic *et al.*, 2009). Although the above techniques are for off-board analysis of images, on board analysis would enable closed-loop control of camera orientation (Zabulis *et al.*, 2008) and the ability to detect and predict upcoming video images that may be of concern to a physician (Wang and Meng, 2009). Such *in situ* video analysis could also be used to help control capsule movement, by increasing or decreasing speed, based on the images collected (Wang and Meng, 2009). Although current vision systems in capsules are good enough for diagnostic tasks, there is little doubt that speed and resolution improvements would be desirable to enhance diagnosis and are necessary to enable future teleoperated robotic capsules.

10.3.2 Telemetry

As mentioned in Section 10.3.1, images obtained from a capsule must be transmitted over a wireless communication link to an external receiver. The objective is to transmit information as quickly as possible using the least amount of power. Currently available commercial capsules are only capable of unidirectional communication (sending images from the capsule). The PillCams accomplish this using telemetry chips produced by Zarlink, Inc. Other custom unidirectional chips (Shen *et al.*, 2005; Thone *et al.*, 2009) are also available which have slightly lower power consumption, but also slower data rates than the Zarlink chip. Because robotic capsules must be able to send and receive commands, bidirectional communication will likely be essential. To this end, Susilo *et al.* (2009) have developed an architecture that incorporates ZigBee (which is based on the IEEE 802.15.4 standard) and a commercial microcontroller to achieve bidirectional communication of control signals. Another promising method of information transfer is electric-field propagation, which is used in the MiroCam capsule by Intromedic Co. It is expected that this technique may have higher data rates and lower power consumption than existing radio frequency (RF) technologies, because the human body is used as the conductive medium for data transmission.

10.3.3 Localization

Because the GI tract is a long, tubular environment lacking obvious landmarks, it is challenging to localize capsule position with respect to the intestine, and thereby determine the location of lesions or other structures of interest seen in capsule images. To provide a means of capsule localization, a number of systems have been explored. One approach, used in the PillCam SB, involves RF triangulation. This technique uses an external sensor array to measure the signal strength of capsule transmissions at multiple points and then estimates the distance the capsule has traveled based on these measurements (Fischer *et al.*, 2004). Unfortunately, this method often returns noisy measurements, resulting in distance estimates having errors of up to 37.7 mm in one study (Wang *et al.*, 2006).

A potentially more accurate approach is to use magnetic tracking of a permanent magnet embedded in the capsule and detected by a skin-mounted magnetoresistive sensor array (Wang *et al.*, 2006). One 3D magnetic system called 3D-MAGMA (Innovent Technology, Germany) uses 27 sensors to determine the location of a magnetic pill and can achieve accuracies of 5 mm in position and 2° in orientation (Hocke *et al.*, 2008). Using biplane fluoroscopy for visualization, Laulicht *et al.* (2011) achieved real-time monitoring and control of a magnetic capsule in the small intestines of rats. Such a system has potential applications for localizing drug delivery capsules (see Section 10.3.6). A similar approach was taken by Carpi *et al.* (2011) who used fluoroscopic imaging in conjunction with a robotic navigation system (Niobe, Stereotaxis, Inc.) originally developed for cardiovascular clinical procedures for 3D localization and steering (see Section 21.3.3) of a magnetic capsule (Carpi *et al.*, 2011). They achieved 3D localization of the capsule with an error of 1 mm.

A simpler localization approach achieved 6° accuracy in estimating capsule orientation using inertial sensing (Ciuti *et al.*, 2010a). Electromagnetic localization using eight small magnetized coils was used to localize an inch-worm robot (see sections 10.3.4 and 10.3.7) and was able to achieve positional errors <10 mm and orientation errors <2° (Li *et al.*, 2008). The InteliSite (Innovative Devices) and Enterion (Phaeton Research and Pharmaceutical Profiles) drug delivery capsules (discussed in more detail in Section 10.3.6) use gamma scintigraphy for localization. This method requires a radioactive agent to be placed inside the capsule, which can then be tracked using gamma cameras (Wilding *et al.*, 2000).

Several noteworthy approaches using computer vision as a means of localizing the capsule have also been developed. One approach achieves 95% accuracy in classifying images as belonging to the upper or lower (that is, the colon) GI tract (Bulat *et al.*, 2007), whereas another classifies different digestive organs based on their unique muscular contraction patterns with 76% accuracy (Lee *et al.*, 2007).

Yet another possible localization approach, which has not yet been tested in the GI tract, uses ultrasonic pulses emitted outside of the body and echoed back by the capsule to determine the capsule location (Arshak and Adepoju,

2006). Another idea drawn from a review of patent literature (Moglia *et al.*, 2008) is the possibility of combining magnetics and X-ray imaging for localization (Kuth *et al.*, 2007).

At the time of writing this chapter, it remains unclear which localization system is likely to be most useful and easily implementable, while providing sufficiently accurate information. However, it is clear that a localization system that can acquire not only the capsule's 3D position in space, but also the distance it has traveled and its position relative to the GI tract would be extremely valuable in both diagnostic and therapeutic applications of WCEs.

10.3.4 Locomotion

Current passive commercial capsules move freely through the GI tract using peristalsis, making their motion erratic and unpredictable, and leading to incomplete evaluations approximately 20% of the time (Westerhof *et al.*, 2009). Active locomotion has the potential to improve capsule imaging consistency and evaluation by enabling the capsule to move forward, backward, or even stop at places of interest (Valdastri *et al.*, 2009). To achieve this, a number of prototype capsules have been developed implementing internal or external locomotion strategies. Internal locomotion involves micromechanisms integrated on board the capsule, while external locomotion utilizes propulsive forces transmitted by an external system, typically a magnetic field.

Internal locomotion

Despite the challenges of designing, manufacturing, and integrating micromechanisms in the limited space available on board a capsule, a number of different internal locomotion systems have been developed over the past few years. One design that is mechanically very simple utilizes vibratory actuation, where a micromotor contains an asymmetric mass on the rotor to create vibrations around its central axis (Ciuti *et al.*, 2011). This vibration aids the forward progression of a capsule by reducing friction with the intestinal wall, but can make orientation control and the acquisition of good images difficult. Another capsule uses two directional friction spirals surrounding the outside ends of the capsule body, combined with two magnets (one that rotates and one that translates), to propel itself forward or backward (Yim and Jeona, 2009).

A few capsule robots that mimic earthworm-like motion have also been developed. Two prototypes developed by Kim and colleagues use cyclic compression/extension of shape memory alloy (SMA) spring actuators to propel the capsule forward relying on directional spines to alternately anchor itself in between cycles (Kim *et al.*, 2005b, 2005c; Kwon *et al.*, 2007). These prototypes were slightly larger in size than the commercial PillCam Colon, but bidirectional motion may not be possible with the directional spines. Another inchworm-like capsule, which is powered by wireless power transmission and localized by electromagnetic localization (see sections 10.3.3 and 10.3.7) has also been developed (Li *et al.*, 2008). This robot, which consists of multiple segments, is a total of 150 mm long, but is connected by gimbals making it flexible enough to traverse the GI tract.

Another bio-inspired approach to locomotion which relies on SMA actuation is a cilia system (intended to mimic biological cells) (Li *et al.*, 2006). This capsule, composed of six units, each with two cilia-like appendages, can achieve bidirectional motion. A disadvantage of both the cilia design and the earthworm design is that SMAs consume significant power as they are heated to induce actuation, and bandwidth is limited because of the time required for heating and cooling. A 'paddling' technique, which uses leg-like fins that travel the length of the capsule body, has also been used for locomotion (Kim *et al.*, 2010). This design enables rapid movement of the capsule through the GI tract, though bidirectional motion was not demonstrated on the first prototype.

Including legs on a capsule is useful for both anchoring and locomotion in the GI tract. An anchoring mechanism is essential for capsules to perform long-term monitoring, as is required in diagnosing GERD. To this end, a 3-legged capsule with compliant feet that can be deployed and retracted has been developed by Tognarelli *et al.* (2009). A prototype similar in intent, though using a different anchoring foot design, is a capsule that uses legs with bio-inspired feet containing adhesives to enhance a capsule's ability to stick to the esophageal wall (Glass *et al.*, 2008). Extending this idea of using micropatterned adhesives, two of these anchoring capsules were combined together to form a six-legged capsule actuated by coil-type SMA wires to mimic a crawling motion (Karagozler *et al.*, 2006).

A series of increasingly sophisticated legged prototypes achieving fully bidirectional motion have been developed over the past 10 years at the Center for Research in Microengineering at Scuola Superiore Sant'Anna, Italy. The first prototype consisted of six SMA-actuated legs (Gorini *et al.*, 2006). The short functional life of the SMA actuators and mechanical complexity of the design prompted a move to miniature DC motors, and designs incorporating four legs (Quirini *et al.*, 2008b), eight legs (Quirini *et al.*, 2007; Quirini *et al.*, 2008a), and 12 legs (Quaglia *et al.*, 2009; Valdastri *et al.*, 2009) have been created. The latest 12-legged design, shown in Fig. 10.4a, can distend tissue in a uniform manner, travel through the colon in a time similar to traditional colonoscopy, and is the size of a commercial camera pill (Valdastri *et al.*, 2009). In addition to tissue distention, legged locomotion also provides the ability to control capsule position and orientation, and anchor and release the capsule as desired. Buselli *et al.* (2009) explored optimizing the design of

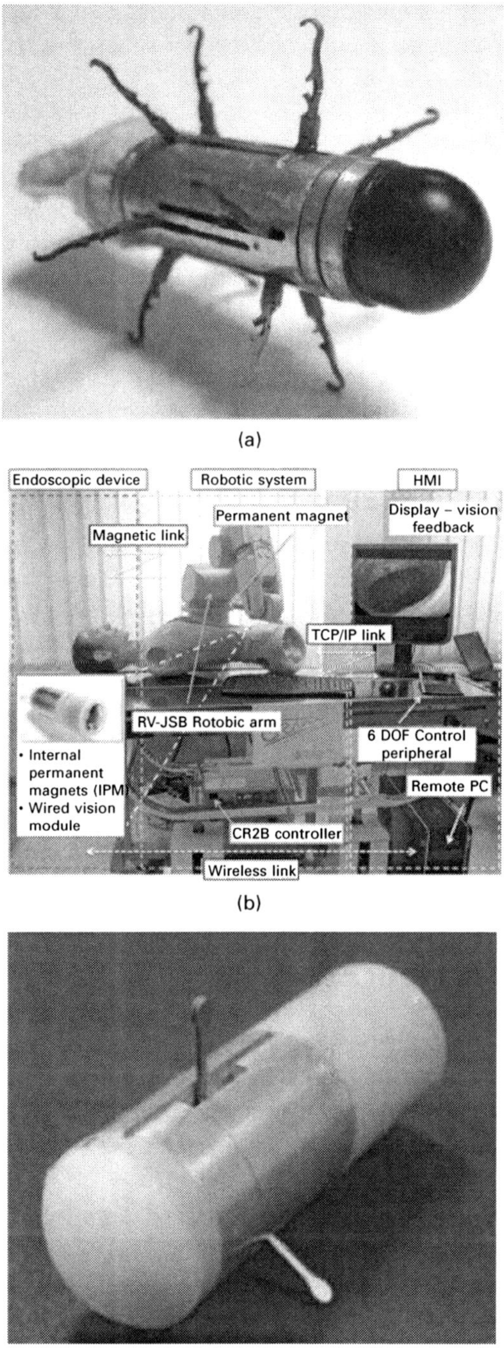

(c)

10.4 For controlled locomotion within the gastrointestinal tract, robotic capsules may use (a) internal mechanisms such as legs (reprinted with permission from Valdastri *et al.* 2009 © 2009 IEEE), (b) external actuation via magnetic field (reprinted with permission from Ciuti *et al.* 2010 © 2009 Georg Thieme Verlag KG), or (c) a combination of both (reprinted with permission from Simi *et al.* 2010 © 2010 IEEE).

superelastic capsule legs as well as adding polymeric microfabricated pillars to capsule legs in order to enhance adhesion and friction forces between the legs and the colon tissue (Buselli *et al.*, 2010).

Because the stomach is an elastic, liquid-filled environment, capsules that can 'swim' have become the most popular form of locomotion for use in this area of the GI tract. One example is a capsule that utilizes propeller propulsion and can steer itself by actuating its propellers according to direction, speed, and rotation (Tortora *et al.*, 2009). Another swimming robot, which is actuated by animal-derived muscle tissue, was proposed by (Herr and Dennis, 2004). Though their current prototype is 12 cm long, the idea of using living muscle tissue for actuation may be beneficial for future capsule endoscopes. A swimming microrobot which uses two pairs of external Helmholtz coils to create a magnetic field that causes a fin-like tail to swing back and forth has also been developed by (Byun *et al.*, 2011), though its applications are not specific to GI capsule endoscopy. Though different in its application, an ingestible wireless capsule designed to release an intragastric balloon for the treatment of obesity has also been developed for use in the stomach (Kencana *et al.*, 2010). Currently, this capsule is too large to be swallowed, though it is capable of inflating a balloon up to a volume of approximately 200 mL.

From earthworm-like motion to crawling to swimming, it is clear that a wide variety of approaches have been taken to provide internal locomotion capabilities to capsules. Other methods that have also been explored (see Swain, 2008) include electrostimulation of GI muscles (Mosse *et al.*, 2001; Woo *et al.*, 2006, 2009) and flagellar swimming (Kosa *et al.*, 2008); while some patents also allude to magnetically actuated propellers (Iddan and Gilad, 2006) and self-propulsion through jets (Iddan, 2006). The advantages of internal locomotion include the ability to obtain precise motion relative to the lumen, while not requiring any external magnetic field generators, and the ability to achieve tissue distention away from the on board camera in some cases. The challenges associated with internal locomotion, however, include designing and manufacturing complex mechanical systems small enough to fit within the space constraints of the capsule, developing more power-efficient mechanisms to run on miniature batteries or other power sources, and to manufacture these capsules cheaply enough to be disposable (which may be preferred) or robust enough to be sterilized.

External locomotion

An alternative to internal locomotion mechanisms on board capsules is to use external systems (primarily magnetic fields) to induce locomotion. External locomotion is being pursued in the research community, and also in the commercial arena by Given Imaging, Inc. and Olympus, Inc. Magnetic fields can be generated outside the patient either by electromagnetic coils or by permanent magnets. Coils can provide electronic control of field strength and direction, whereas permanent magnets typically generate higher fields in smaller form factors.

One of the earliest groups to utilize magnetic fields for capsule locomotion was the Norika Project team, who developed a capsule controlled by external coils embedded in a jacket worn by the patient (Moglia *et al.*, 2007; Uehara and Hoshina, 2003). Olympus has also been developing a bidirectional magnetically actuated capsule that has an internal magnet which interacts with a varying, controllable, rotating field created by three pairs of external magnets (Moglia *et al.*, 2007). Using an Olympus magnetic capsule endoscope and a Siemens magnetic guidance system, Rey *et al.* (2010) showed that magnetically navigated capsules can accomplish gastric examinations. Given Imaging, Inc. has taken a slightly different approach to using magnetic fields, using an external hand-held plate magnet to manipulate a magnetic capsule under gastroscopic visualization (Keller *et al.*, 2011; Swain *et al.*, 2010). Feasibility studies using the hand-held magnetic system suggest that remote manipulation of the capsule is feasible in both the esophagus and stomach (Keller *et al.*, 2011; Swain *et al.*, 2010).

A custom-designed magnetic capsule navigation system using a pair of electromagnets has been developed and tested in both simulation and in a small-scale physical setup by (Lam and Mintchev, 2009). Incorporating diamagnetic materials in the capsule casing to provide finer control and stabilization of on board magnets is also being explored (Lam and Mintchev, 2009). Yet another approach uses a rotating external magnetic field to move a variable diameter capsule that contains an internal magnet and a spiral fin around its body (Zhang *et al.*, 2010). Controlling a magnetic field by fixing a permanent magnet to a Cartesian robot was proposed by Kim *et al.* (2005a). This idea was studied in more depth by Ciuti *et al.* (2010), who exploited the precise control of a six degree-of-freedom (DOF) robotic manipulator with a permanent magnet fixed to its end effector to control capsule locomotion (Fig. 10.4b). Using this system, robotic control for magnetic steering of capsule endoscopes was demonstrated to be more precise and reliable than manual operation (Ciuti *et al.*, 2010a).

An innovative approach utilizing two commercially available technologies, the Niobe System by Stereotaxis, Inc. and the PillCam SB by Given Imaging, Inc. was proposed by Carpi *et al.* (2006, 2011) and Carpi and Pappone (2009). In this system, a magnetic sleeve was created to fit around the PillCam SB, whose orientation was then controlled using the Niobe system. Omnidirectional steering accuracy of 1° was achieved. Using magnetic fields to directly steer the camera of a capsule has also been proposed by Valdastri *et al.* (2010). In this work, a remote controlled capsule, known as the magnetic internal mechanism (MIM) capsule, uses two internal permanent magnets fixed to a toothed gear, which rotates when a motor is activated. When placed in an external magnetic field, the internal magnets remain aligned with the external magnetic field, causing the entire capsule to pivot about a single point, enabling fine adjustment of the camera orientation (Valdastri *et al.*, 2010).

The primary advantage of external locomotion, in comparison with internal locomotion, is a reduction in components on board the capsule, enabling a larger diagnostic or therapeutic payload. The drawback is the requirement of a large and complex system outside the patient to generate the magnetic field. Methods to determine the necessary field characteristics for a given desired capsule motion or force application are also open research areas (Abbott *et al.*, 2007; Ciuti *et al.*, 2010b). One other challenge in using magnetic locomotion is that the deflated intestine significantly impedes their motion (this is why many of the existing prototypes are tested in conjunction with endoscopy, which can control insufflation during the test). Recently, wireless insufflation has been proposed to overcome this obstacle (Toennies *et al.*, 2010; Toennies and Webster, 2009). It is also possible to combine internal and external locomotion in a hybrid capsule (Fig. 10.4c) which is primarily magnetically actuated but uses legs to assist with locomotion and tissue distention as needed (Simi *et al.*, 2010). Another hybrid approach uses a spiral ridge which is rotated by a micromotor as its primary source of locomotion and uses external magnetic fields to provide assisting force and increase speed as needed (Wang *et al.*, 2010).

10.3.5 Diagnostic systems

Many different sensing systems have been developed for wireless capsules. An example is a swallowable pH-sensing capsule that uses voltage differences to measure pH and half-ring electrodes for impedance monitoring, developed for diagnosis of GERD (Gonzalez-Guillaumin *et al.*, 2007). This capsule is held to the esophageal wall by an external magnet near the throat.

Several capsules have been developed that can measure temperature in the GI tract. Examples include the VitalSense ingestible telemetric physiological monitoring system, which uses thermistor-based sensing, and the CorTemp pill system, which measures crystal oscillations for temperature sensing, (McKenzie and Osgood, 2004). Other capsules that can measure both temperature and pressure include the Philips IntelliCap (www.philips.com) (also discussed in Section 10.3.6) (Forgione, 2009) and a design by van der Schaar and colleagues that can expel a small amount of liquid (Moglia *et al.*, 2008). Two other sensing capsules reviewed in (Twomey and Marchesi, 2009) include the Lab-on-a-Pill capsule (Johannessen *et al.*, 2004) which can sense pH, conductivity, and oxygen levels, and the Standford Endocapsule (Allison *et al.*, 2006), which has optical, chemical, temperature, and pH measuring capabilities. Moglia *et al.* (2008) also review other recent patents on capsule-based biosensors.

Optical biopsy may also be a useful diagnostic tool for capsule endoscopes, because traditional biopsies often require multiple samples to be taken from the same site and analyzed within 1–2 h of extraction. Unlike traditional biopsies, optical biopsies rely on the properties of light for diagnosis (Sauk and Itzkowitz, 2011). One example of a capsule system that detects lesions or internal bleeding within the GI tract was developed by (Liu *et al.*, 2010) and another was described in a patent by (Schostek *et al.*, 2007). Other promising techniques include fluorescence endoscopy, optical coherence tomography, confocal microendoscopy, light-scattering spectroscopy, raman spectroscopy, and molecular imaging, all of which are discussed in detail by Wang and Van Dam (2004).

10.3.6 Intervention

Perhaps the most compelling aspect of robotic capsules is their potential to both diagnose and treat lesions they encounter *in situ*. Although current commercial capsules have significantly improved physicians' ability to see areas deep within the GI tract, they are still passive devices and subsequent surgery is often required in order to perform an intervention. Compared with many of the other robotic modules discussed in this chapter, interventional capabilities of capsules are still in their infancy. Despite this, a few innovative designs have been developed which include a clip deployment capsule, drug delivery capsules, and biopsy sampling.

The first therapeutic capsule of its kind, recently developed by Valdastri *et al.* (2008), can deploy a single preloaded SMA clip at the site of a lesion, based on a wirelessly transmitted command. This capsule (Fig. 10.5) also

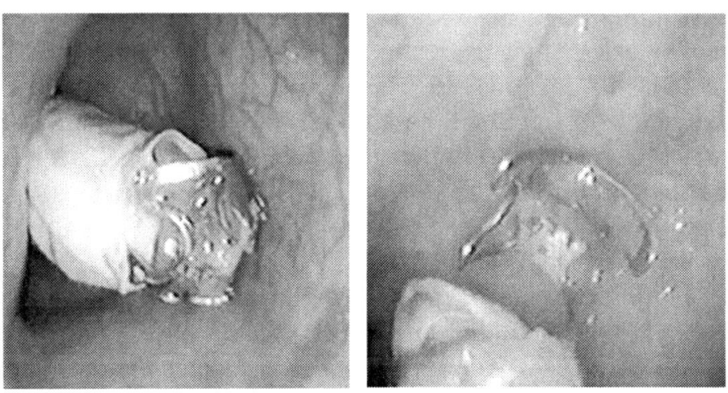

(a) (b)

10.5 This interventional capsule (a) uses magnetic locomotion to position itself near a lesion and then (b) deploys a clip to stop the bleeding (reprinted with permission from Valdastri *et al.* 2008, © 2009 Georg Thieme Verlag KG).

has permanent magnets embedded inside of it, enabling active locomotion via an external magnetic field so that the capsule can be properly aligned with the site of interest.

Other therapeutic capsules have also been designed to deliver topical drugs to an area of interest. It is hoped that delivering drugs directly at the site of interest will lower the dosage levels required for treatment and lower the time required for healing to begin. The InteliCap, under development at Philips, Inc., can measure and transmit temperature and pH levels (as mentioned in Section 10.3.5) in addition to delivering a treatment agent on command. As mentioned in Section 10.3.3, Laulicht *et al.* (2011) are developing a magnetic localization platform that allows a user to adjust a capsule's location within the GI tract in order to optimize the release of drugs in the area of greatest absorption or therapeutic action. Yet another drug delivery capsule uses a novel micromachined thruster that converts chemical energy into propulsion energy which produces sufficient pressure to empty a drug reservoir on board the capsule (Pi *et al.*, 2010). Other drug delivery capsules include the InteliSite capsule (Innovative Devices) which uses SMA wires to line perforated inner and outer sleeves to disperse a drug through holes and the Enterion capsule (Phaeton Research and Pharmaceutical Profiles), which uses a piston/spring system to deliver a treatment agent (Wilding *et al.*, 2000). Both Twomey and Marchesi (2009) and Wilding *et al.* (2000) provide further in-depth discussions of drug delivery capsules.

As mentioned in Section 10.3.5, conventional biopsy procedures often require taking multiple samples from one location and then having these samples analyzed within 1–2 h of extraction. Although optical biopsy from a capsule platform has been proposed, a biopsy device which uses a rotational razor for cutting tissue has been implemented on board a capsule and was successful in extracting a tissue sample in an *ex vivo* animal intestine (Kong *et al.*, 2005). It is unknown yet whether this type of capsule is able to take multiple samples as required in traditional biopsy for accurate histological analysis. A few patent disclosures (Moglia *et al.*, 2008) also suggest other ideas for therapeutic and interventional capsules including capsules housing ultrasonic transducers (Miyake, 2006; Taniguchi, 2005) and a dual-capsule camera biopsy system (Swain, 2007).

Interventional capsules are one of the most compelling aspects of endoscopic capsule research from the perspectives of reducing invasiveness and costs of treatment. Endowing capsules with interventional capabilities, however, is challenging due to the intelligent and miniaturized mechanisms that are required for both diagnosis and treatment. Such capabilities, however, will likely propel capsule endoscopes into becoming truly robotic devices.

10.3.7 Power

The need for an energy-dense power source is the greatest challenge facing researchers developing mobile robotic surgery platforms today. For vision alone, commercial GI capsules rely on two silver oxide coin cell batteries which take up almost half of the space available on board (Moglia *et al.*, 2009). In general, batteries do not scale down well to the mesoscale, primarily because the batteries that are small enough to fit within a robotic capsule are not energy-dense enough to power robotic mechanisms for very long. Lithium ion polymer (LiPo) batteries are the best source of electrical power available today because they can source peak currents up to 20 times their nominal current. Furthermore, they can be shaped or slightly bent for optimal placement within a capsule. Valdastri *et al.* (2009) elaborate on the power requirements of their actively locomoting 12-legged capsule, which they estimated would require 430 mW, plus an additional 180 mW for real-time vision. They determined that the smallest (10 mm in diameter × 30 mm in length) battery available to power their 12-legged capsule was a 100 mA h battery. This battery is almost the same size as those used in commercial capsule endoscopes. Thus, future advancements in battery technology are needed to enable completely wireless robots with complex mechanisms.

One alternative is wireless power transfer via inductive coupling, which uses internal coils on board a capsule to derive power from a magnetic field established by an external solenoid coil. This approach was used in the intracorporal video probe (Lenaerts and Puers, 2007) and was also used in powering a propeller-driven capsule, shown in Fig. 10.6 (Carta *et al.*, 2009). Further, the Norika project team proposed using inductive coupling to power a capsule by having a patient wear a vest that had coils embedded in it for both power transmission and direction control (Uehara and Hoshina, 2003). Wireless power transmission was also used to power an inchworm-like robot (Li *et al.*, 2008), where the maximum applied power was 35 W, and the average received power was 490 mW. By using electromagnetic localization and synthesis of the magnetic field vector, a wireless power system that can automatically tune the power-transmitting coils and can regulate the output power based on the capsule's need was developed (Li *et al.*, 2010).

One potential alternative to electrical energy is fluid power. Fluid power involves the phase transition of a liquid fuel to a gas, which generates pneumatic pressure. This concept was initially demonstrated in a prosthetic arm by Goldfarb *et al.* (2003), where experiments indicated that it could improve an energetic figure of merit (a metric that encompasses energy density, conversion efficiency, and actuator power density) by an order of magnitude. Based on this, the idea of utilizing fluid power for capsule robots has also been proposed (Toennies *et al.*, 2010; Toennies and Webster, 2009), where initial experiments for wireless insufflation were performed as

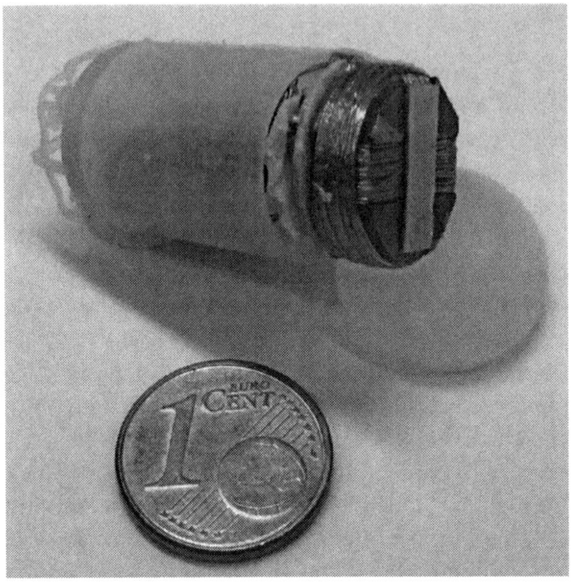

10.6 A propeller-driven capsule (Carta *et al.* 2009), which uses inductive coupling for wireless power transmission. The internal coils on board the capsule derive power from an external magnetic field to propel the capsule throughout the stomach.

a first step toward using fluid power to actuate more complex mechanisms. These feasibility studies suggest that it is possible for a capsule to carry a sufficient volume of fluid to generate sufficient gas to significantly enhance visualization. At this point, it is unclear which form of power generation is most efficient for robotic capsules. It is clear, however, that capsule robots require enhanced batteries or alternative sources of power such as inductive coupling, fluid power, or other novel technologies to be developed at the scales, power levels, and current sourcing capacities required to achieve their full potential.

10.4 Future trends in mobile surgical devices

Future innovations in several aspects of robotic capsules will open the door to many new surgical applications. The most important need is a highly energy dense power supply. Also extremely useful would be miniature wireless cameras capable of high-definition imaging and high frame rates. This will be enabled by advancements in flexible electronics and 3D packaging of integrated electronics and optics components. Design of miniature, high-performance mechanisms is the key to enabling biopsy and interventional capabilities.

As the technologies described in each of the preceding sections evolve, mobile surgical robots are poised to become increasingly useful diagnostic and interventional devices in the GI tract and in abdominal surgery. As the robotic technologies described in previous sections are combined, miniaturized, and made more power-efficient, mobile surgical robots will take on increasingly complex tasks in many different kinds of surgery.

Future systems can be expected to evolve along several different parallel trajectories. First, mobile robots containing cameras (the first few examples of which have already appeared in academic laboratories, as discussed earlier in this chapter) will provide physicians with many new view angles on existing surgical sites. This will enable image-processing techniques to provide even more information to the physician, including 3D reconstructions of anatomical information, and augmented reality interfaces. Other sensors can also be integrated onto mobile platforms to enable *in situ* diagnosis of disease (e.g. by spectroscopy or chemical sensors).

To overcome the power issue, early generations of mobile surgical platforms will be 'softly tethered', meaning that they incorporate very small and lightweight tethers to provide power and other capabilities. Magnets can be used in conjunction with soft tethers to enable several robots to work cooperatively to perform laparoscopic surgery. The natural progression as advances in each aspect of mobile surgical robots are made will be to cut the cord and remove these tethers. Wireless interventional capsules have already been demonstrated in the GI tract, although much work is needed before they become clinically available, and many new designs will be needed to address different pathologies.

Microscale mobile robots are also an active area of research as reviewed in chapters 8, 9 and 11. They are particularly useful as the target environment becomes smaller (e.g. eye, blood vessels). In terms of manufacturing, microscale robots typically require micromanufacturing techniques and/or integration of biological components. In contrast, mesoscale robots can often be fabricated using high-precision, but fundamentally standard manufacturing processes.

Looking to the future, rather than converging to one single device that can do everything, it is likely that specific robot systems will be designed for specific surgical indications. Also, teams of mobile robots will probably collaborate to meet surgical objectives. These devices or teams of devices will make surgery less invasive and more effective, enabling physicians to see, diagnose, and apply proper therapy, simultaneously.

10.5 Conclusion

In this chapter, we have reviewed the state-of-the art in mesoscale mobile robots. We have focused on robotic capsules for endoscopy within the GI tract, because this is the most accessible location in the human body to capsule robots, and has thus served as the proving ground for many current devices. Although passive imaging capsules have rapidly become the gold standard for diagnosis within the small intestine, robotic capsules have yet to be implemented clinically due to the many challenges associated with miniaturizing internal mechanisms and the lack of an energy-dense power source. Despite this, many robotic capsules are currently being developed and enabling technologies are being explored to overcome the current challenges in applying capsule robots in surgery. In the future, it is likely that these technologies will propel capsules into clinical implementation and enable them to see, diagnose, and treat diseases within the human body from a mobile, minimally invasive platform.

10.6 References

Abbott, J. J., Ergeneman, O., Kummer, M. P., Hirt, A. and Nelson, B. (2007), 'Modeling magnetic torque and force for controlled manipulation of soft-magnetic bodies', *IEEE Transactions on Robotics*, **23**, 1247–1252.

Allison, E., Kiraly, Z., Springer, G. and Dam, J. (2006), 'Endocapsule'. Patent Number WO/2006/045011.

Arshak, K. and Adepoju, F. (2006), 'Capsule tracking in the GI tract: a novel microcontroller based solution', *IEEE Sensors Applications Symposium, Houston, TX, USA*, pp. 186–191.

Bang, S., Park, J., Jeong, S., Kim, Y., Shim, H., Kim, T., Lee, D. and Song, S. (2009), 'First clinical trial of the 'MiRo' capsule endoscope by using a novel transmission technology: electric-field propagation', *Clinical Endoscopy*, **69**, 253–259.

Bejakovic, S., Kumar, R., Dassopoulos, T., Mullin, G. and Hager, G. (2009), 'Analysis of Crohn's disease lesions in capsule endoscopy images', *IEEE International Conference on Robotics and Automation*, Kobe, Japan.

Britannica (2009), 'Human digestive system'. http://www.britannica.com/. Accessed May 2011.

Bulat, J., Duda, K., Duplaga, M., Fraczek, R., Skalski, A., Socha, M., Turcza, P. and Zielinski, T. (2007), 'Data processing tasks in wireless GI endoscopy: image-based capsule localization and navigation with video compression', *Proceedings of IEEE/EMBS*, Lyon, France, pp. 2815–2818.

Buselli, E., Pensabene, V., Castrataro, P., Valdastri, P., Menciassi, A., and Dario, P. (2010), 'Evaluation of friction enhancement through soft polymer micro-patterns in active capsule endoscopy', *Measurement Science and Technology*, **21**, 105802 (7pp).

Buselli, E., Valdastri, P., Quirini, M., Menciassi, A. and Dario, P. (2009), 'Superelastic leg design optimization for an endoscopic capsule with active locomotion', *Smart Materials and Structures*, Pisa, Italy **18**, 015001 (8 pp).

Byun, D., Choi, J., Cha, K., Park, J. and Park, S. (2011), 'Swimming microrobot actuated by two pairs of Helmholtz coils system', *Mechatronics*, **21**, 357–364.

Carpi, F., Galbiati, S. and Carpi, A. (2006), 'Magnetic shells for gastrointestinal endoscopic capsules as a means to control their motion', *Biomedicine and Pharmacotherapy*, **60**, 370–374.

Carpi, F., Kastelein, N., Talcott, M. and Pappone, C. (2011), 'Magnetically controllable gastrointestinal steering of video capsules', *IEEE Transactions on Biomedical Engineering*, **58**, 231–234.

Carpi, F. and Pappone, C. (2009), 'Magnetic maneuvering of endoscopic capsules by means of a robotic navigation system', *IEEE Transactions on Biomedical Engineering*, **56**, 1482–1490.

Carta, R., Tortora, G., Lenaerts, B., Thone, J., Valdastri, P., Menciassi, A., Puers, R. and Dario, P. (2009), 'Wireless powering for a self-propelled and steerable endoscopic capsule for stomach inspection', *Biosensors and Bioelectronics*, **25**, 845–851.

Cavallotti, C., Merlino, P., Vatteroni, M., Valdastri, P., Abramo, A., Menciassi, A. and Dario, P. (2011), 'An FPGA-based versatile development system for endoscopic capsule design optimization', *Sensors and Actuators A*, **172**, 301–307.

Cavallotti, C., Piccigallo, M., Susilo, E., Valdastri, P., Menciassi, A. and Dario, P. (2009), 'An integrated vision system with autofocus for wireless capsular endoscopy', *Sensors and Actuators A*, **156**, 72–78.

Cave, D., Fleischer, D., Gostout, C., Faigel, D., Leighton, J., Heigh, R., Sharma, V., Mergener, K., Bhattacharya, K., Rajan, E., Foley, A., Lee, M., Knipschield, M. and Hibberd, P. (2007), 'A multi-center randomized comparison of the EndoCapsule: Olympus Inc and the PillCam SB: Given Imaging in patients with obscure GI bleeding [abstract]', *Gastrointestinal Endoscopy* **65**, AB125.

Chen, X., Zhang, X., Zhang, L., Li, X., Qi, N., Jiang, H. and Wang, Z. (2009), 'A wireless capsule endoscope system with low-power controlling and processing ASIC', *IEEE Transactions on Biomedical Circuits and Systems*, **3**, 11–21.

Ciuti, G., Donlin, R., Valdastri, P., Arezzo, A., Menciassi, A., Morino, M. and Dario, P. (2010a), 'Robotic versus manual control in magnetic steering of an endoscopic capsule', *Endoscopy*, **42**, 148–152.

Ciuti, G., Pateromichelakis, N., Sfakiotakis, M., Valdastri, P., Menciassi, A., Tsakiris, D. P., and Dario, P. (2011), 'A wireless module for vibratory motor control and inertial sensing in capsule endoscopy', *Sensors and Actuators A: Physical*, doi: 10.1016/j.sna.2011.12.024.

Ciuti, G., Valdastri, P., Menciassi, A. and Dario, P. (2010b), 'Robotic magnetic steering and locomotion of microsystems for diagnostic and surgical endoluminal procedures', *Robotica*, **28**, 199–207.

Drossman, D. A., Grimm, I. and Shaheen, N. (2005), *Handbook of gastroenterologic procedures – fourth edition*, Lippincott Williams and Wilkins, Philadelphia, PA.

Eliakim, R., Yassin, K., Niv, Y., Metzger, Y., Lachter, J., Gal, E., Spaznikov, B., Konikoff, F., Leichtmann, G., Fireman, Z., Kopelman, Y. and Adler, S. N. (2009), 'Prospective multicenter performance evaluation of the second-generation colon capsule compared with colonoscopy', *Endoscopy*, **41**, 1026–1031.

Ergeneman, O., Dogangil, G., Kummer, M. P., Abbott, J. J., Nazeeruddin, M. K. and Nelson, B. J. (2008), 'A magnetically controlled wireless optical oxygen sensor for intraocular measurements', *IEEE Sensors Journal of the American Chemical Society*, **8**, 29–37.

Fischer, D., Schreiber, R., Levi, D. and Eliakim, R. (2004), 'Capsule endoscopy: the localization system', *Gastrointestinal Endoscopy Clinics of North America*, **14**, 25–31.

Forgione, A. (2009), 'In vivo microrobots for natural orifice transluminal surgery. current status and future perspectives', *Surgical Oncology*, **18**, 121–129.

Given Imaging, Inc. www.givenimaging.com. Accessed May 2011.

Glass, P., Cheung, E. and Sitti, M. (2008), 'A legged anchoring mechanism for capsule endoscopes using micropatterned adhesives', *IEEE Transactions on Biomedical Engineering*, **55**, 2759–2767.

Goldfarb, M., Barth, E., Gongola, M. and Wehrmeyer, J. (2003), 'Design and energetic characterization of a liquid-propellant-powered actuator for self-powered robots', *IEEE/ASME Transactions on Mechatronics*, **8**, 254–262.

Gonzalez-Guillaumin, J., Sadowski, D., Kaler, K. and Mintchev, M. (2007), 'Ingestible capsule for impedance and pH monitoring in the esophagus', *IEEE Transactions on Biomedical Engineering*, **54**, 2231–2236.

Gorini, S., Quirini, M., Menciassi, A., Pernorio, G., Stefanini, C. and Dario, P. (2006), 'A novel SMA-based actuator for a legged endoscopic capsule', *IEEE/RAS-EMBS International Conference on Biomedical Robotics and Biomechatronics*, Pisa, Italy pp. 443–449.

Hasan, M. and Wallace, M. (2009), 'Image-enhanced endoscopy', *American Society for Gastrointestinal Endoscopy*, **16**, 1–5.

Heresbach, D., Leray, E., d'Halluin, P. N., Cholet, F., Lapalus, M. G., Gaudric, M., Ben Soussan, E., Gaudin, J. L., Vahedi, K., Quentin, V., Filoche, B., Saurin, J. C., Chaussade, S. and Ponchon, T. (2010), 'Diagnostic accuracy of esophageal capsule endoscopy versus conventional upper digestive endoscopy for suspected esophageal squamous cell carcinoma', *Endoscopy*, **42**, 93–97.

Herr, H. and Dennis, R. (2004), 'A swimming robot actuated by living muscle tissue', *Journal of NeuroEngineering and Rehabilitation*, **1**, 6.

Hocke, M., Schone, U., Richert, H., Gornert, P., Keller, J., Layer, P. and Stallmach, A. (2008), 'Every slow-wave impulse is associated with motor activity of the human stomach', *American Journal of Physiology Gastrointestinal and Liver Physiology*, **296**, 709–716.

Iddan, G. (2006), 'Self propelled device'. US Patent Number 2006/0030754 A1.

Iddan, G. and Gilad, Z. (2006), 'Motor for an in-vivo device'. Patent Number WO 2006/070350 A2.

Jinshan Science and Technology Group, Ltd., Co. http://www.omom.us/main.php?sLAN=en.

Johannessen, E. A., Wang, L., Cui, L., Tang, T. B., Ahmadian, M., Astaras, A., Reid, S. W. J., Yam, P. S., Murray, A. F., Flynn, B. W., Beaumont, S. P., Cumming, D. R. S. and Cooper, J. M. (2004), 'Implementation of multichannel sensors for remote biomedical measurements in a microsystems format', *IEEE Transactions on Biomedical Engineering*, **51**, 525–535.

Karagozler, M., Cheung, E., Kwon, J. and Sitti, M. (2006), 'Miniature endoscopic capsule robot using biomimetic micro-patterned adhesives', *IEEE/RAS-EMBS International Conference on Biomedical Robotics and Biomechatronics*, Pisa, Italy pp. 105–111.

Keller, J., Fibbe, C., Volke, F., Gerber, J., Mosse, A. C., Reimann-Zawadzki, M., Rabinovitz, E., Layer, P., Schmitt, D., Andresen, V., Rosien, U. and Swain, P. (2011), 'Inspection of the human stomach using remote-controlled capsule endoscopy: a feasibility study in healthy volunteers (with videos)', *Gastrointestinal Endoscopy*, **73**, 22–28.

Kencana, A. P., Rasouli, M., Huynh, V. A., Ting, E. K., Lai, J. C. Y., Huy, Q. D. Q., Tan, S. L., Wong, K. J. and Phee, S. J. (2010), 'An ingestible wireless capsule for treatment of obesity', *32nd Annual International Conference of the IEEE EMBS Conference*, pp. 963–966.

Kim, B. K., Park, J. O. and Hong, Y. S. (2005a), 'Capsule type endoscope control system', Korean Institute of Science and Technology. Patent Number WO/2005/122866.

Kim, B., Lee, S., Park, J. H. and Park, J. O. (2005b), 'Design and fabrication of a locomotive mechanism for capsule-type endoscopes using shape memory alloys (SMAs)', *IEEE/ASME Transactions on Mechatronics*, **10**, 77–86.

Kim, B., Park, S., Yoon, S. J. and Jee, C. Y. (2005c), 'An earthworm-like locomotive mechanism for capsule endoscopes', *IEEE/RSJ International Conference on Intelligent Robots and Systems*, Edmonton, Alberta, Canada pp. 2997–3002.

Kim, H. M., Yang, S., Kim, J., Park, S., Cho, J. C., Park, J. Y., Kim, T. S., Yoon, E., Song, S. Y. and Bang, S. (2010), 'Active locomotion of a paddling-based capsule endoscope in an in vitro and in vivo experiment (with videos)', *Gastrointestinal Endoscopy*, **72**, 381–387.

Kolar, A., Pinna, A., Romain, O., Viateur, S., Ea, T., Belhaire, E., Graba, T. and Granado, B. (2009), 'A multishutter time sensor for multispectral imaging in a 3-D reconstruction integrated sensor', *IEEE Sensors Journal*, **9**, 478–484.

Kong, K., Cha, J., Jeon, D. and Cho, D. (2005), 'A rotational micro biopsy device for the capsule endoscope', *IEEE/RSJ International Conference on Intelligent Robots and Systems*, Edmonton, Alberta, Canada pp. 1839–1843.

Kosa, G., Jakb, P., Hata, N., Jolesz, F., Neubach, Z., Shoham, M., Zaaroor, M. and Szekely, G. (2008), 'Flagellar swimming for medical micro robots: theory, experiments, and application', *IEEE/RAS-EMBS International Conference on Biomedical Robotics and Biomechatronics*, Scottsdale, AZ USA pp. 258–263.

Kuth, R., Reinschke, J. and Roeckelein, R. (2007), 'Method for determining the position and orientation of an endoscopy capsule guided through an examination object by using a navigating magnetic field generated by means of a navigation device'. German patent, DE102005032370.

Kwiatek, M. A. and Pandolfino, J. (2008), 'The Bravo(TM) pH capsule system', *Digestive and Liver Disease*, **40**, 156–160.

Kwon, J., Park, S., Park, J. and Kim, B. (2007), 'Evaluation of the critical stroke of an earthworm-like robot for capsule endoscopes', *Proceedings of the IMechE Part H: Journal of Engineering in Medicine*, **221**, 397–405.

Lam, M. and Mintchev, M. (2009), 'Diamagnetically stabilized levitation control of an intraluminal magnetic capsule', *Physiological Measurement*, **30**, 763–777.

Laulicht, B., Gidmark, N. J., Tripathi, A. and Mathiowitz, E. (2011), 'Localization of magnetic pills', *Proceedings of the National Academy of Science*, **108**, 2252–2257.

Lee, J., Oh, J., Shah, S., Yuan, X. and Tang, S. (2007), 'Automatic classification of digestive organs in wireless endoscopy videos', *Proceedings of the ACM Symposium on Applied Computing*, Seoul, Korea, pp. 1041–1045.

Lehman, A., Dumpert, J., Wood, N., Redden, L., Visty, A., Farritor, S., Varnell, B. and Oleynikov, D. (2009), 'Natural orifice cholecystectomy using a miniature robot', *Surgical Endoscopy*, **23**, 260–266.

Lenaerts, B. and Puers, R. (2007), 'An inductive power link for a wireless endoscope', *Biosensors and Bioelectronics*, **22**, 1390–1395.

Li, H., Yan, G. and Gao, P. (2010), 'A method for improving the wireless power transmission efficiency of an endoscopic capsule based on electromagnetic localization and synthesis of magnetic field vector', *Proceedings of the IMechE Part C: Journal of Mechanical Engineering Science*, **224**, 1463–1471.

Li, H., Yan, G. and Ma, G. (2008), 'An active endoscopic robot based on wireless power transmission and electromagnetic localization', *International Journal of Medical Robotics and Computer Assisted Surgery*, **4**, 355–367.

Li, W., Guo, W., Li, M. and Zhu, Y. (2006), 'A novel locomotion principle for endoscopic robot', *IEEE International Conference on Mechatronics and Automation, Luoyang*, China pp. 1658–1662.

Lin, M. C., Dung, L. R. and Weng, P. K. (2006), 'An ultra-low-power image compressor for capsule endoscope', *BioMedical Engineering OnLine*, **5**, 14.

Liu, H., Wang, G., Wei, K., Pi, X., Zhu, L., Zheng, X. and Wen, Z. (2010), 'An intelligent electronic capsule system for automated detection of gastrointestinal bleeding', *Journal of Zheijiang University SCIENCE B*, **11**, 937–943.

Martel, S., Felfoul, O., Mathieu, J.B., Chanu, A., Tamaz, S., Mohammadi, M., Mankiewicz, M. and Tabatabaei, N. (2009), 'MRI-based medical nanorobotic platform for the control of magnetic nanoparticles and flagellated bacteria for target interventions in human capillaries', *International Journal of Robotics Research*, **28**, 1169–1182.

McKenzie, J. and Osgood, D. (2004), 'Validation of a new telemetric core temperature monitor', *Journal of Thermal Biology*, **29**, 605–611.

Metzger, Y., Adler, S., Shitrit, A., Koslowsky, B. and Bjarnason, I. (2009), 'Comparison of a new PillCam SB2 video capsule versus the standard PillCam SB for detection of small bowel disease', *Medical Imaging*, **2**, 7–11.

Miyake, K. (2006), 'Capsule ultrasonic endoscope and capsule ultrasonic endoscope system'. Japanose Patent JP325874.

Moglia, A., Menciassi, A. and Dario, P. (2008), 'Recent patents on wireless capsule endoscopy', *Recent Patents on Biomedical Engineering*, **1**, 24–33.

Moglia, A., Menciassi, A., Dario, P. and Cuschieri, A. (2009), 'Capsule endoscopy: progress update and challenges ahead', *Natural Reviews in Gastroenterology and Hepatology*, **6**, 353–362.

Moglia, A., Menciassis, A., Schurr, M. and Dario, P. (2007), 'Wireless capsule endoscopy: from diagnostic devices to multipurpose robotic systems', *Biomed Microdevices*, **9**, 235–243.

Mosse, A., Mills, T., Appleyard, M., Kadirkamanathan, S. and Swain, P. (2001), 'Electrical stimulation for propelling endoscopes', *Gastrointestinal Endoscopy*, **54**, 79–83.

Nagy, Z., Harada, K., Fluckiger, M., Susilo, E., Kaliakatsos, I. K., Menciassi, A., Hawkes, E., Abbott, J. J., Dario, P. and Nelson, B. J. (2009), 'Assembling reconfigurable endoluminal surgical systems: Opportunities and challenges', *International Journal of Biomechatronics and Biomedical Robotics*, **1**, 3–16.

Olympus, Inc. www.olympus.com. Accesed May 2011.

Patronik, N., Ota, T., Zenati, M. and Riviere, C. (2009), 'A miniature mobile robot for navigation and positioning on the beating heart', *IEEE Transactions on Robotics*, **25**, 1109–1124.

Philips, Inc. www.philips.com. Accessed May 2011.

Pi, X., Lin, Y., Wei, K., Liu, H., Wang, G., Zheng, X., Wen, Z. and Li, D. (2010), 'A novel micro-fabricated thruster for drug release in remote controlled capsule', *Sensors and Actuators A*, **159**, 227–232.

Platt, S., Hawks, J. and Rentschler, M. (2009), 'Vision and task assistance using modular wireless in vivo surgical robots', *IEEE Transactions an Biomedical Engineering*, **56**, 1700–1710.

Quaglia, C., Buselli, E., Webster III, R. J., Valdastri, P., Menciassi, A. and Dario, P. (2009), 'An endoscopic capsule robot: a meso-scale engineering case study', *Journal of Micromechanics and Microengineering*, **19**, 105007, 11p.

Quirini, M., Menciassi, A., Scapellato, S., Dario, P., Rieber, F., Ho, C. N., Schostek, S. and Schurr, M. (2008a), 'Feasibility proof of a legged locomotion capsule for the GI tract', *Gastrointestinal Endoscopy*, **67**, 1153–1158.

Quirini, M., Menciassi, A., Scapellato, S., Stefanini, C. and Dario, P. (2008b), 'Design and fabrication of a motor legged capsule for the active exploration of the gastrointestinal tract', *IEEE/ASME Transactions on Mechatronics*, **13**, 169–179.

Quirini, M., Scapellato, S., Valdastri, P., Menciassi, A. and Dario, P. (2007), 'An approach to capsular endoscopy with active motion', *IEEE/EMBS, Lyon, France*, pp. 2827–2830.

Rentschler, M., Dumper, J., Platt, S., Iagnemma, K., Oleynikov, D. and Farritor, S. (2006), 'Modeling, analysis, and experimental study of in vivo wheeled robotic mobility', *IEEE Transactions on Robotics*, **22**, 308–321.

Rey, J. F., Ogata, H., Hosoe, N., Ohtsuka, K., Ogata, N., Ikeda, K., Aihara, H., Pangtay, I., Hibi, T., Kudo, S. and Tajiri, H. (2010), 'Feasibility of stomach exploration with a guided capsule endoscope', *Endoscopy*, **42**, 541–545.

Sauk, J. and Itzkowitz, S. (2011), 'Optical enhancements in diagnosis and surveillance of colorectal neoplasia', *Current Colorectal Cancer Reports*, **7**, 24–32.

Schostek, S., Rieber, F., Ho, C. and Schurr, M. (2007), 'Device for hemorrhage detection'. US Patent Number 11/772603.

Shen, M. W., Lee, C. Y. and Bor, J. C. (2005), 'A 4.0-mW 2-Mbps programmable BFSK transmitter for capsule endoscope applications', *IEEE Asian Solid-State Circuits Conference*, Hsinchu, Taiwan.

Simi, M., Valdastri, P., Quaglia, C., Menciassi, A. and Dario, P. (2010), 'Design, fabrication, and testing of a capsule with hybrid locomotion for gastrointestinal tract exploration', *IEEE/ASME Transactions on Mechatronics*, **15**, 170–180.

Simi, M., Tolou, N., Valdastri, P., Herder, J. L., Menciassi, A. and Dario, P. (2012), 'Modeling of a compliant joint in a magnetic levitation system for an endocscopic camera', *Mechanical Sciences*, **3**, 5–14.

Susilo, E., Valdastri, P., Menciassi, A. and Dario, P. (2009), 'A miniaturized wireless control platform for robotic capsular endoscopy using advanced pseudokernel approach', *Sensors and Actuators A: Physical*, **156**, 49–58.

Swain, C. P. (2007), 'Method, system and device for in-vivo biopsy'. Patent Number EP1757099.

Swain, P. (2008), 'The future of wireless capsule endoscopy', *World Journal of Gastroenterology*, **14**, 4142–4145.

Swain, P., Toor, A., Volke, F., Keller, J., Gerber, J., Rabinovitz, E. and Rothstein, R. I. (2010), 'Remote magnetic manipulation of a wireless capsule endoscope in the esophagus and stomach of humans (with videos)', *Gastrointestinal Endoscopy*, **71**, 1290–1293.

Taniguchi, Y. (2005), 'Intracoelomic mobile body, and capsule-type ultrasonic endoscope'. Patent Number US20050119577.

Thone, J., Radiom, S., Turgis, D., Carta, R., Gielen, G. and Puers, R. (2009), 'Design of a 2 Mbps FSK near-field transmitter for wireless capsule endoscopy', *Sensors and Actuators A*, **156**, 43–48.

Toennies, J. L., Ciuti, G., Smith, B. F., A., M., Valdastri, P. and Webster III, R. J. (2010), 'Toward tetherless insufflation of the GI tract', Proceedings of the *IEEE Engineering in Medicine and Biology Conference (EMBC)*, pp. 1946–1949.

Toennies, J. L., Tortora, G., Simi, M., Valdastri, P. and Webster III, R. J. (2010), 'Swallowable medical devices for diagnosis and surgery: the state of the art', *Proceedings of the IMechE, Part C: Journal of Mechanical Engineering Science*, **224**, 1397–1414.

Toennies, J. L. and Webster III, R. J. (2009), 'A wireless insufflation system for capsular endoscopes', *ASME Journal of Medical Devices*, **3**(2), 27514.

Tognarelli, S., Quaglia, C., Valdastri, P., Susilo, E., Menciassi, A. and Dario, P. (2009), 'Innovative stopping mechanism for esophageal wireless capsular endoscopy', *Procedia Chemistry*, **1**, 485–488.

Tortora, G., Valdastri, P., Susilo, E., Menciassi, A., Dario, P., Rieber, F. and Schurr, M. (2009), 'Propeller-based wireless device for active capsular endoscopy in the gastric district', *Minimally Invasive Therapy and Allied Technologies*, **18**, 280–290.

Turcza, P., Zielinski, T. and Duplaga, M. (2008), 'Hardware implementation aspects of new low complexity image coding algorithm for wireless capsule endoscopy', *International Conference on Computational Science*, **5101**, 476–485.

Turgis, D. and Puers, R. (2005), 'Image compression in video radio transmission for capsule endoscopy', *Sensors and Actuators A*, **123–124**, 129–136.

Twomey, K. and Marchesi, J. R. (2009), 'Swallowable capsule technology: current perspectives and future directions', *Endoscopy*, **41**, 357–362.

Uehara, A. and Hoshina, K. (2003), 'Capsule endoscope NORIKA system', *Minimally Invasive Therapy and Allied Technologies*, **1**, 227–234.

Valdastri, P., Quaglia, C., Buselli, E., Arezzo, A., Di Lorenzo, N., Morino, M., Menciassi, A. and Dario, P. (2010), 'A magnetic internal mechanism for precise orientation of the camera in wireless endoluminal applications', *Endoscopy*, **42**, 481–486.

Valdastri, P., Quaglia, C., Susilo, E., Menciassi, A., Dario, P., Ho, C. N., Anhoeck, G. and Schurr, M. O. (2008), 'Wireless therapeutic endoscopic capsule: in vivo experiment', *Endoscopy*, **40**, 979–982.

Valdastri, P., Webster, III, R. J., Quaglia, C., Quirini, M., Menciassi, A. and Dario, P. (2009), 'A new mechanism for mesoscale legged locomotion in compliant tubular environments', *IEEE Transactions on Robotics*, **25**, 1047–1057.

Vatteroni, M., Covi, D., Cavallotti, C., Clementel, L., Valdastri, P., Menciassi, A., Dario, P. and Sartori, A. (2010), 'Smart optical CMOS sensor for endoluminal applications', *Sensors and Actuators A*, **162**, 297–303.

Vatteroni, M., Valdastri, P., Sartori, A., Menciassi, A. and Dario, P. (2011), 'Linear–logarithmic CMOS pixel with tunable dynamic range', *IEEE Transactions on Electron Devices*, **58**, 1108–1115.

Wang, T. D. and Van Dam, J. (2004), 'Optical biopsy: a new frontier in endoscopic detection and diagnosis', *Clinical Gastroenterology and Hepatology*, **2**, 744–753.

Wang, X. and Meng, M. (2009), 'In situ analysis of capsule endoscopy images and preliminary results', *IEEE/RSJ International Conference on Intelligent Robots and Systems*, pp. 5737–5742.

Wang, X., Meng, M. and Hu, C. (2006), 'A localization method using 3-axis magnetoresistive sensors for tracking of capsule endoscope', *Proceedings of IEEE/EMBS*, New York, NY USA pp. 2522–2525.

Wang, X., Meng, M. Q. H. and Chen, X. (2010), 'A locomotion mechanism with external magnetic guidance for active capsule endoscope', 32nd Annual International Conference of the IEEE EMBS Conference pp. 4375–4378.

Westerhof, J., Weersman, R. and Koornstra, J. (2009), 'Risk factors for incomplete small-bowel capsule endoscopy', *Gastrointestinal Endoscopy*, **69**, 74–80.

Wilding, I., Hirst, P. and Connor, A. (2000), 'Development of a new engineering-based capsule for human drug absorption studies', *Pharmaceutical Science and Technology Today*, **3**, 385–392.

Woo, S. H., Jang, J. Y., Jung, E. S., Lee, J. H., Moon, Y. K., Kim, T. W., Won, C. H., Choi, H. C. and Cho, J. H. (2006), 'Electrical stimuli capsule for control moving direction at the small intestine', *Proceedings of IASTED International Conference on Biomedical Engineering*, Innsbruck, Austria.

Woo, S. H., Kim, T. W., Lee, J. H., Kim, P. U., Won, C. H. and Cho, J. H. (2009), 'Implemented edge shape of an electrical stimulus capsule', *International Journal of Medical Robotics and Computer Assisted Surgery*, **5**, 59–65.

Yim, S. and Jeona, D. (2009), 'Capsular microrobot using directional friction spiral', *IEEE International Conference on Robotics and Automation*, pp. 4444–4449.

Zabulis, X., Argyros, A. and Tsakiris, D. (2008), 'Lumen detection for capsule endoscopy', *IEEE/RSJ International Conference on Intelligent Robots and Systems*, Nice, France pp. 3921–3926.

Zhang, Y. S., Jiang, S. Y., Zhang, X. W., Yu, H. H., Wang, D. L. and Guo, D. M. (2010), 'Dynamic characteristics of an intestine capsule robot with variable diameter', *Chinese Science Bulletin*, **55**, 1813–1821.

11
Real-time software platform using MRI for *in vivo* navigation of magnetic microrobots

K. BELHARET, D. FOLIO and A. FERREIRA,
Laboratoire PRISME, Ecole Nationale Supérieure d'Ingénieurs de Bourges, France

Abstract: A magnetic resonance imaging system is described for (MRI) navigation of microrobots for targeted therapy in cardiovascular systems. The software architecture of the robotic platform is presented, the MRI constraints are discussed, and a linear model of the microrobotic system is examined for navigating in vessels. A navigation path planning method is presented, which has ferromagnetic imaging recognition, and ferromagnetic tracking. Microrobot control is discussed and multiple simulation results are presented.

Key words: magnetic resonance imaging, robotics, targeted therapy, minimally invasive surgery.

11.1 Introduction

Microrobots designed to perform targeted therapy by navigating in the cardiovascular system are a prolific research area for minimally invasive surgeries (Ishiyama *et al.*, 2002; Abbott *et al.*, 2007) and the efficiency of treatments through early diagnosis of diseases (Cavalcanti *et al.*, 2009). Cardiovascular problems are generally correlated with obesity, human sedentary lifestyle, or hereditary characteristics. When microrobots are propelled in body fluids, particularly in the blood circulatory system, a very large number of remote locations in the human body become accessible. However, because the diameters of the blood vessels in the human body may vary from approximately 25 mm (aorta) down to 0.010 mm (capillaries), it is obvious that propelling such wireless microdevices in the human cardiovascular system with existing technologies represents a great technical challenge (Abbott *et al.*, 2009). Because the method of propulsion should allow such a microrobot to navigate through the cardiovascular system, the use of the normal blood flow itself must be considered only as a complementary means of propulsion when the travel path is in the direction of the blood flow.

These untethered microrobots have been mainly developed according to three different designs: magnetic bead pulling (Abbott *et al.*, 2007), biomimetic flagellated robot (Behkam and Sitti, 2006) and magnetotactic bacteria (Martel *et al.*, 2009). Furthermore, navigation requires observation of the scene in order either to plan the trajectory by offline mapping, or to correct online the microrobot's pose error between the planned and the observed trajectory. Recently, medical micro-/nanorobotic platforms using magnetic resonance imaging (MRI) have been investigated to reach deep locations in the human body while enhancing targeting efficacy. A recent breakthrough in interventional MRI-guided *in vivo* procedures demonstrated that real-time MRI systems can offer a well-suited integrated environment for the imaging, tracking, and control of a ferromagnetic device, which was done in the carotid artery of a living pig (Chanu *et al.*, 2008). These successful experiments pointed out critical challenges in terms of real-time imaging, tracking and navigation for future therapeutic applications, such as controlled targeted drug delivery in brain (Park *et al.*, 2008), navigable magnetic carriers for implantable biosensors (Cavalcanti *et al.*, 2009) or controlled ultrasensitive imaging for early diagnosis and treatment of diseases (Abbott *et al.*, 2009). An intravascular ultrasound (IVUS) medical-imaging technique coupled to preoperational images of computerized tomography (CT) (Park and Park, 2008), rendered possible three-dimensional (3D) navigation in blood vessels. Based on these path-planning techniques, only explorative two-dimensional (2D) control strategies have been adopted so far using a simple proportional-integral-derivative (PID) controller (Tamaz *et al.*, 2008). In Felfoul *et al.* (2008), the authors demonstrate a new concept of magnetic signature selective excitation tracking (MS-SET) providing high position update rate (Sabra *et al.*, 2005).

The challenges in MRI-based microrobot navigation are: to plan an efficient pathway in the cardiovascular networks; to recognize and track the microcarrier location; and to guide it robustly against the MRI constraints to the targeted area. Therefore, the main objective of this chapter is to propose an automated technique based on image processing and control algorithms for path finding, tracking and navigation control of a ferromagnetic microrobot using a clinical MRI system. The MRI-based control of a ferromagnetic microcapsule presented here is dedicated to microscale navigation, which focuses on conveying the device in vessels such as arteries and arterioles. The chapter is organized as follows. We first introduce the MRI-based navigation system by providing a common MRI platform overview and the MRI constraints, and then describing a simple model of the microrobotic system navigating in vessels. Secondly, we present the MRI-based microrobot navigation by focusing on the challenges presented. Various applications are described to show the validation of the proposed path planning, image processing and control algorithms.

11.2 Magnetic resonance imaging (MRI) navigation

A clinical magnetic resonance imaging (MRI) platform is used here to track and propulse a microdevice within the vascular network. The propulsion of the ferromagnetic microcapsule in the cardiovascular system is realized through the induction of force from magnetic gradients provided by the MRI. This MRI system guides the microcarrier *in vivo* through vascular networks to a targeted area. The overview of the system architecture is depicted in Fig. 11.1. The designed MRI-based navigation system requires observation of the scene in order to:

- plan the navigation pathway by offline mapping thanks to the navigation path-planner module;
- to track the microdevice position online using the artifact tracking module; and
- to drive its pose between the planned and the observed path through the navigation control module.

In particular, it is necessary, to ensure a robust and smooth conveyance of the capsule to its destination, while avoiding collisions and the risk of being trapped in wrong pathways; navigation performance is affected by external perturbations and MRI technological constraints, and sensing capabilities. In the next section, we explain the main MRI platform constraints.

11.2.1 MRI navigation constraints

As previously mentioned navigation in blood vessels requires observation of the scene in order either to plan the path by offline mapping, or to correct

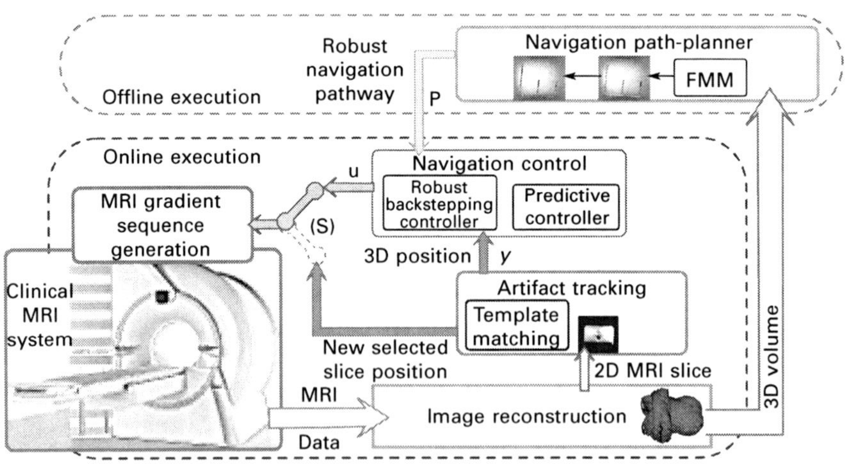

11.1 MRI-based navigation system overview.

online the microrobot pose error between the planned and the observed path. To ensure a smooth conveyance of the microcapsule to its destination, avoiding collisions and the risk of being trapped by the endothelium, optimal navigation performance is affected by external perturbations and MRI technological constraints such as:

- Non-negligible pulsatile flow, whose variations in waveform, amplitude, and frequency exist from one vessel to another (such as arteries and arterioles);
- MRI overheating avoidance leading to limitations on the MRI duty cycle, which tends to increase the disproportional scaling between magnetic forces used for control purpose and perturbation forces (drag forces and net buoyancy forces);
- limitations on the magnetic gradient amplitude in available clinical MRI devices;
- a significant delay in the image-processing algorithms that renders the navigation control unstable; and
- magnetic gradients, used both for observation and control purposes in a time-multiplexed sequence, require different trade-offs in terms of refresh rate, duty cycle of the propulsion gradients, and repetition time of the tracking sequence.

In particular, the overall concept of the *in vivo* MRI tracking system is based on the fact that both tracking and propulsion are possible with the gradient coils of the MRI system. Software based upgrading of a clinical MRI system is the least expensive approach to convert a platform that is used for imaging to an effective interventional platform. Nevertheless, at any instant only one of the functions can be applied (i.e. either tracking or propulsion), but both are executed over the same MRI interface. The MRI system has therefore to be shared, as illustrated with the switch 'S' in Fig. 11.1, and a time-division-multiple-access scheme for it has been developed (Belharet *et al.*, 2011). Moreover, Fig. 11.2 shows an overview of the real-time sequence with time-multiplexed positioning and propulsion phases introduced by Felfoul *et al.* (2008). The main aspects relevant to the controller's performance are: the duty cycle $T_{\text{Prop}}/T_{\text{s}}$ that stands for the ratio between the propulsion time and the time between two successive position requests, and the synchronization event delay T_{Sync} that stands for the minimum time allowed for image processing and real-time control feedback.

First, the duty cycle should be adapted to apply sufficient magnetic propulsion gradients during a predefined propulsion time T_{Prop} to prevent the microrobot from drifting away from the path. Second, a large time delay T_{Sync} produces oscillations as the microrobot approaches the reference path P leading to position instabilities. Such limitations have been pointed out by Tamaz *et al.* (2008) when implementing a simple proportional-integral-

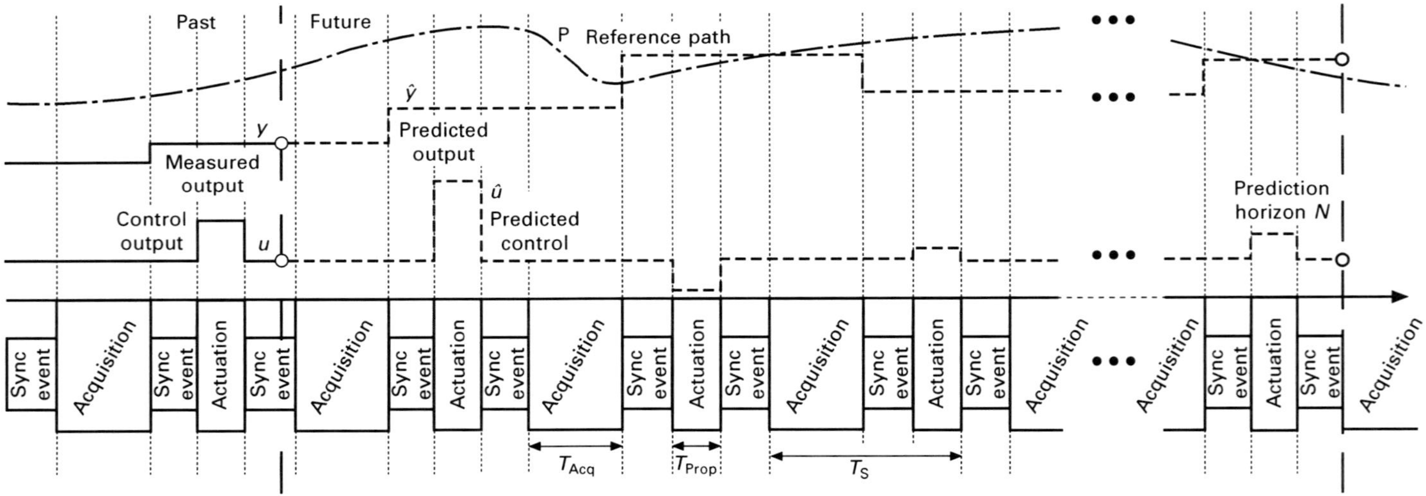

11.2 Timeline of acquisition and control prediction.

derivative (PID) controller. In Belharet *et al.* (2010a, 2011) are proposed to use predictive control strategies including the microrobot's motion and dynamics with estimation of the pulsative blood flow and time-multiplexed positioning. Predictive path-tracking controls consider a prediction window (cf. Fig. 11.2). The propulsion phase starts during T_{Prop} at the same initial condition as the prediction phase, recording the performance of the system according to a prediction horizon. After this phase, the system ends after an imaging–propulsion sequence at a final position y which is set as the new initial condition of the next prediction output $\hat{y}$. The proposed predictive controller offers stability by design and allows the designer to trade-off performance for (computation) speed; stability margins vary according to the MRI application and technological requirements (Camacho and Bordons, 2004), as described detailed in Section 11.3.3.

11.2.3 Model description of a microrobot in a viscous fluid

The purpose of this section is to present a simplified 3D model of the ferromagnetic microrobot in a blood vessel. The dominant forces exerted on a single microparticle in a blood vessel are (Fig. 11.3): the controlled magnetic force $\vec{F}_{\text{m}}$, the blood-flow drag force $\vec{F}_{\text{d}}$ and apparent weight $\vec{W}_{\text{a}}$ (see also Section 11.5). The magnetic forces $\vec{F}_{\text{m}}$ generated by the MRI coils on the ferromagnetic particles immersed in a fluid such as blood is formulated as:

$$\vec{F}_{\text{m}} = \mu_0 V_{\text{m}} (\vec{M}\nabla)\vec{H} \qquad [11.1]$$

Where μ_0 is the permeability of free space, V_{m} is the magnetic volume of the ferromagnetic material, $\vec{M}$ its magnetization, $\vec{H}$ is the magnetic field and ∇ the gradient operator. If the microrobot moves sufficiently slowly (i.e. with a Reynolds number $Re \ll 1$) the hydrodynamic drag force acting on the particle can then given by Stokes' law, and $\vec{F}_{\text{d}}$ of the microdevice in the aqueous medium is defined as:

$$\vec{F}_{\text{d}} = -6\pi\eta r(\vec{v} - \vec{v}_{\text{f}}) \qquad [11.2]$$

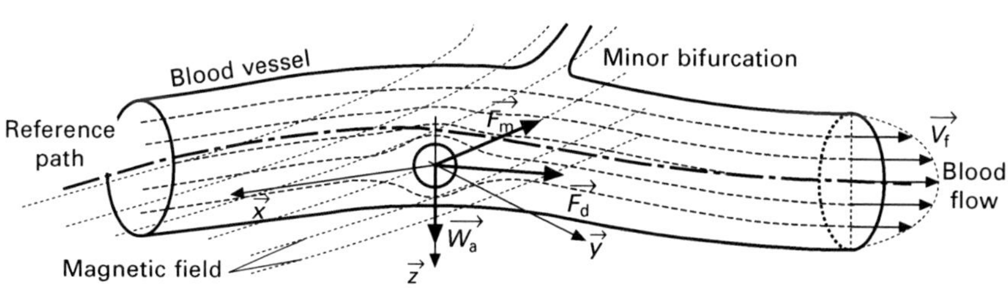

11.3 Forces applied on microrobot navigating in blood vessel.

where η denotes the fluid viscosity; r the spherical radius of the microcarrier; $\vec{v}$ the velocity of the microrobot; and $\vec{v}_f$ is the fluid velocity. The apparent weight considering the gravitational force on the microrobot in a viscous fluid is expressed as

$$\vec{W}_a = V_m(\rho - \rho_f)\vec{g} \qquad [11.3]$$

Where ρ is the density of the microrobot in the liquid medium, ρ_f the density of the liquid medium, and $\vec{g}$ the acceleration owing to gravity. Therefore, the force balance equation for the microdevice in the aqueous solution in the presence of external magnetic field can be formulated as:

$$\vec{F}_m + \vec{F}_d + \vec{W}_a = m_p \frac{dv}{dt} \qquad [11.4]$$

where m_p is the mass of the microcarrier modeled by a ferromagnetic sphere with a high saturation magnetization. The projection of the forces on the $(\vec{x}, \vec{y}, \vec{z})$ plane leads to:

$$\begin{cases} m_p\ddot{x} = \vec{F}_{dx} + \vec{F}_{mx} \\ m_p\ddot{y} = \vec{F}_{dy} + \vec{F}_{my} \\ m_p\ddot{z} = \vec{F}_{dz} + \vec{F}_{mz} + \vec{W}_a \end{cases} \qquad [11.5]$$

If $\vec{v}_f = (v_{fx}, v_{fy}, v_{fz})$ denotes the blood flow velocity, and (x, y, z) the robot location in the blood vessel with respect to a given frame $F(O, \vec{x}, \vec{y}, \vec{z})$ (Fig. 11.3), the linear model can be written as follow:

$$\begin{cases} \ddot{x} = \alpha_1(\dot{x} - v_{fx}) + \alpha_2 u_x \\ \ddot{y} = \beta_1(\dot{y} - v_{fy}) + \beta_2 u_y \\ \ddot{z} = \gamma_1(\dot{z} - v_{fz}) + \gamma_2 u_z \end{cases} \qquad [11.6]$$

where the following parameters α_i, β_i and γ_i and the magnetic gradients considered as control inputs u_x, u_y and u_z that is:

$$\begin{cases} \alpha_1 = -4.5\,\frac{\eta \cos\varphi \sin\theta}{r^2\rho}, & u_x = \left\|\vec{\nabla}\beta_x\right\| \\ \beta_1 = -4.5\,\frac{\eta \cos\varphi \sin\theta}{2} & u_y = \left\|\vec{\nabla}\beta_y\right\| \\ \gamma_1 = -4.5\,\frac{n \sin\varphi}{r^2\rho}, & u_z = \left\|\vec{\nabla}\beta_z\right\| \\ \alpha_2 = \beta_2 = \gamma_2\,\frac{m}{\rho} \end{cases} \qquad [11.7]$$

where $\boldsymbol{B} = (B_x, B_y, B_z)^T$ is the magnetic field generated by the MRI system, $\theta = (\overrightarrow{Ox}, \overrightarrow{Fd}$ and $\varphi = (\overrightarrow{Oz}, \overrightarrow{Fd})$.

Finally, the state-space representation is deduced from equation [11.6]:

$$(S)\begin{cases}\dot{x} = v_x \\ \dot{v}_x = \alpha_1 v_x - \alpha_1 v_{fx} + \alpha_2 u_x \\ \dot{y} = u_y \\ \dot{v}_y = \beta_1 v_y - \beta_1 v_{fy} + \beta_2 u_y \\ \dot{z} = v_z \\ \dot{v}_z = y_1 v_z - \beta_1 v_{fz} + \gamma_2 u_z\end{cases} \qquad [11.8]$$

where $\vec{v} = (v_x, v_y, v_z)^T$ denotes the robot velocity along $\vec{x}$-axis, $\vec{y}$-axis and $\vec{z}$-axis. Assuming that the microrobot location (x, y, z) can be measured thanks to the MRI system (cf. Section 11.3.2), we denote by $y = (x, y, z)^T$ the process measure.

11.3 Microrobot navigation

As previously mentioned, to design an efficient and reliable MRI-based microrobot navigation platform we have to:

- plan an efficient pathway in the cardiovascular networks;
- to recognize and track the microcarrier location; and
- to guide it robustly against the MRI constraints to the targeted area.

These three different aspects are discussed in the following subsections.

11.3.1 Navigation planning

To allow the microdevice to navigate properly within a tubular structure network we need to find a valid pathway between the initial and final states. Classically, a navigation pathway could be defined as a geodesic linking two points, that globally minimizes an energy functional weighted by a potential. Finding a navigation path within the endovascular network is then an essential, primary, and important step that must be addressed. This problem has received considerable attention in the computer-vision and medical-imaging communities (Kirbas and Quek, 2004). Hence, several types of methods have been proposed to find a path from a set of medical imaging, such as tracking methods (Felfoul *et al.*, 2008; Reuzé *et al.*, 1993; Tokuda *et al.*, 2010), path extraction methods (Deschamps, 2001; Wink *et al.*, 2000) and so on. For instance Sabra *et al.* (2005) proposed a path-planning method based on 3D potential fields and enhanced breath-first search algorithms based on MRI.

However, most works based on *in vivo* MRI tracking methods usually need many user-defined way points as the input of a controller module for the navigation computation. A major drawback in general remains when the user must define many points (e.g. way or fiducial points) manually. Hence, for a complex structure (e.g. a colon or small vessels) the required interactivity can be very tedious. Belharet *et al.* (2010a) and Belharet *et al.* (2010b)), proposed a framework to allow a *minimal centered navigation path* to be found, building upon the fast marching method (FMM) firstly introduced by Sethian (1999). The FMM needs a very simple initialization and leads to global minimum of a snake-like energy, thus avoiding local minima. Moreover, it is fast and accurate. In the FMM framework the path finding problem is solved through the computation of the minimal action map u: $c \rightarrow \mathbb{R}^+$, associated with an initial state x_0 on the domain $c \subset \mathbb{R}^3$. Moreover, the map u satisfies the Eikonal equation:

$$\begin{cases} \|\nabla u(x)\| = \omega(x), & \forall x \in c \\ u(x_0) = 0 \end{cases} \qquad [11.9]$$

where the isotropic cost function ω: $x \in c \rightarrow \omega(x) \in \mathbb{R}^+$ is a metric or a potential map of the state x; and the map u is a weighted distance map to the source x_0. Specifically, u may be regarded as the arrival time of a front propagation from the source with velocity $1/\omega(x)$. This map u has only one local minimum: either the initial point x_0 or the final point x_f. The minimal path can be therefore be retrieved with a simple gradient descent on u from a targeted seed x_f to x_f. The key challenge of the FMM is then to define an appropriate and efficient cost function $\omega(x)$ to drive the front propagation efficiently. A basic idea is to design such a cost function on a spatial consideration that leads to:

$$\omega_{VSL}: x \in c \rightarrow \text{Enhance}(x) \in \mathbb{R}^+ \qquad [11.10]$$

Where c is the input MRI data, and Enhance(x) is a vesselness enhancement function. Classically, to design the Enhance(x) function, we use some *a priori* knowledge about vessels' shape and intensity in the MRI data. Hence, a typical cost function ω_{VSL} could be simply designed by using a multiscale analysis based on geometric properties of the image retrieved from the Hessian matrix. Such a filter, proposed by Frangi *et al.* (1998) or Sato *et al.* (1998) for instance, allows us to compute for a voxel the pseudoprobability of belonging to a vessel structure. We have applied this approach to different sets of data, in 2D (Belharet *et al.*, 2010b) as well as in 3D (Belharet *et al.*, 2010a). Figure 11.4 illustrates the process of obtaining a centerline navigation path.

Recently (Folio *et al.*, 2011), this approach has been extended to obtain a robust pathway against the sensing uncertainty. Indeed, there are several important sources of uncertainty that should be considered in MRI-based navigation planning. These include uncertainty in MRI data acquisition

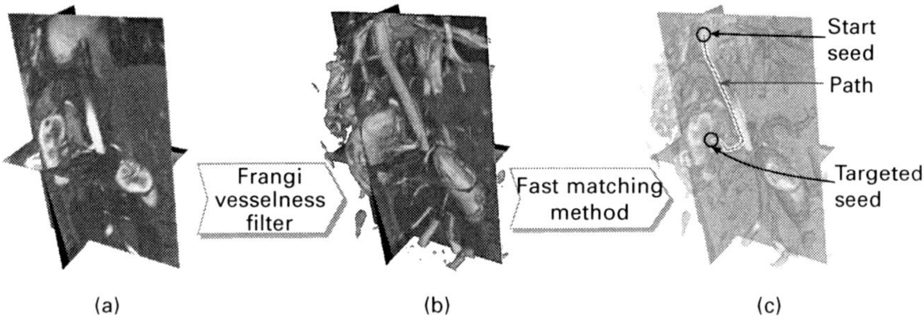

11.4 3D navigation centerline extraction: (a) original (input) 3D MRI data; (b) vesselness enhancement function using Frangi filter; and (c) extracted navigation pathway between the start and end (targeted) seeds using the fast marching method.

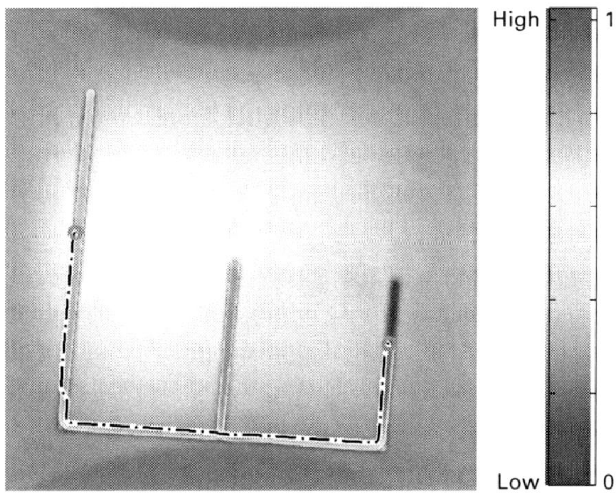

11.5 Robust navigation path extracted using the information gain cost function.

and processing, carrier model and position tracking. Failure to account for these uncertainty sources in the planning method could result in trapping the device in a wrong tube segment. Therefore, another cost function ω_{Bel} that maps the system's belief in its position x is required. A sensor model as been proposed as follows (Folio *et al.*, 2011):

$$\omega_{\text{Bel}}: x \in c \rightarrow l(x) \in \mathbb{R}^{+} \qquad [11.11]$$

where $l(x)$ is defined as the expected information gain (or, equivalently, the expected entropy reduction). The expected information gain $l(x)$ is computed, given the observed data y and a sensing model, from the difference in Shannon entropy of the prior and posterior distributions (Cover *et al.*, 1991). Figure 11.5 shows an expected information gain $l(x)$ and the resulting navigation path for a 0.7 mm steel ball tracking sequence. The pathway obtained between the selected points (the circles) is then the one that minimizes the sensing uncertainty during the navigation.

11.3.2 MRI-based sensing

Since the introduction of MRI, the occurrence of magnetic susceptibility artifacts has been studied. In clinical practice, the focus is usually on avoiding artifacts and producing correct images of anatomical structure (Port and Pomper, 2000). In the targeted system, susceptibility artifacts caused by the ferromagnetic microrobotic device are exploited for position determination. For this purpose, the imaging parameters and artifact formation principles have been investigated.

Imaging parameters and artifacts

The image acquisition procedure applied in MRI relies on the presence of a strong homogeneous main magnetic field $\boldsymbol{B}_0$ and three well-defined gradient fields. Insertion of magnetic material into the field of view clearly violates the assumption of homogeneity. This has two mainly effects:

- *intravoxel dephasing:* spins inside a single voxel are dephased owing to field inhomogeneity, leading to a damping or loss of signal; and
- *Spatial misregistration:* the spatial coding scheme is corrupted and signals are registered incorrectly, causing bright fringes around metallic objects.

In practice, the artifact shape depends on several factors related to the magnetic object and the imaging sequence. Saturation magnetization and object volume are the most important object-specific parameters. For small aspect ratios, object shape is of minor importance. The most important sequence-dependent parameters are echo type (gradient echo or spin echo) and echo time. Generally, gradient echo sequences produce much larger artifacts than spin echo sequences, in terms of affected volume. This is because of their inability to compensate for temporally constant field inhomogeneities.

Wortmann *et al.* (2010) studied the imaging parameters by experiment using a General Electric Signa 3*T* clinical MRI scanner. A representative selection of imaging sequences has been tested: conventional *gradient echo (GE)*, conventional *spin echo (SE)* and the real-time sequence *single-shot fast spin echo (SSFSE)*. Sample scans taken from the imaging experiments and the segmentation results for the GE sequence are shown in Fig. 11.6. The artifact observed in the GE sequence shows the greatest dimensions. Highest signal peaks are found using the conventional SE sequence. SSFSE produces the least severe artifacts. It has to be noted, that the artifact dimensions

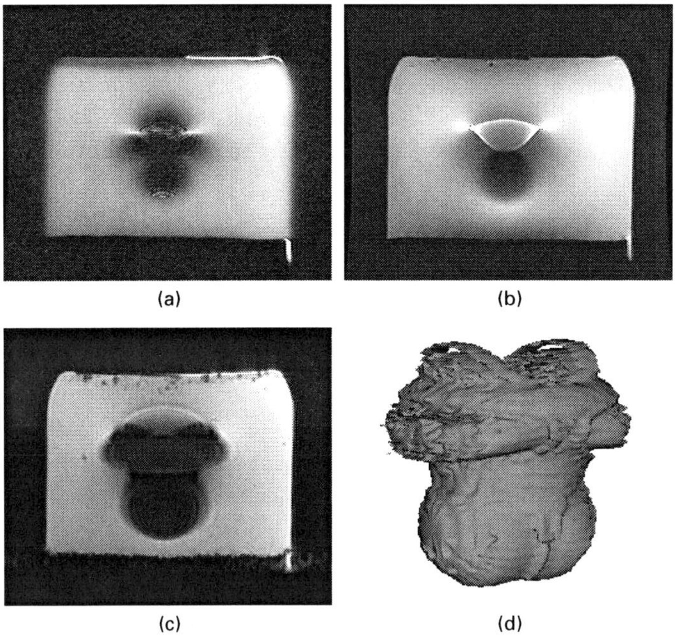

11.6 MRI susceptibility artifact imaging for a 2.5 mm steel sphere, embedded into agarose gel: (a) SSFSE sequence, (b) conventional SE, (c) conventional GE; and (d) reconstructed artifact volume of GE.

are orders of magnitude above the object dimensions. From the segmented susceptibility artifacts centroid, the object location can be concluded using a fixed offset vector.

Ferromagnetic device tracking

Efficient and reliable tracking of the untethered microdevice is a critical requirement for the success of MRI guided intervention. Several methods have been developed, categorized as passive or active (Felfoul *et al.*, 2008). Passive MRI tracking is simpler but commonly slower than active methods. Aboussouan *et al.* (2006) proposed a rapid passive MRI-tracking of the magnetic device dubbed magnetic signature selective excitation tracking (MS-SET), which is based on selective excitation of magnetic equipotential curves. On three acquired k-space lines, correlation is applied for position determination. In experiments using a 0.293 mm pixel size, an average error of 0.064 mm was achieved for a static particle, corresponding to 0.22 pixels. For dynamic particles, the average error was 1.2 mm or 4.1 pixels. Felfoul *et al.* (2008), recorded a 0.5 pixel precision. However, the poor position accuracy of the MS-SET tracking technique induces navigation or trajectory control errors over preplanned paths (Sabra *et al.*, 2005).

Furthermore, owing to the characteristic shape of the artifact (Fig. 11.6), the microcarrier could also be located in the image in most cases by executing template matching (Folio *et al.*, 2011), achieved during the recognition phase, by extracting a template that is subsequently used for tracking. The template-matching approach chosen is based on correlation. With a template T and the input image I in the 2D case:

$$C(x_p, y_p) = \Sigma_{x=0}^{x_t} \Sigma_{y=0}^{y_t} I(x_p + x, y_p + y) T(x, y) \qquad [11.12]$$

The position of the artifact depicted in the template is then derived from the maximum position inside the correlation matrix: $C(x_{object}, y_{object}) = \max(C)$. The position of the maximal value in the correlation matrix corresponds to the position of the tracked object, and the center of gravity of the object can be calculated. In order to determine the 3D position y of the artifact corresponding to the microdevice, a correlation is applied with a template stack to deliver the third dimension co-ordinate. The approach used involves multiple correlation templates, which are subsequently used to determine the best match. To evaluate the efficiency of this 3D tracking algorithm, experiments were carried out in a clinical MRI system. For this, steel balls of different sizes were fixed and repeatedly scanned for static particles. The imaging sequences used for this were a HASTE sequence and a FLASH sequence. The results for the experiment are summarized in Table 11.1, which shows that, the standard deviation (std) of the extracted positions is mostly better when using the FLASH sequence. No clear dependence on size is observed. Generally, the std is less than 0.2 voxels, which in this case with the voxel spacings from the sequence parameters delivers a std well below 200 μm.

11.3.3 MRI-based microrobot control

To ensure a robust and smooth conveyance of the capsule to its destination, it is necessary to control its position between a planned and the observed

Table 11.1 Standard deviations in X [std(x)] and Y [std(y)] directions for the tracking algorithm

Size (mm)	Sequence	Std(*x*) (voxels)	Std(*y*) (voxels)	Std(*x*) (mm)	Std(*y*) (mm)
0.7	HASTE	0.080	0.043	0.100	0.053
1.5	HASTE	0.127	0.127	0.159	0.159
2.0	HASTE	0.116	0.098	0.144	0.123
3.0	HASTE	0.042	0.044	0.053	0.055
0.7	FLASH	0.036	0.054	0.042	0.063
1.5	FLASH	0.036	0.054	0.042	0.063
2.0	FLASH	0.047	0.061	0.055	0.071
3.0	FLASH	0.166	0.158	0.194	0.185

trajectory by means of a navigation control module. To our knowledge, most feedback controller schemes designed in the scope of microrobotics facing drag are simple PID approaches (Mathieu *et al.*, 2007; Tamaz *et al.*, 2008). Efforts have mostly focused on fine modeling, feasibility and sizing of these various designs, but a few studies deal with advanced control and observation of these non-linear systems. However, observation problems have not been studied. Tamaz *et al.* (2008) report instabilities and important oscillations around the equilibrium, especially when the blood stream is modeled as a pulsatile flow. They also indicate a lack of robustness to noise and unmodeled dynamics. It is clear that non-linear control techniques can improve the tracking, both at the control and at the observation point of view. Arcèse *et al.* (2009, 2011), the authors proposed to design a controller based on the backstepping approach that ensures Lyapunov stability. Because backstepping can be regarded as a pre-compensation of the model's non-linearities, working with a more accurate model is a real improvement. Since determination of Lyapunov functions is generically a challenging issue, it is preferable to use Lyapunov control functions in a backstepping control approach (Kenellakopoulos *et al.*, 1992; Krstic *et al.*, 1995). Thus, from equation [11.8] we can obtain a system in a triangular form as follow:

$$\begin{cases} \dot{x} = v \\ \dot{v} = f(x, v) + u \\ y = x \end{cases} \qquad [11.13]$$

Where $x = (x, y, z)$, $v = (v_x, v_y, v_z)$, and $f(x, v)$ is a function of the full state obtained from the microrobot model (cf. Section 11.2.3). Denoting x^*, $\dot{x}^*$ and $\ddot{x}^*$, respectively, the desired reference trajectory, velocity and acceleration, the control law equation for the system given by equation [11.13] can be expressed as (Arcèse *et al.*, 2009):

$$u = \ddot{x}^* + (k_1 + k_2)\dot{x}^* + (1 + k_1k_2)x^* - (1 + k_1k_2)x - (k_1 + k_2)v - f(x, v) \qquad [11.14]$$

where k_1 and k_2 are the strictly positive backstepping gains.

However, such a control scheme could be regarded as a low-level controller that is guaranteeing local stability. It is then difficult to overcome the MRI time-multiplexing constraint using only such robust control strategies. Therefore, we could use such a low-level control scheme together with a higher control level such as predictive control strategies (cf. Fig. 11.7) as proposed by Belharet *et al.* (2010b, 2011), and previously mentioned in Section 11.2.2

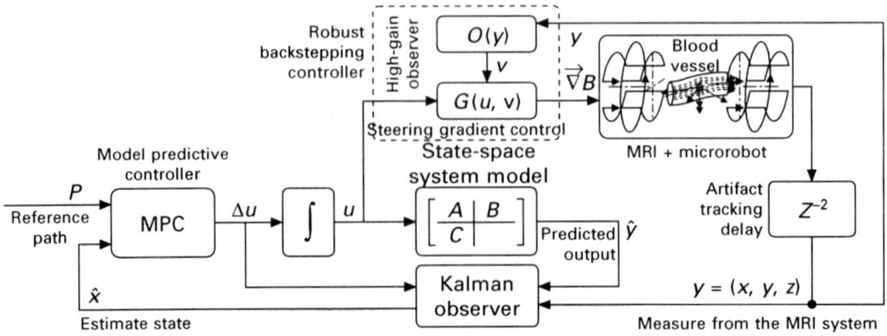

11.7 MRI-based navigation control module.

Predictive control

Predictive control has become an area of significant research interest over the past twenty years. This interest has been powered by a stream of successful industrial applications (Qin and Badgwell, 2003). When focusing on linear (and unconstrained) discrete time transfer function models and quadratic cost functions, some of the best known approaches include the generalized predictive control (GPC) introduced by Clarke *et al.* (1987), and the inner loop stabilizing stable predictive control (Kouvaritakis *et al.*, 1992). In particular, in a more general way, model predictive control (MPC) refers to a class of predictive control algorithms that use an explicit process model to predict the future response of the system. One way to design MPC is to use an extended state–space representation, which is classically given by:

$$\begin{cases} \ddot{x}_{k+1} = AX_k + B\Delta u_k \\ y_k = Cx_k \end{cases} \quad [11.15]$$

where $\Delta u_k = u_k - u_{k-1}$ is the discrete difference operator; and the different matrices A, B, and C can be simply retrieved from equation [11.8]. The predicted state vector at time $k + i$ is then computed (Camacho and Bordons, 2004):

$$\hat{x}_{k+i/k} = A^i x_{k/k-1} + \Sigma_{j=0}^{i-1} A^j B u_{k-j-1} \quad [11.16]$$

The future outputs $y_{k+j/k}$ are than computed based on the real system for future times starting at time k using a recursion procedure, defined by:

$$\hat{y}_{k+i/k} = C(A^i x_k + \Sigma_{j=1}^{i} A^{i-j-1} B u_{k+i-j/k}) \quad [11.17]$$

The design criterion is defined for a certain interval of predictions (several steps in the future). It includes the part of the control error, in which the model of the system is covered (insertion of equations of prediction [11.17]) and the part of control actions, where the input energy (control actions) is weighted. The latter part redistributes control errors to individual steps of predictions and provides coupling within intervals of predictions. The usual form of the criterion for predictive design is written as:

$$J_k = \Sigma_{j=N_1+1}^{N_2}(y_{k+j}W_{k+j}^T Q_y y_{k+j} W_{k+j}) + \Sigma_{j=1}^{N_u}(u_{k+j-1}^T Q_u u_{k+j-1}) \qquad [11.18]$$

The criterion is expressed in step k, $N = N_2 - N_1$ is a horizon of prediction, N_u is the control horizon, Q_y and Q_u are output and input penalizations, and y_{k+j} and u_{k+j-1} are output and input (full or incremental) values. Finally, let us note how to construct the real control actions by an incremental algorithm: after computing a vector for the whole horizon, only the first control u_k is used; then, to obtain the full control actions, the second line of equation [11.15] is applied. When using MPC in the state–space formulation, and, in general for the use of other state–space controls, it is necessary to solve the question of availability of the state of the system (state vector). If this is not available, and only system output from the measurement are known, then some state–space estimation has to be considered. A suitable well-known solution for such an estimation is the state–space observer based on the Kalman filter.

Application and results

In practice, MRI systems are able to generate magnetic gradients with an intensity of some tens of mT m^{-1}. Let us note that this limitation is additionally affected by the gradient coils duty cycle and by the time-multiplexing sequence (T_{Prop}/T_s) needed both for controlling and observing sequences. In order to make sure that the amplitude of the control inputs remains bounded by the physical actuators limits u_{umax}, and to protect the system, we applied a simple time-scaling factor defined by $u_i/k(t)$, with $k(t) = \max\{1, u_i/u_{i,max}\}$. The following set of simulations corresponds to a microcapsule radius of $r = 300$ µm and a time-scaling settled at $k(t) = 0.55$. Various cases are considered to illustrate and to validate the performance of the proposed MRI-based controller schemes.

The proposed control strategy has been validated on a 3D endovascular navigation path $\mathcal{P}$ extracted from MRI data with the previously presented path-planning method (Section 11.3.1), and to evaluate the efficiency of the proposed MRI-based controller, some tests have been performed with a white Gaussian noise on the system output measure y. Figure 11.8 describes the navigation path followed by the microrobot and Fig. 11.9 presents the relative error norm between the current position y and the reference path $\mathcal{P}$, for a time horizon $N = 5$. As shown, the system output y follows perfectly the reference $\mathcal{P}$. In particular, the microdevice is able to quickly reach the navigation path, in spite of a gap between the initial position y and P. The

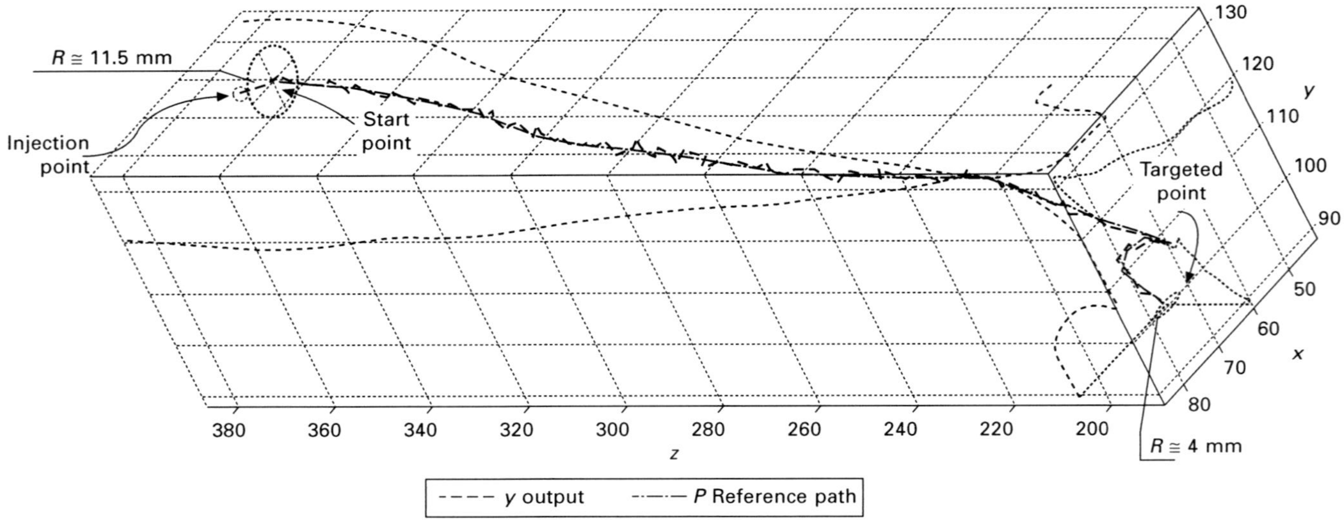

11.8 3D MRI-based microrobot endovascular navigation ($N = 5$, in mm).

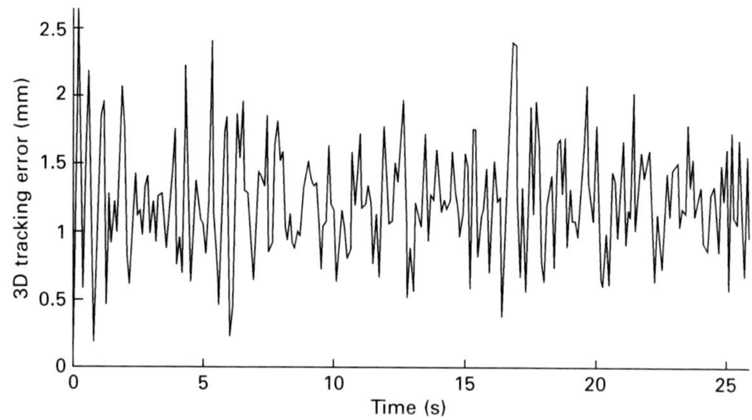

11.9 3D tracking error: $\| y - P \|$ for $N = 5$ (in mm).

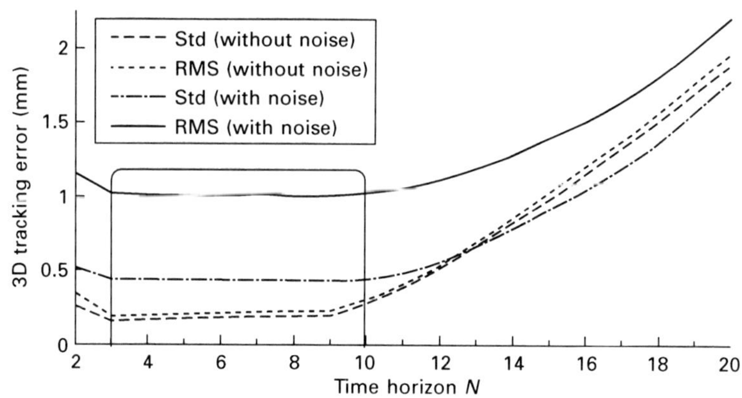

11.10 Tracking error statistics for different time horizons N (in mm).

3D tracking is not overly affected by the Gaussian noise because position standard deviation (std) and root mean square (RMS) error are acceptable. Figure 11.10 simulates the impact of the time horizon N on the system tracking error for optimized time horizon values between $3 \leq N \leq 10$.

Comparing the error statistics, the nature of anticipation of the predictive controller scheme is well illustrated; important values of N improve greatly the anticipation nature of the path behavior but, at the same time, the path tracking error increases. Hence, a large value of N does not necessarily guarantee good performances, and classically increases the complexity of the scheme. Furthermore, to evaluate the robustness of our control strategies, we have also applied an external disturbance which represents the pulsatile blood flow behavior. Hence, we have modeled the blow flow as a time-sinusoidal profile with spatial parabolic form $\sigma_{\text{flow}}(t)$. For an artery, to model the action of flow (positive) and reflux of blood (negative) $\sigma_{\text{flow}}(t)$ were moved up, leading to:

$$\sigma_{\text{flow}}(t) = 0.025\left[1 + 1.15\sin\left(2\pi t + \frac{\pi}{8}\right)\right] \qquad [11.19]$$

Where amplitude of 0.025 is representative of the maximum blood flow speed. Moreover, the performance and stability of the predictive controller with respect to physiological parameters variations are demonstrated in Fig. 11.11. It appears that the system is robust for uncertain physiological parameters (disturbance applied at $t = 13$s) because the 3D position tracking error norm is bounded to 0.2%. Finally, we have evaluated the robustness of our controller for different duty cycle values: 25, 50 and 75%, respectively. The error curves and statistics for the three scenarios are illustrated in Fig. 11.12. For a duty cycle of 50%, the MRI system propels during the first half-period, and acquires 3D images during the other half-period; the path tracking is acceptable, corresponding to the real-time navigational and trajectory control constraints reported by Tamaz *et al.* (2008). Nevertheless for a duty cycle of 25% (i.e. the MRI propels during the first quarter and the image is taken during the remaining three quarters of the cycle), the microrobot can not properly track the reference path ω leading to a large

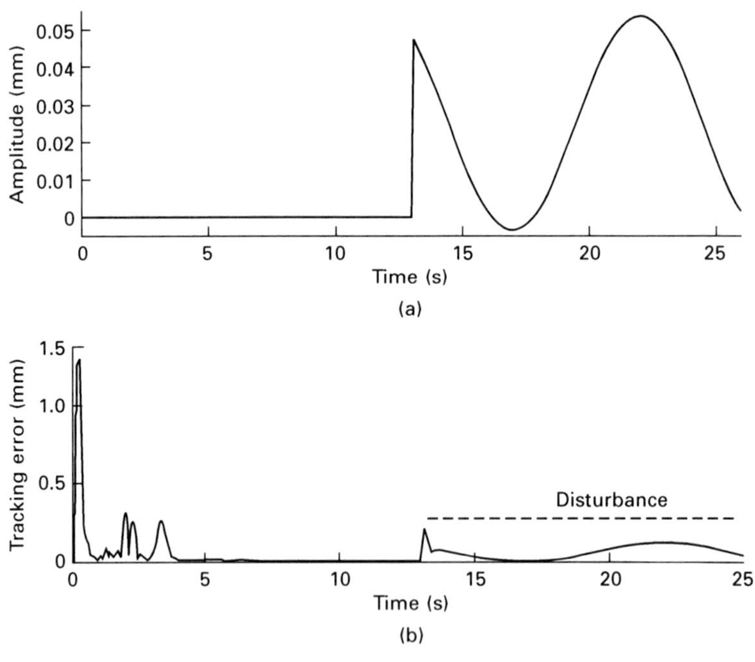

11.11 MRI-based navigation with blood flow disturbance: (a) blood flow disturbance $\sigma_{\text{flow}}(t)$; (b) tracking error (in mm).

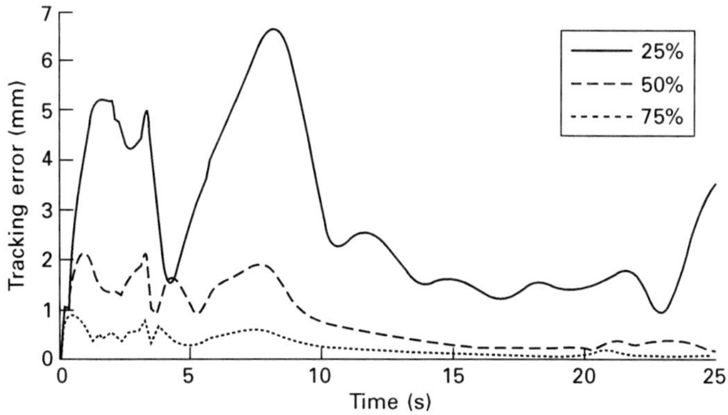

	25%	50%	75%
Std	1.5871	0.6860	0.2563
RMS	3.2023	0.9697	0.3628

11.12 Tracking error for various values of duty cycle (in mm).

tracking error. The time-multiplexing duty cycle is optimized for a value around 40%. Optimally, the simulated predictive behavior of the MPC controller suggests better tracking results compared with those obtained by Tamaz *et al.* (2008) that should be confirmed by experimentation.

11.4 Conclusions and future trends

In this chapter, we describe a framework that allows a microdevice to navigate correctly within the vascular network using a conventional MRI system. After a brief description of the overall system, and the main constraints related to the use of a clinical MRI platform, the main challenges are described: path planning and ferromagnetic device tracking and control. These three challenging aspects are necessary for efficiently autonomously guiding and the microrobot to reach deep locations in human body for various therapy and treatment applications. The results illustrate the ability to plan the navigation pathway and to recognize, track and control the microcarrier in the cardiovascular system to the targeted area, against the system constraints.

The main drawback of MRI-based navigation stems from the strong limitations on the magnetic gradient amplitude of available clinical MRI devices. As magnetic forces used for propelling are volumetric, whereas the drag force is, at best, dependent on the area of the microcapsule; the smaller the capsule, the higher the required control forces with respect to hydrodynamic perturbations. Consequently, this approach is well suited for microcapsules whose radius is up to a few dozen micrometers using actual MRI devices.

MRI targeting aims at using ferromagnetic microcarriers (for drug delivery for instance) and stopping them through embolization at the arterioles entry close to the targeted area. Then possible releasing mechanisms could rely on biodegradable polymer and techniques used in hyperthermia where aggregates of nanocapsules can be heated to melt polymer. The current state of our work has shown that a clinical MRI system can be used to generate magnetic forces able to displace magnetized microdevices in the cardiovascular system. Future studies will be aimed at magnetic aggregation of the particles placed within the magnetic field of the MRI system in order to identify the parameters that can be used to influence the geometry, volume and density of the magnetic aggregates, and to extend the study to aggregates of nanocapsules.

11.5 Sources of further information and advice

This chapter gives an overview of a proposed framework for the navigation of a microcarrier for targeted therapy using a clinical MRI platform. What follows is a briefly annotated selection of titles that provide useful further reading and reference.

- Model predictive control

  Fletcher, R (1987), *Practical methods of optimization*. John Wiley & Son Ltd.

  Maciejowski, J M (2002) *Predictive control with constraints*. Pearson Education.

- Model and control of a ferromagnetic device in a viscous fluid

  Arcèse L, Fruchard M, and Ferreira A (2009), Nonlinear modeling and robust controller-observer for a magnetic microrobot in a fluidic environment using MRI gradients, in *IEEE/RSJ International Conference on Intelligent Robots and Systems*, St. Louis, USA, pp. 534–539.

  Arcèse L, Cherry A, Fruchard M and Ferreira A (2010), High gain observer for backstepping control of a MRI-guided therapeutic microrobot in blood vessels, in *IEEE/RAS–EMBS International Conference on Biomedical Robotics and Biomechatronics*, Tokyo, pp. 349–354.

  These report precise modeling and controller/observer for a magnetic microdevice navigating inside a vessel.

- Navigation planning

  Sethian J A (1999), *Level set methods and fast marching methods: evolving interfaces in computational geometry, fluid mechanics, computer vision, and materials science*, Cambridge University Press, Cambridge, UK.

This book is the main reference about the fast marching methods, and a good review of the fast marching in 3D together with some applications can be found in:

Deschamps T and Cohen L D (2001), Fast extraction of minimal paths in 3D images and application to virtual endoscopy, *Medical Image Analysis*, **5**(4) 281–299.

11.6 References

Abbott J J K, Peyer E, Lagomarsino M C, Zhang L, Dong L X, Kaliakatsos I K, and Nelson B J (2009), 'How should microrobots swim?' *Int. J. Robot. Res.*, doi: 101177/0278364909341658.

Abbott J, Nagy Z, Beyeler F, and Nelson B (2007), 'Robotics in the small,' *IEEE Robot. Automat. Mag.*, 92.

Aboussouan E, Felfoul O, Mathieu J, Beaudoin G, and Martel S (2006), 'Real-time projection based technique for tracking ferromagnetic devices,' in *Int. Soc. Magn. Reson. Med.*, 637.

Arcèse L, Fruchard M, and Ferreira A (2009), 'Nonlinear modeling and robust controller–observer for a magnetic microrobot in a fluidic environment using MRI gradients,' in *IEEE/RSJ International Conference on Intelligent Robots and Systems*, St. Louis, MO, USA, pp. 534–539.

Arcèse L, Fruchard M, and Ferreira A, and Nelson B J (2011), 'Adaptive backstepping and MEMS force sensor for an MRI-guided microrobot in the vasculature,' in *IEEE International Conference on Robotics and Automation*, Shanghai, China.

Behkam B, and Sitti M (2006), 'Design methodology for biomimetic propulsion of miniature swimming robots,' *ASME J. Dyn. Syst. Meas. Control*, **128**, 36–43.

Belharet K, Folio D, and Ferreira A (2010a), '3D MRI-based predictive control of a ferromagnetic microrobot navigating in blood vessels,' in *IEEE RAS & EMBS International Conference on Biomedical Robotics and Biomechatronics*, Tokyo, Japan.

Belharet K, Folio D, and Ferreira A (2010b), 'Endovascular navigation of a ferromagnetic microrobot using MRI-based predictive control,' in *IEEE/RSJ International Conference on Intelligent Robots and Systems*, Taipei, Taiwan, doi:10.1109/IROS.2010.5650803.

Belharet K, Folio D, and Ferreira A (2011), 'Three-dimensional controlled motion of a microrobot using magnetic gradients,' *Adv. Robot.*, **25**(8), 1069–1083.

Camacho E, and Bordons C (2004), *Model predictive control*. Springer Verlag.

Cavalcanti T A, Shirinzadeh B, and Ikeda S (2009), 'Nanorobot for brain aneurysm,' *Int. J of Robot Res.*, **28**(4), 558–570.

Cavalcanti T A, Shirinzadeh B, and Ikeda S (2009), 'Nanorobot for brain aneurysm,' *Int. J. Robot. Res.*, **28**(4), 558–570.

Chanu A, Felfoul O, Baudoin G, and Martel S (2008), 'Adapting the clinical MRI software environment for real-time navigation of an endovascular untethered ferromagnetic bead for future endovascular interventions,' *Magn. Reson. Med.*, **59**, 1287–1297.

Clarke D, Mohtadi C, and Tuffs P (1987), 'Generalized predictive control – Part I & II,' *Automatica*, **23**, 137–160.

Cover T, Thomas J, and Wiley J (1991), *Elements of information theory*. Wiley Online Library, **306**.

Deschamps T (2001), 'Curve and shape extraction with minimal path and level-sets techniques: applications to 3D medical imaging,' PhD dissertation, University of Paris.

Felfoul O, Mathieu J, Beaudoin G, and Martel S (2008), 'In vivo MR-tracking based on magnetic signature selective excitation,' *IEEE Trans. Med. Imag.*, **27**(1), 28–35.

Folio D, Dahmen C, Wortmann T, Zeeshan M, Shou K, Pané S, Nelson B, Ferreira A, and Fatikow S (2011) 'MRI magnetic signature imaging, tracking and navigation for targeted micro/nano-capsule therapeutics,' in *IEEE/RSJ International Conference on Intel. Robots and Systems*, San Francisco, USA.

Frangi A, Niessen W, Vincken K, and Viergever. M (1998), 'Multiscale vessel enhancement filtering,' *Lect. Notes Comp. Sci.*, **1496**, 130–137.

Ishiyama K, Sendoh M, and Arai K I (2002), 'Magnetic micromachines for medical applications,' *J. Magn. Magn. Mater.* **242–245**, 41–46.

Kanellakopoulos I, Kokotovic P, and Morse A (1992), 'A toolkit for nonlinear feedback design' *Syst. Contr. Lett.*, **18**(2), 83–92.

Kirbas C and Quek F (2004), 'A review of vessel extraction techniques and algorithms,' *ACM Comput. Surv.*, **36**(2), 81–121.

Kouvaritakis B, Rossiter J, and Chang A (1992), 'Stable generalised predictive control: an algorithm with guaranteed stability,' *IEE Proc. Part D Contr. Theory Appl.*, **139**(4), 349–362.

Krstic M, Kanellakopoulos I, and Kokotovic P (1995), *Nonlinear and adaptive control design.* Wiley, New York, **222**.

Martel S, Mohammadi M, Felfoul O, Lu Z, and Pouponneau P (2009), 'Flagellated magnetotactic bacteria as controlled MRI-trackable propulsion and steering systems for medical nanorobots operating in the human microvasculature,' *Int. J. Robot. Res.*, **28**(4), pp. 571–582.

Mathieu J, and Martel S (2007), 'In vivo validation of a propulsion method for untethered medical microrobots using a clinical magnetic resonance imaging system,' in *IEEE/RSJ International Conference on Intel. Robots and Systems.* IEEE, pp. 502–508.

Park J, von Maltzahn G, Zhang L, Schwartz M, Ruoslahti E, Bhatia S, and Sailor M (2008), 'Magnetic iron oxide nanoworms for tumor targeting and imaging,' *Adv. Mater.*, **20**(9), 1630–1635.

Park S, and Park J-O (2008), 'Frontier research program on biomedical robot for intravascular therapy,' *2nd IEEE/RAS-EMBS International Conference on Biomedical Robotics and Biomechatronics*, 360–365.

Port J, and Pomper M (2000), 'Quantification and minimization of magnetic susceptibility artifacts on GRE images,' *Neuroradiology*, **24**, 958–964.

Qin S, and Badgwell T (2003), 'A survey of industrial model predictive control technology,' *Cont. Eng. Pract*, **11**(7), 733–764.

Reuzé P, Coatrieux J, Luo L, and Dillenseger. J (1993), 'A 3D moment based approach for blood vessel detection and quantification in MRA,' *Technol Health Care*, 1, 181–188.

Sabra W, Khouzam M, and Martel S (2005), 'Use of 3D potential field and an enhanced breath-first search algorithms for path-planning of microdevices propelled in the cardiovascular system,' *27th IEEE EMBS Annual International Conference*, pp. 3916–3920.

Sato Y, Nakajima S, Atsumi H, Koller T, Gerig G, Yoshida S, and Kikinis R (1998), 'Three-dimensional multi-scale line filter for segmentation and visualization of curvilinear structures in medical images,' *Med. Image Anal.*, **2**(2), 143–168.

Sethian J A (1999), *Level set methods and fast marching methods: evolving interfaces in computational geometry, fluid mechanics, computer vision, and materials science.* Cambridge University Press, Cambridge.

Tamaz S, Chanu A, Mathieu J-B, Gourdeau R, and Martel S (2008), 'Real-time MRI-based control of a ferromagnetic core for endovascular navigation,' *IEEE Trans. Bio-Med. Eng.*, **55**(7), pp. 1854–1863.

Tokuda J, Fischer G S, DiMaio S P, Gobbi D G, Csoma C, Mewes P W, Fichtinger G, Tempany C M, and Hata N (2010), 'Integrated navigation and control software system for MRI-guided robotic prostate interventions,' *Comput. Med. Imag. Graph.*, **34**(1), 3–8.

Wink O, Niessen W J, and Viergever M A (2000), 'Minimum cost path determination using a simple heuristic function,' *International Conference on Pattern Recognition*, **3**, p. 7010.

Wink O, Niessen W, Verdonck B, and Viergever M (2001), 'Vessel axis determination using wave front propagation analysis,' *Med. Image Comput. Comput. Assist Interv*, 2208, 845–853.

Wortmann T, Dahmen C, and Fatikow S (2010), 'Study of MRI susceptibility artifacts for nanomedical applications,' *J. Nanotechnol. Eng. Med.*, **1**(4), 041002.

12
Robotic surgery and ethical challenges

N. SHARKEY and A. SHARKEY, University of Sheffield, UK

Abstract: The various types of surgical robotic systems are reviewed and a range of ethical problems is discussed. Topics include the patient experience of such techniques, how robotic systems are marketed, training and the balance of cost versus access, as well as challenges relating to remote robotic surgery and automated hospitals and applications of specific systems such as da Vinci and RoboDoc.

Key words: robotic surgery, ethics, da Vinci, RoboDoc.

12.1 Introduction

Surgical robotics is poised to revolutionise the way that operations are performed. There is much to suggest that the technology will be of great benefit over the coming years. There are claims that robotically assisted surgery can facilitate minimally invasive operations, and thereby reduce blood loss and the length of time spent in hospital following surgery, resulting in less pain and fewer postoperative complications. The problems caused by surgeons' fatigue and hand tremors could be reduced or eliminated, and their view of the procedures is much improved. Robotic surgical systems may greatly expand the scope of minimally invasive systems, 'allowing dexterity beyond his [the surgeon's] natural physical limitations, thereby broadening the scope and skill of surgical interventions' (Diodato *et al.*, 2004). Robotic systems could potentially perform routine operations with greater accuracy and repeatability. In the future, telesurgery could enable battlefield or roadside operations and surgery in remote locations.

A large and growing number of surgeons are being trained to perform robotically assisted surgery. Some want to train because of the novelty value of a new technology with the potential to innovate and, possibly, revolutionise surgery. Some believe that it is the best tool available at present for laparoscopic surgery. Others train because it is required by their hospitals because they have invested in the technology. There is also a growing number of patients who want robot surgery because they believe that it produces better outcomes with less pain and fewer complications than other types of surgery. Hospital managers in the US are increasingly keen to install robot surgical systems because of the risk that patients may go elsewhere if they do not have them.

However, we must not let the promise of revolutionary new technology blind us to the difficulties and ethical issues involved in the early stages of developing such technologies. As Moore (2000) succinctly wrote in discussing surgical innovation in general, 'The surgeon should be aware of the fact that patients threatened by severe illness display a surprising and sometimes alarming readiness to accept uncertainty and reach out for something new. The surgical scientist must avoid exploiting this willingness of patients to try something new in a desperate situation'. There are always teething problems and side effects with any new technology as well as ethical issues to resolve.

Morgenstern (2006) provides an insightful discussion of the ethics of surgical innovation in general. He points to the difficulty of achieving a reasonable balance between overregulation stifling surgical innovation, and underregulation creating harmful and dangerous practices. His view agrees with the three criteria proposed by Moore (2000) to make 'surgical innovation acceptable':

- First, sufficient laboratory experience is required before conducting an innovative procedure.
- Second, the 'field strength', or intellectual and technical expertise available in the institution where the work is to be done is important.
- Third, good 'institutional stability' based on its resources, support systems and staff should be in place.

An innovative technique such as robotic surgery must satisfy these criteria if it is to be beneficial and meet the expectations of patients.

As yet, there has been only limited discussion of the ethical applications of robotically assisted surgery. Weber (2008) presents a detailed case study of the RobotDoc surgical system whereas others have considered the ethics of robot surgery only in the wider context of healthcare robotics (Datteri and Tamburrini, 2009) or for conducting surgery at a distance using telesurgery (Dickens and Cook, 2006; van Wynsberghe and Gastmans, 2008). In this chapter, we address these concerns by first defining the types of robotic surgery available before going on to discuss a range of ethical issues:

- the patient experience of robotic surgery;
- the marketing of this technology;
- training challenges; and
- costs versus benefits.

Then we discuss ethical issues specifically relating to the use of remote robotic surgery as well as the potential future emergence of automated hospitals.

12.2 Types of robotic surgery

When considering the ethical issues in robot surgery, it is first important to establish how the robot is controlled. Two main types are discussed in this chapter:

- *automatic* (sometimes called *active*) systems that perform surgery directly after being programmed by the surgeon and/or other human operators; and
- *controlled* (sometimes called *passive*) systems that are entirely dependent on the actions of the surgeon.

The ethical concerns about each of these differ to an extent, although there are some problems that are common to both as will become apparent.

12.2.1 Automatic systems

Automatic systems should not be confused with autonomous systems, which make choices dependent on sensor activity, whereas automatic machines follow precise preprogrammed instructions planned by a surgeon. Several of the first tranche of robot surgery devices were automatic systems adapted from industrial robots. For example, the CyberKnife uses an adapted KUKA industrial robot with six degrees of freedom for high-precision non-invasive irradiation of cancerous cells (Adler *et al.*, 1997). With multiple beams of high-dose radiation from a variety of angles, CyberKnife can be used to treat tumours in difficult positions, such as near the spine or the brain. The robotic manipulator automatically follows a fixed preplanned path around the patient, but this path can be modified on the basis of patient displacement information, resulting in a degree of autonomy. Imaging software provides a continuous update of the patient's position, and allows the robotic manipulator to correct for changes in patient position during treatment. The system is frameless, and does not require the head-mounted frames needed for other radiosurgical systems such as the Gamma Knife.

A second example is the Robodoc system based on a 5-DoF SCARA robot. Robodoc is used for total knee arthroplasty, and total hip arthroplasty. The surgeon plans the implant location and orientation using three-dimensional (3D) data from a CT scan of the patient and then Robodoc executes the plan. PROBOT is another automatic system that is used for prostate removal after the surgeon analyses the target and surrounding organs and plans the actions needed for the intervention. Although the process is monitored and can be stopped to change parameters, the robot rather than the surgeon does the cutting.

The use of such technology can be problematic for some surgeons. Rodriguez y Baena and Davies (2010) report that the surgeons using PROBOT 'felt unease at being just observers of a procedure that was largely in the control of the robot programmer'. They suggest that surgeon training leads to an expectation of continual interaction with the patient that requires a 'hands-on robot in which the surgeon interacted with the robot as if it were an intelligent tool under his direct command'. This led to the development of the semiautomatic Acrobot orthopaedic surgical robot. Rather than executing a preprogrammed plan, the robot actively constrains the surgeon to cut accurately within a safe region by means of a force-controlled handle.

The neuroArm robot acts to constrain the movements of the neurosurgeon performing brain surgery. neuroArm can genuinely be used in areas where humans cannot go. It sits inside an iMRI machine, so that the surgeon can see 3D images of the patient's brain in near real time. The surgeon can set up a surgical 'corridor' such that any attempt to move outside the corridor receives force feedback. neuroArm has been used successfully in a relatively small number of procedures but it is potentially one of the most promising surgically assistive robots to date. The empirical comparisons with conventional brain surgery have not yet been made, but this system appears to represent a considerable step in the right direction for future robot surgical devices.

12.2.2 Controlled systems

Controlled systems are the most popular among patients and doctors. The da Vinci system by Intuitive Surgical is a good example of a 'hands-on' robot designed for soft-tissue surgery in the abdominal cavity. The two robotic arms, equipped with various instruments, are teleoperated by a surgeon, who observes and controls all of the robot movements from a console. The Zeus system is similar, although its arms have fewer DoF. Such systems represent extensions or developments of minimally invasive surgical procedures.

12.3 The patient experience of robotic surgery

One problem that would at first appear relevant for robot surgery is the loss or reduction in human contact. In previous studies we have argued that robots cannot form adequate replacements for human carers of either the very young, (Sharkey and Sharkey, 2010) or the frail elderly (Sharkey and Sharkey, 2012). Others have also argued that increased use of robots could lead to serious neglect of the elderly, and a reduction in the amount of human interaction they receive (Sparrow and Sparrow, 2006). Surgery is different. Anaesthetised patients are not aware that they are in the company of machines rather than humans and so there is little need for hand-holding and sympathy. Caring human contact is, however, required pre- and postoperatively for assurance and anxiety reduction. This will need further consideration as more autonomy is introduced in the future (Sharkey, 2008) and for telesurgery (van Wynsberghe and Gastmans, 2008). One aspect that raises ethical issues is the trend to design robots with human features and responses to encourage people to treat them as human (Sharkey and Sharkey, 2010; Sharkey and Sharkey, 2011).

Dignity is a major concern for robot care, particularly when it comes to elderly people with dementia. However, it does not present obvious ethical issues for current robot surgery. In a sense, patients may lose some of their dignity by just being in hospital and being the 'object' of an operation. But this is no different for robotically assisted surgery than for conventional surgery. It makes little difference to an anaesthetised patient. It is possible that there could be more objectification with telesurgery (van Wynsberghe and Gastmans, 2008) and, consequently, a greater loss of dignity but not enough is known about the impacts yet for further discussion.

12.4 The marketing of robotic surgery

The reporting and marketing of robotic surgery raises a number of ethical problems, particularly about the claimed benefits compared with conventional techniques. Many press reports have been highly favourable. Because it the most commonly used system of its type, the da Vinci surgical robotics system was, for example, featured on the cover of the *U.S. News & World Report's* 'Best Hospitals' issue in the summer of 2011. A surgical robotics system even appeared on the TV show *Grey's Anatomy* and President Barack Obama has been photographed trying his hand at one such system during a visit to a clinic in Cleveland, Ohio.

The benefits of robotic surgery are highlighted on manufacturers' websites. As an example, the Intuitive Surgical Website (http://www.intuitivesurgical.com/specialties/) includes two video clips on the home page relating to its da Vinci robotic surgery system. The first is a number of testimonials from people who have had da Vinci surgery. The second presents the testimonials of a number of surgeons, starting off with 'I am a da Vinci surgeon because ...' and then they give their reasons for using robotic surgery. Examples include:

- 'I believe that women deserve the best surgery possible ... it's changing the lives of women and approving their outcome ... patients get better results'
- 'patients get better results ultimately in terms of their functional results',
- 'the surgical field is evolving. This is a cutting edge that gives my patients the best care ... they can get their life back a lot quicker';
- 'I can offer patients a minimally invasive approach when in the past I had to offer them an open abdominal approach';

- 'there is no doubt on my mind that I get better results ... less morbidity complications';
- 'it's better for my patients, it's better for me and it makes me be a better doctor'; and
- 'it's obvious to me that this is an improvement, a paradigm shift if you will, a leap forward in our ability to take care of my patients. There's no doubt in my mind that I get better results using da Vinci.'

The site does not make it clear how representative these views are of those surgeons who have used the da Vinci system, nor does it highlight wider studies of the effectiveness of robotic surgery. The bottom of each page of the website includes the following disclaimer: 'While clinical studies support the effectiveness of the *da Vinci* Surgical System when used in minimally invasive surgery, individual results may vary. There are no guarantees of outcome. All surgeries involve the risk of major complications'

A number of concerns have been raised about how accurately this kind of advertising represents the scope and benefits of robotic surgery, its risks and how well it compares with conventional surgery. In 2001, the FDA issued two warning letters to Intuitive Surgical about claims that they were making on their websites, saying: 'The materials on these sites make misleading claims for Intuitive's da Vinci™ Surgical System (da Vinci™) ...' It also stated: 'Additionally your web page, titled, 'Clinical Applications' at intusurg.com/html/clinicalapps.html, by its presentation, implies that the da Vinci™ system has broader uses than have been cleared by the agency.'

Similar concerns have been raised about the way hospitals promote the Da Vinci system. Jin *et al.* (2011) conducted a systematic analysis of 400 randomly selected US hospital websites in June of 2010; 41% of hospital websites described robotic surgery, 37% of these had robot surgery on their homepage with 33% including links to the manufacturer's website. The authors stated that as many as 86% of the websites made statements about the clinical superiority of surgical robotics. They concluded that: 'Materials provided by hospitals regarding the surgical robot overestimate benefits, largely ignore risks and are strongly influenced by the manufacturer.'

It has been noted that use of the Da Vinci system increased by 400% in US hospitals between 2006 and 2010. Given its widespread employment in the US, some hospital staff are also concerned about the way that the da Vinci robot has been marketed to hospitals. 'There's a medical arms race', according to Phil Levy, executive of Beth Israel Deaconess Medical Center in Boston. He told the *Wall Street Journal* that, because he saw no reliable evidence that da Vinci was better for patients, he resisted buying one. However, he felt he had to give in when the hospital was losing business to competitors who had robots. 'Technologies are being adopted and becoming widespread based on the marketing prowess of equipment makers and suppliers, not necessarily on the public good.' (Carreyrou, 2010). Urologist

Dr Jeffrey Cadeddu made similar comments to the *New York Times*. He had been conducting traditional laparoscopic prostatectomy for many years. 'But now, patient after patient is walking away. They do not want that kind of surgery. They want surgery by a robot.' 'They say: 'Do you use the robot? OK, well, thank you.' And they leave' (Kolata, 2010).

Another concern is that the promotion of the benefits of surgical robotic systems such as Da Vinci by manufacturers, hospitals and others does not reflect the evidence on how the new technology compares in practice with conventional techniques. It has led some patients to assume greater benefits from robotic surgery than is supported by available studies comparing different techniques. To explore these concerns in more depth, a number of these studies are reviewed in the next section.

12.5 Comparing robotic surgery with other types of surgery

There have been a number of studies comparing robotic surgery with more conventional surgical techniques. The RoboDoc system has been used extensively in Germany where about 10 000 RoboDoc operations were conducted between 1994 and 2004 (Grund, 2004). In a comparison of RoboDoc total hip arthroplasty (THA) operations with manual THA, Bargar *et al.* (1998) found that they resulted in similar outcomes, but that RoboDoc operations took longer and caused more blood loss. In January 2007, a patient of the ACE Arthro Clinic in Essen made a successful claim against the clinic because the doctors did not provide sufficient information about the risks of an operation using RoboDoc, particularly the risk of muscle damage (Weber, 2008). There have also been claims about mismanagement of postoperative complications (Grund, 2004).

The original clinical trial for the da Vinci surgical robotics system, a three-month study at Hospital Torre Medica in Mexico City in 1999, consisted of 129 laparoscopic cholecystectomies and laparoscopic fundoplications using this system: 'The study objective was to demonstrate device equivalence in safety and effectiveness to the control of standard laparoscopic equipment in performance of general laparoscopic tasks, including grasping, cutting, blunt and sharp dissection, approximation, ligation, electrocautery and suturing.' (Summary minutes of the General and Plastic Surgery Devices Panel, 1999). This trial, which suggested the da Vinci surgical robotics system was at least equivalent to standard laparoscopic surgery, subsequently led to premarket approval by the Federal Drugs Administration (FDA).

Subsequently, there have been a number of recent US studies comparing robotic surgery and other methods. A population study carried out by Hu *et al.* (2009) used the Medicare records for 8837 men who underwent radical prostatectomy between 2003 and 2007. The study concluded that although those undergoing minimally invasive radical prostatectomy (MIRP) experienced a shorter length of stay and fewer respiratory and miscellaneous surgical complications and strictures, they were more likely to have genitourinary complications, incontinence and erectile dysfunction. The authors admitted that the data did not allow separation between conventional laparoscopic surgery and robotically assisted surgery. Although this was a weakness, they quite reasonably inferred that in the region of 50 to 70% of the data was likely to be from robot-assisted surgery as this was the percentage of robot-assisted laparoscopic surgery at the time. This suggested a similar level of performance between robot-assisted laparoscopic surgery and conventional laparoscopic surgery.

Another extensive review of the comparative effectiveness of robotic surgery, which considered 111 studies, rated robot-assisted radical prostatectomy among patients with clinically localized, low-risk prostate cancer as 'unproven with potential', pending further long-term controlled studies (Institute for Clinical and Economic Review, 2009). More recent studies include Barocas *et al.* (2010). They compared the recurrence-free survival rates of 1904 patients with clinically localised prostate cancer; 25.9% of the patients underwent open radical prostatectomy and 74.1% underwent robot assisted laparoscopic prostatectomy. For both groups, experienced urological surgeons at the same institution performed the surgery. Direct comparison showed no significant difference between the effectiveness of conventional methods and robot-assisted laparoscopic approaches. A paper by Jin *et al.* (2011) examined the findings from eight studies using randomised-control trials in general surgery procedures. Seven of the studies, published between 2001 and 2009, showed no patient benefit from the use of robotics technology. Only one of the studies demonstrated a decreased length of stay in hospital following surgery.

What seems clear from these comparisons is that, whilst robotic surgery can be as effective as conventional surgery, there is far less evidence that it is, as yet, better than traditional techniques. Those who make such claims, and encourage patients to opt for robotic surgery as inherently better, are potentially misleading them. It is important that any claims are based on the best evidence available, that they are balanced and do not exaggerate potential benefits at the expense of potential risks. This reinforces the point made by Moore (2000) that there needs to be the right level of experience to prove the real effectiveness of a new procedure.

12.6 The need for training

One major area of risk in a new technology such as robotic surgery is the training required to carry out surgery successfully. This picks up the point made by Moore (2000) about the need for 'field strength', i.e. having the right level of intellectual and technical expertise to support a new procedure. The importance of appropriate expertise is illustrated by the example of Sherry Long, a 42 year old woman from Rochester in the US who was told by her surgeon at the Wentworth–Douglas hospital that robotics would be used for her hysterectomy. She was told that it would be less invasive than other methods, but she was not told that the surgeon performing the operation was a trainee who was insufficiently experienced with the da Vinci surgical system robot. The result was that Sherry Long had both her ureters cut, an error that could cause her kidneys to shut down. She required four more procedures to correct the problem. In May 2010, the law firm Swartz and Swartz filed the first malpractice suit in New Hampshire for a botched robotics surgical procedure (Angueira, 2010).

The *Wall Street Journal* (Carreyrou, 2010) reported that two other female patients undergoing gynaecological surgery had their bladders lacerated in similar circumstances. Retired Air Force Colonel David Antoon filed a similar suit to Sherry Long in 2010 after complications arising from a robot-assisted laparoscopic prostatectomy, claiming that the operation had been carried out by a surgeon with insufficient experience in robotic surgery without proper supervision by a more experienced colleague.

Such cases illustrate the need for adequate training in a new procedure. When Intuitive Surgical was given premarket approval for the da Vinci surgical system from the FDA, training was certainly a feature of the discussion with the approving panel. When Dr Barry Gardiner MD, the principal investigator for the Mexico City premarket trials for Intuitive Surgical testified to the FDA panel about the learning curve for the surgical robot, he said, 'Having been involved in the development of choloresection, for example, laparoscopically, it took me 65 or 70 cases before I was really comfortable that I could do those operations with equal facility to open surgery. Now, I don't think it is going to take anywhere near that degree of training on this device. It is pretty clear to me that you are safe and effective sitting down and operating with it initially, but there is no question you are going to get better as you go – I don't know, 10 or 15 cases maybe' (Summary minutes of General and Plastic Surgery Devices Panel, 1999).

Other users of robotic surgery have suggested that considerably more training is required. Dr Jim Hu, a surgeon at Brigham and Women's Hospital in Boston who has done more than 1000 surgeries, told the *Wall Street Journal* that it takes a urologist anywhere from 250 to 700 cases to master it (Carreyrou, 2010). Dr Ashutosh Tewari from Weill Cornell Medical College, who has carried out more than 3000 robot-assisted operations, told the *New York Times* that it takes 200 to 300 operations to become highly proficient (Kolata, 2010).

At the FDA premarket approval meeting for the da Vinci surgical systems, concerns about training were raised. Ms Dubler, a bioethicist on the panel, said, 'I fear we need more data on risk, which would be related in my mind to the dimension of the training that will be required. People who are not sufficiently trained could, in fact, pose a risk using this procedure'. Given the lack of information on such a new procedure at the time, the panel was unable to agree what level of training might be appropriate. In the end, the FDA approved the da Vinci surgical system for use on condition that that the sponsors provide a detailed description of the training they endorse for use of their product. Our understanding in the case of the Da Vinci system is that Intuitive Surgical provides two days' training on pigs and cadavers for two staff as part of the agreement to supply the system and can then schedule cases proctored by a surgeon who has performed at least 20 robotically assisted laparoscopic procedures. If this is the case, it would seem to underestimate the amount of training required before full proficiency is achieved.

12.7 Costs versus benefits

Social justice relates to the rights of all citizens to life, health and wellbeing and access to the best means possible to fulfil these rights. The means of access to healthcare varies between countries and this gives rise to different ethical issues. For example, in the USA, hospitals are generally private with payments for surgery being made either by insurance companies or the patients' own funds. This puts hospitals in a competitive relationship for patient recruitment. It can put pressure on hospitals to oversell robot surgery and to put pressure on surgeons to use the kit, sometimes without adequate training.

The FDA discussed the issue of cost in the premarket approval meeting (FDA, 1999). Bioethicist Nancy Dubler pointed out the important ethical issue but it went no further:

> I just want to followup on one discussion and the cost-benefit analysis is the basis for it. We have talked about individual benefit, and there is a school of ethical analysis these days that argues the following: that it is, in fact, unethical to approve new technologies that will add to the cost of medicine, given the number of people without health insurance and access to health care, unless there is a measurable benefit that proceeds from that technology.
>
> Now, I think we have been told that we can't assess that benefit at this point, and we can't produce the cost-benefit analysis, but I would simply like to register my discomfort that we may be adding a substantial cost without commensurate benefit. (FDA, 1999)

In the European Union, Article 35 of the Charter of Fundamental Rights grants all citizens the right to access health care and it insists that 'A high level of human health protection shall be ensured in the definition and implementation of all Union policies and activities'. In the UK, hospitals are generally funded by the taxpayer and so everyone has the right to the same treatment. Unfortunately, this means that in the UK, the best treatment for certain diseases may sometimes not be offered because of cost.

Questions about access to robot surgery have already begun to arise in the UK. Access to robot surgical systems such as CyberKnife or da Vinci is not always provided by the National Health Service (NHS) even when patients want it. Sutcliffe *et al.* (2006) report five hospitals with da Vinci systems installed in the UK, but they are not necessarily made available to patients on the NHS. Similar problems have been found by patients hoping to be given access to CyberKnife sterotactic robotic radiosurgery.

A UK national newspaper reported a refusal by NHS to fund robotic radiosurgery treatment using CyberKnife for a woman in Sussex (Donnelly, 2011). The article pointed out that the treatment apparently costs about £10 000, but that, although almost £9 million has been spent buying the robotic technology for three NHS hospitals, various NHS Primary Care Trusts have been rejecting referrals. The woman received the treatment only after raising charitable funding. Such controversies illustrate the difficult balance that needs to be found between an individual's right to the best treatment, the fair distribution of limited resources, and about the likely outcomes of a given system.

How much better would robot surgery have to be to make the extra cost worth it? In the UK, the National Centre for Health and Clinical Excellence (NICE) has to make many difficult decisions about which patients should have access to what procedures or whether procedures are cost-effective. If robot surgery could truly demonstrate better outcomes, dramatic decreases in hospital bed occupation and considerably less aftercare and complications, then there would be an ethical imperative to use it.

12.8 Ethical issues relating to remotely operated surgery

In 2001, Dr Jacques Marescaux in New York conducted 'Operation Lindbergh', the world's first transatlantic telesurgery. He operated on the gall bladder of a woman in Strasbourg using the Zeus robotic surgical system. The operation was the most expensive intervention of this kind. It cost \$1.5 million in equipment, \$150 million in research and development by France Telecom over 2.5 years to achieve the necessary telecommunication speed and 80 people were needed to monitor the integrity of the equipment and signal (Marohn and Hanly, 2004). It was a demonstration that long distance telesurgery was now a possibility. We can at last see the potential for conducting operations in third world countries where there may be very few, if any, high quality surgeons. At the same time, the prohibitive cost argues against the likelihood of such methods being accessible to people in places such as Africa for some time into the future.

Telesurgery also carries with it a number of ethical risks that will need to be monitored as the technique develops. Privacy of patient data could become an issue as telesurgery develops, as data may have to be shared with more people than usual and possibly across national boundaries. Different countries have differing privacy laws and data that may be protected in one country may be more available to commercial interests in another. Caution and care is needed to ensure that patient data is protected in a way that would be expected in the patient's home country of origin or perhaps international agreements need to be negotiated.

Responsibility for errors would also need to be ensured for operations that cross national borders. A clear chain of accountability would need to be established in advance. The issue was broached in 1999 when da Vinci was given premarket approval. One member of the committee, Dr Ferguson, commented, '... again looking at the future, I don't know how you do this but I would like to be assured somehow that the surgeon who is responsible for the case is in the room, and not removed to another telesituation, and also that he was able to get to the patient and get in, in case of a severe emergency'.

Telesurgery would also bring an increased need for security protection – with safeguards and checks put in place to prevent hackers from interfering with operations. There are no absolutely hacker safe applications; a computer is only secure until someone breaks into it. It can be made safer with considerable data encryption, but this is at the cost of delays in the control of a robot. Hackers would not have to know how to control a robot surgeon, they could simple intercept and interfere with its operation. Just one unexpected movement of remote controlled tools could be lethal. Time will tell, but it may be that such concerns, and the problems of cost and speed may hold up extensive use of remote surgery.

Van Wynsberghe and Gastman (2008) discuss the effect that telesurgery might have on the patient–physician relationship. They suggest that it is likely to diminish or disrupt it, although they acknowledge that in such drastic situations as those found in a battlefield this reduction in care may not seem important. Their concerns that interactions with a remote surgeon may diminish the level of care received by the patient are related to the concern often raised in the context of robotics, namely the loss, or reduction in human contact.

However, despite these ethical dangers telesurgery holds great promise as a means for conducting emergency procedures in difficult conditions such as disasters or emergencies. Being able to load a portable telesurgery system into an ambulance could help to prevent deaths. For example, many people die on the way to hospital following a serious car accident. A prototype proof of this concept, the *trauma pod*, has been developed by SRI in California, USA (where the original da Vinci research was carried out). This was a portable covered operating table for performing surgical procedures near the battlefield with surgeons at a considerable distance. A wounded soldier could be sealed in a hygienically prepared pod for remote surgical intervention; cleanliness is one of the great difficulties of surgery in the field.

12.9 The automated hospital

Although it may seem like science fiction, many of the elements are now in place to be able to create totally automated hospitals. With the touted robotics revolution in elder care in Japan and the introduction of 'smart homes' in the UK, the possibility of the 'smart hospital' is worth considering. Initial consultations between surgeon and patient could be conducted by a remote doctor via a telepresence robot. Robot receptionists and nurses could conduct hospital admissions. Robot porters could deliver their meals, and robots could do the cleaning. We are already beginning to see the automation of some hospital functions such as automated pharmacy and drug delivery.

The new Forth Valley Royal Hospital in Scotland opened in July, 2011 is using robots to deliver meals, sort hospital mail, move bed linen, and dispose of clinical waste through a dedicated network of corridors beneath the hospital. In further developments, we can imagine that patients might be transported to the operating theatre by means of a robotic bed and so on. Subsequent ward rounds checking up on their recovery could again be conducted by remote telepresence robots. Clearly, benefits could result such as considerably cleaner, more hygienic hospitals and more prompt meal delivery. Children might be able to use their companion robot to say goodnight to their parents (Sharkey and Sharkey, 2010).

In terms of automating surgery, Duke University in the USA, for example, is developing a robot arm that is controlled by a computer program on the basis of ultrasound data with the aim of guiding a biopsy plunger device to take samples. Ultimately, this could prove to be more economical, and could reduce waiting times by enabling such routine operations to be performed without surgeon fatigue.

On the downside, the increasing use of robots could reduce the amount of human contact experienced by patients. The families of patients might increasingly opt for virtual rather than real visits. Parents might stop sleeping by their child's bedside, and use a robot to check in with them. Patients might not even have the small human contact afforded by the hospital cleaner, or porter if such tasks were performed by uncomplaining, and unpaid robots. Vallor (2011) makes the interesting point that in such a situation, not only would the patient's experience of care be greatly reduced, but those who might have provided the care, the caregivers, will also have missed out on the benefits to be obtained from caring.

Sympathetic interactions with fellow human beings are likely to positively affect recovery times, and it is worth considering the possible consequences that could arise if hospitals were to become too enthusiastic about replacing humans with robots in the areas surrounding the operating theatre. Clearly, we wish to avoid a future in which hospitals become production lines where patients are fed into conveyer belt autonomous surgery and then retrieved and bedded by robot nurses.

12.10 Conclusions

There is a law widely attributed to Roy Amara, the first President of the Institute of the Future. Amara's law states, 'We tend to overestimate the effect of a technology in the short run and underestimate the effect in the long run'. This may well apply to robotic surgery. Manufacturers, hospitals and patients have been guilty of overstating the advantages of robotic surgery in the short-term, a failure compounded by initial infrastructural weaknesses such as the level of training required. There is a particular responsibility on both the industry and health professionals to resist commercial and other pressures, including pressure from patients themselves, and provide a balanced account of benefits and drawbacks, drawing on the best evidence available. The current ethical issues may prove to be teething problems. However, we must learn from the lessons of today and stay ethically vigilant for the new surgery of tomorrow.

12.11 References

Adler Jr., J. R., Chang, S. D., Murphy, M. J., Doty, J., Geis, P., and Hancock, S. L. (1997). The Cyberknife: a frameless robotic system for radiosurgery. *Stereotactic and Functional Neurosurgery*, **69**: 1–4, Pt. 2, 124–128.

Angueira, D. P. (2010) Robotics surgery botched procedure. Available from http://massinjurylawyerblog.com/?p=62, last accessed 24th July 2011.

Bargar, W., Bauer, A, and Borner, M. (1998) Primary and revision total hip replacement using the Robodoc system, *Clinical Orthopaedics and Related Research*, **354**, 82–91.

Barocas, D. A., Salem, S., Kordan, Y., Herrell, D., Chang, S. S., Clark, P. E., Davis, R., Baumgartner, R., Philips, S., Cookson, M. S., and Smith Jr, J. A. (2010) Robotic assisted laparoscopic prostatectomy versus radical retropubic prostatectomy for clinically localized prostate cancer: comparison of short-term biochemical recurrence-free survival, *Journal of Urology*, **183**, 990–996.

Carreyrou, J. (2010) Surgical robot examined in injuries, *Wall Street Journal*, May 4, 2010 accessed online at: http://on.wsj.com/kWfUMw, last accessed 24th July, 2011.

Datteri, E., and Tamburrini, G. (2009) Ethical reflections on health care robotics, in R. Capurro and M. Nagenborg (eds.), Ethics and robotics, IOS Press/AKA, Amsterdam–Heidelberg, 35–48.

Dickens, B. and Cook, R. (2006) Legal and ethical issues in telemedicine. *International Journal of Gynaecology and Obstetrics*, **94**: 73–78.

Diodato, M. D., Prosad, S. M., Klingensmith, M. E., and Damiano, R. J. (2004) Robotics in surgery. *Current Problems in Surgery*, **41**: 9, 752–810.

Donnelly, L. (2011) Cancer patients denied last hope robot surgery. *Daily Telegraph* 3rd April 2011. Available from http://www.telegraph.co.uk/health/healthnews/8423891/Cancer-patients-denied-last-hope-robot-surgery.html, last accessed 18th July 2011.

FDA (1999) Food and Drug Administration, General and Plastic Surgery Devices Panel, Medical Devices Advisory Committee, Open Session, Gaithersburg Hilton, Maryland, Wednesday, June 16, 1999.

Grund, J. (2004) Wissenschaftlicher Fortschritt im Operationssaal. Strukturelle Probleme in der experimentellen Phase. Beispiel: Robodoc. *Patientenrechte*, **3**, 63–68.

Hu, J. C., Gu, X., Lipsitz, S. R., Barry, M. J., D'Amico, A. V., Weinberg, A. C., and Keating, N. L. (2009) Comparative effectiveness of minimally invasive vs open radical prostatectomy, *Journal of the American Medical Association*, **302**(14), 1557–1564.

Institute for Clinical and Economic Review (2009) Active surveillance and radical prostatectomy for the management of low-risk, clinically-localized prostate cancer. Final appraisal document. Accessed online at www.icer-review.org/index.php/asrpfinal.html.

Jin, L. X., Ibrahim, A. M., Newman, N. A., Makarov, D. V., Pronovost, P. J., and Makary, M. A. (2011) Robotic surgery claims on United States Hospital websites, *Journal for Healthcare Quality*, **33**(6), 48–52, DOI: 10.1111/j.1945-1474.2011.00148.x.

Kolata, G. (2010) Results unproven, robotic surgery wins converts, *New York Times* Health Section, February 13, 2010 accessed at http://www.nytimes.com/2010/02/14/health/14robot.html

Marohn, M. R. and Hanly, E. J. (2004) Twenty-first century surgery using twenty-first century technology: surgical robotics. *Current Surgery*, **61**(5), 466–473.

Morgenstern, L. (2006) Innovative surgery's dilemma, *Surgical Innovation*, **13**(1), 73–74.

Moore, F. D. (2000) Ethical problems special to surgery: surgical teaching, surgical innovation, and the surgeon in managed care. *Archives of Surgery*, **135**, 14–16.

Rodriguez, Y., Baena, F. and Davies, B. (2010) Robotic surgery: from autonomous systems to intelligent tools. *Robotica*, **28**, 163–170.

Sharkey, A. and Sharkey, N. (2011) Children, the elderly, and interactive robots. *IEEE Robotics and Automation Magazine*, **18**(1), 32–38.

Sharkey, N. (2008) Don't dismiss robot surgeons, *The Guardian*, 26 August 2008. Accessed online at http://www.guardian.co.uk/commentisfree/2008/aug/26/health.robertwinston

Sharkey, N. and Sharkey, A. (2012) The Eldercare Factory. *Gerontology*, **58**, 282–288.

Sharkey, N. E. and Sharkey, A. J. C. (2010) The crying shame of robot nannies: an ethical appraisal. *Interaction Studies*, **11**(2), 161–190.

Sparrow, R. and Sparrow, L. (2006) In the hands of machines? The future of aged care. *Mind and Machine*, **16**, 141–161.

Summary minutes of the General and Plastic Surgery Devices Panel (1999) Summary minutes of the General and Plastic Surgery Devices Panel of the Medical Devices Advisory Committee open session, June 16, Gaithersburg Hilton.

Sutcliffe, P., Czoski-Murray, C., Chattle, M., Ayiku, L., and Parry, G. (2006) Emerging technology briefing paper on the use of robots in surgery, April, 2006, Presented to the Interventional Procedures Advisory Committee (IPAC) and experts attending a meeting at the National Institute for Health and Clinical Excellence (NICE) on the 24th May 2006.

Vallor, S. (2011) Carebots and caregivers: sustaining the ethical ideal of care in the twenty-first century. *Philosophy and Technology*, DOI 10.1007/s13347-011-0015-x.

Van Wynsberghe, A., and Gastmans, C. (2008) Telesurgery: an ethical appraisal. *Journal of Medical Ethics*, **34**, e22.

Weber, J. (2008) Robotic surgery. In Capurro, R., Tamburrini G., and Weber, J. (eds.), Techno-ethical case-studies in robotics, bionics, and related AI agent technologies, Technical Report 5, April 2008, VI Framework Programme Project ETHICBOTS, pp. 60–84.

Index

accordion effect, 24
ACROBOT/Sculptor, 92, 94, 101–2, 108–9
  alignment error and functional improvement for robotics and UKA surgeries, 102
  illustration, 101
Acrobot Sculptor Robotic System, 25
ACS TriPort system, 214
active constraint robots, 94
adjustable cutting blocks, 136–8
  adjustable blocks use, 138
  navigation system directions, 137
adrenalectomy, 213
Agile Patency System, 226–7
ankle centre, 128
  digitisation, 129
apex robotic technology (ART), 126–38, 153
  components, 126
  intelligent instrumentation, 135–8
  software, 127–35
appendectomy, 213
ARTHROBOT, 10
articulated robotic MedProbe (ARM), 84
Ascension, 53
Atracsys, 48
Aurora system, 53
automated cochleostomy, 179–80
automated endoscope system for optimal positioning (AESOP), 11, 161–2
automated hospital, 288–9
automatic systems, 278–9

balloon aortic valvuloplasty (BAV), 80
Biosense Webster, 53, 54
BoneMorphing, 129–35
  customisable computer-assisted surgical protocol, 134–5
    operating room, surgical and tourniquet time comparison, 135
  3D implant planning and visualisation, 131
    virtual femoral surgery, 132
  femoral positioning and sizing, 131–2
    posterior referencing, 133
  gap balancing, 132–4
    CAS ligament balancing software, 134
  imageless anatomical registration, 130

Calypso-Varian system, 54, 56
CardioARM, 22
cardiovascular interventions, 78–87
  future trends, 87
  heart conditions and the evolving role of cardiac surgeons and cardiologists, 78–81
  proposed novel robots, 82–7
    concentric tube robot, 83
    HeartLander, 86
    highly articulated robotic probe, 83
    hybrid snake robot, 85–6
    millimetre-scale active catheters, 87
    serpentine robot consists of series of rigid links, 83
    shape-memory alloy continuum robot, 85
    surgical continuum robots, 84–5
    surgical serpentine robots, 84
    worm-like organ-mounted robots, 86

surgical robot requirements and availability, 81–2
Carto-3, 54
cellphone test, 53
Certus, 48
charge coupled device (CCD), 227
cholecystectomy, 213
chopstick technique, 214
chorioallantoic membrane (CAM), 205–6
cilia system, 234
clinical accuracy, 140–3
clinical study methods, 140–1
postoperative overall, individual femoral and tibial component alignment, 141
results, 141–3
complications and failures, 143
intraoperative and computer data and radiographic data, 142
overall leg alignment and individual component alignment, 141–2
patient factor effect on efficiency, 143
postoperative overall limb alignment, 142
colectomy, 213
compact bevel-geared robot for advanced surgery (CoBRASurge), 12
complementary metal oxide semiconductor (CMOS), 227
computer-assisted surgery (CAS), 113–15
computer numerical control (CNC), 172–80
concentric tube robot, 83, 85
controlled systems, 279
conventional surgery, 117–19
surgical approaches and muscle exposure in conventional TKA, 118
CorTemp pill system, 238
CyberKnife, 9, 51, 278

da Vinci surgical system, 210–11, 279, 281
minimally invasive surgery (MIS), 212–13
da Vinci telemanipulator, 165–7
Defense Advanced Research Projects Administration (DARPA), 212
degrees of freedom, 189
diagnostic system, 238–9
direct cochlear access (DCA), 172–7
direct cochlear access results comparison, 178
ENT robot system, 176
Euclidian distance errors, 178
Kuka KR3 robotic system, 175
location of facial nerve and chorda tympani in the conventional mastoidectomy, 173
main error sources between standard IGS and DCA goal, 174
Direct-Drive Endoscopic System, 217
duty cycle, 255–6

ear, nose and throat (ENT) surgery
computer numerical control (CNC), 172–80
image-guided interventions, 167–72
medical robotics, 159–81
overview
advantages and disadvantages of human and robot capabilities, 161
technology, 159–60
telemanipulator, 160–7
Eikonal equation, 260
electrode array insertion, 180
automatic advance off-stylet electrode insertion tool, 181
EndoCapsule, 227
EndoSAMURAI, 217
endoscope holder
functional endoscopic sinus surgery (FESS), 160–2
custom-built ORL robot with an endoscope attachment, 16
EndoWrist, 13, 211, 213
Ensite-NavX, 54
Enterion capsule, 240
epiretinal membrane, 191
ESO2, 225
EtherCAT protocol, 203
ethics
robotic surgery, 276–89
automated hospital, 288–9
costs vs benefits, 285–6
ethical issues in relation to remotely operated surgery, 286–8

marketing, 280–2
patient experience, 279–80
training need, 283–5
types, 278–9
vs other surgery types, 282–3
European Union, Article 35 of Charter of Fundamental Rights, 285–6

fast marching method (FMM), 260
Federal Drugs Administration (FDA), 282
femoral component, 149–52
flexible software and a robotic cutting guide fit adjustment, 150
intraoperative assessment of fit tightness, 151
intraoperative femoral component fit, 151
ferromagnetic device tracking, 263–4
standard deviations for tracking algorithm, 264
field-programmable gate array (FPGA), 230
Food and Drug Administration, 212, 227
forbidden-region virtual fixtures (FRVF), 27–8
force sailing, 71
functional endoscopic sinus surgery (FESS)
endoscope holder, 160–2
custom-built ORL robot with an endoscope attachment, 16
navigate control application, 170–1

gastric banding, 213
gastrointestinal minimally invasive surgery
mesoscale mobile robots, 224–44
commercial gastrointestinal wireless capsule endoscopes, 225–7
future trends in mobile surgical devices, 242–3
robotic capsule module, 227–42
GelPoint access port, 214
GelSeal Cap, 214
General Electric Signa 3T clinical MRI scanner, 262
generalised predictive control (GPC), 266
German Aerospace Centre (DLR), 17
gradient echo (GE), 262
guidance virtual fixtures (GVF), 27–8

Hall-effect sensors, 51
Hansen Medical catheters, 82
hearing aid implantations, 172–80
HeartLander, 20, 86
highly articulated robotic probe (HARP), 22, 83
hip centre, 127–8
human–machine interface (HMI), 164
hybrid coronary revascularisation (HCR), 80
hybrid snake robot, 85–6
hysterectomy, 213

i-Snake, 24
iBlock, 92, 106–8
illustration, 107
image-guided intervention, 167–72
accuracy importance, 167–9
major error sources, 168
registration process, 170
variability of manual screw and semiautomatic localisation, 169
FEE navigate control application, 170–1
mastoidectomy, 171–2
navigate control, 169–70
Image Guided Technologies Flashpoint, 47
implant bed milling, 177, 179
robotic manipulator assist, 179
infrared emitting diodes (IRED), 43, 48
Instatrak system, 53
instrument manipulation, 163–5
MicroMan device positioning accuracy testing, 163
RobOtol device kinematics, 165
InteliCap, 240
InteliSite capsule, 240
intervention, 239–40
interventional capsule, 239
intravoxel dephasing, 262
ISG viewing wand, 47

knee centre, 128–9
KneeAlign, 123
KUKA industrial robot, 278

Lab-on-a-Pill capsule, 238
laparoendoscopic single-site surgery (LESS), 213

Laservibrometer, 205
learning curve, 140–3
  clinical study methods, 140–1
    postoperative overall, individual femoral and tibial component alignment, 141
  results, 141–3
    complications and failures, 143
    effect and efficiency, 142–3
    intraoperative and computer and radiographic data, 142
    overall leg alignment and individual component alignment, 141–2
    patient factor effect on efficiency, 143
    postoperative overall limb alignment, 142
    tourniquet time by case group, 143
light-emitting diodes (LEDs), 230
light endoscope robot (LER), 16
localisation, 231–3
locomotion, 233–8
  external, 236–8
  internal, 233–6
    robotic capsules may use internal mechanisms and external actuation, 235

macro–micro architecture, 93
3D-MAGMA, 232
magnetic internal mechanism (MIM), 237–8
magnetic resonance imaging (MRI), 253–9
  model description of microrobot in viscous fluid, 257–9
    forces applied on microrobot navigating in blood vessel, 257
  navigation constraints, 254–7
    acquisition and control prediction timeline, 256
  navigation system overview, 254
magnetic signature selective excitation tracking (MS-SET), 263
MAKOplasty, 25
master and slave translumenal endoscopic robot (MASTER), 217–18
master console, 193–8
  force feedback, 194–6
    backdrivability, 195
    high stiffness, 195
    low friction, 195
    low inertia and moving mass, 195
    zero backlash, 196
  mechanical design, 196–8
    haptic interface characteristics, 198
    range of motion of ϕ and Ψ DoF, 197
    two 5-DoF haptic interfaces and kinematic chain scheme, 196
  system layout, 193–4
    intuitive working environment, 194
mastoidectomy, 171–2
MATLAB/Simulink, 204
MAZE procedure, 80
medical position sensors
  localisation and tracking technologies, 41–57
    dynamic referencing, 46
    future trends, 57
  requirements for position sensors, 42–6
    co-ordinate system for tracking system, 44
  types, 46–56
    effect of tip bending on tip displacement accuracy, 50
    electromagnetic tracking systems, 51–4
    fibre optic tracking systems, 55–6
    GPS-based systems, 56
    hybrid systems, 56
    impedance-based tracking systems, 54–5
    in-bore MRI tracking, 55
    mechanical linkages, 46–7
    optical systems, 47–51
    sensor coils for electromagnetic tracking system, 52
    sound-based systems, 51
    video matching, 55
medical robotics, 119–26
  clinical studies on active robotic systems used in total knee arthroplasty, 119
  ear, nose and throat (ENT) surgery, 159–81
    computer numerical control (CNC), 172–80
    image-guided interventions, 167–72

overview, 159–60
telemanipulator, 160–7
Galileo miniature robot for TKA, 123
orthopaedic surgery, 90–109
orthopaedic robotic systems, 92–5
orthopaedic surgical robots impact evaluation, 95–109
Precision Freehand Sculptor (PFS), 122
Robotic Arm Interactive Orthopaedic system, 121
mesoscale mobile robots
gastrointestinal minimally invasive surgery, 224–44
commercial gastrointestinal wireless capsule endoscopes, 225–7
future trends in mobile surgical devices, 242–3
robotic capsule module, 227–42
MicroMan, 163
microrobot navigation, 259–71
application and results, 267–71
3D MRI-based microbot endovascular navigation, 268
3D tracking error, 269
MRI-based navigation with blood flow disturbance, 270
tracking error for various duty cycle values, 271
tracking error statistics for different time horizons, 269
MRI-based microrobot control, 264–71
module, 266
predictive control, 266–7
MRI-based sensing, 262–4
ferromagnetic device tracking, 263–4
imaging parameters and artifacts, 262–3
MRI susceptibility artifact imaging, 263
navigation planning, 259–62
3D navigation centreline extraction, 261
path extracted using the information gain cost function, 261
microscale mobile robots, 243
millimeter-scale active catheters, 87
Minerva, 63
minimally invasive surgery (MIS), 117–19, 187, 211–16
da Vinci surgical system, 212–13
single-incision surgery, 213–16
prototype, 215
surgical console prototype for robotic SILS, 216
surgical approaches and muscle exposure in conventional TKA, 118
MIRO robots, 17
MiroCam Capsule, 227
MicroSurge, 17
mobile adjustable-focus robotic camera (MARC), 220
mobile endoluminal robot, 220
model predictive control (MPC), 266
motion sailing, 71
MRBot, 11
multi-turn, tension-stiffening catheter, 84
multifunctional dexterous robot, 221

Nathanson liver retractor, 211
National Centre for Health and Clinical Excellence (NICE), 286
National Health Service (NHS), 286
natural orifice transluminal endoscopic surgery (NOTES), 33, 216–21
miniature surgical robots, 219–21
in vivo miniature robot, 220
navigate control, 169–70
application in FESS, 170–1
navigation system, 119–26
Orthalign, 124
NavX system, 54
NDI Optotrak 3020, 48
neck/larynx dissection, 167
nephrectomy, 213
neuroArm, 15, 63, 279
NeuRobot telecontrolled system, 15
NeuroMate, 9, 63
neurosurgery, 59–75
evolution of neurosurgical robots, 61–4
three robotic system designs, 62
future trends, 74–5
human-machine interface (HMI), 65–74
audio, 69
hazards related to introduction of robotics into neurosurgery, 66

humanising haptics, 72–4
neuroArm end effector, 71
neuroArm manipulators holding bipolar forceps, 73
neuroArm workstation, 68
Shadow Dexterous Hand, 73
tactile, 69–72
vision, 66–9
maintaining operator control, 64–5
progression, 59–61
timeline of historical progress of neurosurgery, 60
Niobe system, 237

Olympus magnetic capsule endoscope, 237
Omega and Delta device, 194
OMOM Capsule, 227
orthopaedic robotic system, 92–5
anatomical interface, 95
controller design, 93–4
design features of commercially available orthopaedic robots, 92
mechanical architecture, 92–3
orthopaedic surgery
medical robotics, 90–109
orthopaedic robotic systems, 92–5
orthopaedic surgical robots impact evaluation, 95–109
orthopaedic surgical robots, 95–109
categories of papers found in literature review, 96
five commercially available robots for orthopaedic surgery, 98
publications by clinical areas of application, 98
publications that focus on technology and evaluation, 97
specific clinical application areas found in literature review, 96

paddling technique, 234
parallel robot, 93
passive arm with dynamic constraints (PADyC), 25
passive toolholders, 93–4
path-planning method, 267
patient-specific instruments, 119–26
position cutting guides, 125
perceptual docking, 25, 27
percutaneous coronary interventions (PCI), 79
percutaneous transluminal coronary angioplasty (PTCA), 79
Phantom, 194
Philips IntelliCap, 238
Philips PercuNav, 53
Picker ViStar system, 51
PillCam Colon, 227
PillCam Colon2, 227
PillCam ESO, 225
PillCam SB, 226–7, 237
PillCam SB2, 226–7
pneumocephalography, 59
Polaris, 48
postoperative alignment
preoperative deformity effect, 144
distribution in 128 robotic-assisted TKA, 145
power, 241–2
propeller-driven capsule, 242
preoperative deformity
effect on alignment, 144
distribution in 128 robotic-assisted TKA, 145
tourniquet time, 144
coronal and sagittal plane deformities effect on robot-assisted TKA surgery, 146
PROBOT, 10, 278
Programmable Universal Machine for Assembly (PUMA), 61
proportional-integral-derivative (PID), 255–6

quad sparing subvastus approach, 147–9
illustration, 148
medial fixation of the robotic cutting guide, 149
Qualysis, 47, 48

radiostereometric analysis (RSA), 47
RAVEN robot, 17
real-time software platform
MRI usage for in vivo navigation of magnetic micro-robot, 252–72
future trends, 271–2
magnetic resonance imaging (MRI) navigation, 253–9

microrobot navigation, 259–71
registration, 127
retinal vein occlusion (RVO), 191
RoboCouch Patient Positioning System, 9
ROBODOC, 9, 92, 93, 98–101, 109, 278
illustration, 99
total hip arthroplasty, 282
robot-assisted microsurgery (RAMS), 17, 63
robot assisted minimally invasive surgery (MIS), 1–34
definitions and development of robotic systems, 4–24
CAD/CAM and assistive systems, 6, 9–12
CAD/CAM systems for surgery, 10
endoscopic camera positioning systems, 13
handheld and mechatronically enhanced surgical tools, 18
i-Snake robot for flexible access surgery, 24
master-slave surgical systems, 12–17
photos of master-slave surgical systems, 14
representative robotic systems for MIS, 7–8
robotically enhanced handheld devices for MIS, 19–20
semiautonomous robots for surgery, 18–24
semiautonomous systems for endoscopic surgery, 21–22
future trends, 32–4
minimally invasive surgery and robotic integration, 2–4
MIS drawbacks and related benefits of robotic integration, 5
perceptual docking for synergistic control, 24–32
dynamic active constraints, 30–1
gaze-contingent motor channelling, 32
synergistic control applications in robot-assisted MIS, 26–7
virtual fixtures, 27–30
robot-assisted vitreoretinal surgery, 185–208
experimental results, 205–6
surgical tasks performed on chicken egg chorioallantoic membrane, 206
user accuracy experiment and haemorrhage caused by pinching veins, 206
future trends, 207–8
initiatives, 186
master console, 193–8
force feedback, 194–6
mechanical design, 196–8
slave robot, 198–203
system layout, 193–4
master control interface, 188
requirements, 187–93
user needs, 190–1
vitreoretinal surgery, 187–90
results, 203–6
slave robot, 198–203
system integration, 203–5
ophthalmic surgeon M. D. de Smet using robotic surgical system, 203
schematic overview, 204
system overview, 191–3
master-slave setup for vitreoretinal eye surgery schematic representation, 192
schematic representation, 192
robot-use time, 140–1
Robotic Arm Interactive Orthopaedic (RIO), 25, 102–4, 109, 120
illustration, 103
robotic-assisted knee replacement surgery, 113–53
apex robotic technology (ART), 126–38
clinical experience, 138–52
clinical accuracy and the learning curve, 140–3
clinical utility in severely deformed knees, 143–4
femoral component fit adjustment, 149–52
Praxim robotic cutting guide, 139
quad sparing subvastus approach, 147–9
future trends, 152–3

overview, 113–26
capital costs and per case cost for passive CAS, 115
robotic capsule module, 227–42
diagnostic system, 238–9
intervention, 239–40
localisation, 231–3
locomotion, 233–8
external, 236–8
internal, 233–6
potential modules required for wireless robotic capsule, 228
power, 241–2
telemetry, 231
vision, 228–31
robotic cutting guide, 135–6
ART, 135
motion control and safety features, 136
robotic laparoscopic single-site (R-LESS), 215
robotic surgery
ethical challenges, 276–89
automated hospital, 288–9
costs vs benefits, 285–6
ethical issues in relation to remotely operated surgery, 286–8
marketing, 280–2
patient experience, 279–80
training need, 283–5
types, 278–9
vs other surgery types, 282–3
types, 278–9
automatic systems, 278–9
controlled systems, 279
robotic systems
cardiovascular interventions, 78–88
future trends, 87
heart conditions and role of cardiac surgeons and cardiologists, 78–81
proposed novel robots, 82–8
surgical robot requirements and availability, 81–2
robotic totally endoscopic coronary artery bypass (TECAB), 80
robotics
minimally invasive surgery and natural orifice transluminal endoscopic surgery, 210–22
future trends, 221–2
minimally invasive surgery (MIS), 211–16
natural orifice transluminal endoscopic surgery (NOTES), 216–21
neurosurgery, 59–75
evolution of neurosurgical robots, 61–4
human-machine interface (HMI), 65–74
maintaining operator control, 64–5
progression, 59–61
RobOtol, 164
root mean square (RMS), 269

Science Accessories Corporation (SAC), 51
semiactive robotic system, 120
Sensei Robotic Navigation System (RNS), 20
serial robot, 93
shape memory alloy (SMA), 233–4
actuators, 23
continuum robot, 85
Siemens magnetic guidance system, 237
single incision laparoscopic surgery (SILS), 33, 211
single-incision surgery, 213–16
prototype, 215
surgical console prototype for robotic SILS, 216
single-shot fast spin echo (SSFSE), 262
slave robot, 198–203
instrument manipulator, 198–200
design characteristics, 200
image, 199
instrument manipulator features, 200–1
slender instrument manipulator design, 201
support system, 201–3
exploded view of modular support, 202
software, 127–35
spatial misregistration, 262
Special Purpose Dexterous Manipulator, 64
spin echo (SE), 262
SpineAssist, 9, 92, 104–6

illustration, 104
studies presenting results for pedicle screw implantations, 105
splenectomy, 213
standard deviation, 269
Stanford Endocapsule, 238
Steady-Hand Eye Robot, 18
Steady-Hand robotic system, 63
Stereotaxis catheters, 82
surgical continuum robots, 84–5
surgical serpentine robots, 84
Swiss cheese technique, 214

tactile guidance system (TGS), 25
telemanipulator, 160–7
telemetry, 231
teleoperator, 94
telepresence, 81
telesurgery, 287
tethered epicardial crawling (TEC) robot, 20
total extraperitoneal inguinal hernia repair, 213
total knee arthroplasty (TKA), 113–116, 116–17
illustration, 116
tourniquet time, 140–1
preoperative deformity, 144
coronal and sagittal plane deformities effect on robot-assisted TKA surgery, 146
transcatheter aortic valve implantation (TAVI), 80
TransPort multichannel access device, 217
triangulation, 216, 221

ultrasonography, 59

VeSPA, 214
Virtual Navigator, 54
vision, 228–31
bleeding lesion from PillCamSB and image of gastric cavity, 229
VitalSense, 238
vitrectomy, 199–200
vitreoretinal surgery, 187–90
human eye anatomy and vitreoretinal instrument, 189
surgeon M.D. de Smet performing vitreoretinal surgery, 190

Watsmart, 47
white Gaussian noise, 267
whole arm manipulation (WAM), 25
wireless capsule endoscopes (WCEs), 225–7
current commercial camera capsules, 226
worm-like organ-mounted robots, 86

Zeus system, 279
Zeus teleoperated surgical robot, 15